Head and Neck Injury Criteria

A Consensus Workshop

Washington, D.C.
March 26–27, 1981

For sale by the Superintendent of Documents, U.S. Government Printing Office
Washington, D.C. 20402

Contents

Page

SESSION 2, PART 2: Physiopathology and Biomechanics of Neck Injury

SESSION 2, PART 3: Closing Comments on Head and Neck Injury

Page

SESSION 2, PART 4: Status of Current Criteria of Head Injury

Preface

A. K. Ommaya, M.D.
Chief Medical Advisor
National Highway Traffic Safety Administration

Injuries to the brain and spinal cord are the most devastating of diseases that afflict humanity, more so than the dread triad of cancer, heart disease and stroke for two significant reasons which are often not deeply understood: First, because neural trauma is the leading cause of mortality and morbidity in the economically most significant segment of the population, i.e., those aged 15 to 45 years; and second, the sequelae of neural trauma including paraplegia and quadriplegia, post-traumatic epilepsy and varying but highly significant disturbances of cognitive and sensory-motor function, extend much longer in time than the suffering and costs of cancer, heart disease and stroke. As one 19-year-old victim of a motor vehicle accident has said, "It is like having unremitting cancer for a life time." The recognition of the human and economic costs of neural trauma should ideally therefore result in a high-priority research and development in the setting of national policies in allotment of resources for public health, certainly much more significantly so than presently available either in terms of overall funding as well as in coordination of existing resources. In this effort two aspects of multi- and interdisciplinary programs have been recognized as different but complementary. One research strategy is *prevention* orientated and has traditionally been conducted as a collaborative effort of engineers, physicians, physiologists and physicians with biomechanics as its primary scientific discipline. The other is *treatment* orientated and although often involving all the specialists mentioned above is much more in the traditional area of the physician and biomedical scientist. Oversimplifying for the sake of our argument one can say that biomechanics-oriented trauma research has been mainly applied in nature and supported to a large extent by the National Highway Traffic Safety Administration (NHTSA) with smaller contributions by other agencies such as Department of Defense (DOD), National Science Foundation (NSF) and National Institutes of Health (NIH). Conversely, therapy-oriented research has been mainly supported by the NIH. As an investigator of neural trauma mechanisms who has worked for over two decades in this field and enjoyed generous support from the NHTSA as well as from NIH and DOD, this author has noted a fundamental problem which has severely handicapped the systematic and long-term pursuit of knowledge in this field. This problem is essentially one of communication between disciplines. To take an extreme example, the engineer seeking to establish a quantitative criterion for head injury will search for the most reliable and simplest model displaying the causation of injury. Pioneering work with this approach begun at Wayne State University over 30 years ago and remains to this day the basis of the current "official" head injury criterion (HIC) which characterizes the threshold for such injury by magnitudes derived from the temporal variation of a single mechanical parameter, the linear acceleration of the head, the description of the impact process to the human head being based on rigid body mechanics, obviously not a satisfactory idealization. Because data on human head tissue injury thresholds are scanty and most reliable only for skull fracture, the current HIC includes the assumption that skull fracture is a good index of brain injury. Although it is undoubtedly true that significant brain injuries can be associated with skull fracture and that in practice useful correlations can be made between the HIC and current indices of injury severity (A.I.S. Levels), there is a disturbing lack of precision in these data.

The biomedical community has not successfully emphasized their data showing the relative independence of neural and vascular tissue component injury mechanisms and thresholds from skull fracture mechanisms and thresholds (especially at lower levels of injury) nor have these data been related to the requirements of the engineer to develop useful models and quantitative tolerance data. Thus the fact that the vast majority of cerebral concussions (Grades I through III) are not associated with skull fracture, that the correlation of even more severe diffuse brain injuries (Cerebral Concussions Grades III through V) with skull fracture is very weak (less than 5%) and that only 50% of patients with one of the most severe and prognostically grave brain lesions, the acute subdural hematoma, have skull fractures are facts that have not been adequately recognized in the continuing improvement of the HIC.

The situation with obtaining a Neck Injury Criterion (NIC) is even worse. Although no "official" NIC exists, attempts have been made to define tolerance levels from human volunteer, cadaver and modelling sources, notably by Mertz and Patrick (see also the reports by W. Goldsmith and A. Burstein in this proceedings). These data are expressed in terms of occipito-condylar torque and movement and obviously require improvement. Again the lack of well-integrated cooperative studies between engineers and biomedical scientists have held back contributions to this field.

The contents of this report initiate the deliberations of a significant group of workers in this field. Members from every major country in which research on Biomechanics is being done are represented and attempts were made by the editor to contact all who have contributed in this field. Any omissions or commissions are the personal responsibility of the editor and apologies are extended to any scientist who may have been overlooked. It is hoped that the contents of this publication will serve as the most comprehensive source book on where data on head and neck injury mechanisms are available and a guide book for exploration of the research and development needs for the prevention of head and neck injuries in humans.

Goals of the Workshop

Diane Steed, Deputy Administrator
National Highway Traffic Safety Administration

Magnitude of Highway Safety Problems

Motor vehicle crashes are the sixth leading cause of death in the Nation and the leading cause of death for those under age 50. "Measured in terms of working life lost, traffic deaths represent a social problem comparable to heart disease and cancer," according to a recent report by the U.S. Congress' Office of Technology Assessment.

Nearly half the people killed in crashes in the last 5 years have been under 25 years of age.

Motor vehicle injuries also cause staggering losses. Motor vehicle crashes are the leading cause of paraplegia and quadriplegia, and a major cause of epilepsy. Each year they cost society $50 billion in medical and rehabilitation costs, lost wages, welfare, and property damages.

Severe head and neck injury caused by automobile accidents is largely irreversible. Victims frequently incur permanent disabilities, with their attendant handicap to the individual and burden on society. Prevention of these injuries is desirable where practical. However, we need knowledge of how to effectively prevent head and neck injuries. This difficult issue is being addressed by this conference.

The most meaningful way of developing vehicle safety features which reduce or prevent injuries is to actually subject a vehicle or vehicle component to a crash impact.

Since human beings obviously cannot be used as subjects in dynamic crash tests, a surrogate must be used to measure the injury potential of the crash. For crash tests of complete vehicles, anthropomorphic test dummies that simulate an actual human being (in size, weight, motion, and response to crash forces) provide the means for measuring the potential for human injury. Dummies which respond like humans in typical vehicle crashes and which predict the potential for various types of injuries are a prerequisite to reliable testing of safety improvements.

The deficiencies in existing dummies have forced the Agency to develop safety standards which require a large number of engineering tests. In most cases, these tests do not involve the use of dummies to measure injury. As a consequence, existing safety standards are numerous, complex, and do not directly measure injury reduction.

In order to improve the effectiveness and reduce the cost of vehicle safety, improved dummies and injury criteria are needed. Improved dummies would encourage manufacturers to use innovation in designing safe cars, because they would afford greater design flexibility than that permitted by existing standards based upon engineering tests. In addition, these improved dummies would permit researchers to develop more effective safety features for the most prevalent injuries in common accident modes. A prerequisite to developing improved dummies is the development of injury tolerance of the human being to impacts like those caused in automobile accidents.

I hope that this workshop will be able to develop a consensus on the best way to proceed with the difficult task of developing more precise injury tolerance for the head and neck.

Lack of biomechanics data on which to base dummy design and injury criteria is one reason many of the existing regulations are not effective. For example, our current side protection standard and steering column standards rely on engineering tests, which are not directly relatable to human injury prevention.

Dummies and injury criteria are crucial to developing effective crash safety programs.

Progress in Biomechanics Research to Date

This Head/Neck Injury Workshop is a valuable step to developing the best possible injury criteria to assist in achieving more effective safety in motor vehicles.

Injury criteria used to date have evolved from years of research. While existing criteria have been generally accepted as the best available at the time it was specified, this criteria should not be considered as cast in stone. As new knowledge and understanding develop, the injury criteria should be upgraded.

The NHTSA Biomechanics research program is charged with the task of continually improving this criteria and of developing improved dummies which, with the criteria, more accurately measure the variety of injuries like those which are occurring everyday on the highways.

The progress toward this end has been relentless, if not as rapid as many would like. Large improvements have been made since the first frontal impact dummy and associated injury criteria were developed.

During the past few years, improved dummies are nearing final development which more accurately simulate human beings when subjected to side impacts. These dummies will be extremely useful in studying the best way to protect vehicle occupants from side impacts.

The NHTSA is also evaluating the frontal impact performance of several advanced dummies for possible application to our safety research program. These evaluations will assist us in determining which dummy to use in our future research. A critical question which must also be answered is what injury criteria should be used with the advanced dummies being evaluated and developed.

I believe that the results of this conference will assist us in answering that question. Communications of the type established in this workshop are important to progress in this difficult area. I would like to thank each of you for your contributions to this workshop, and I encourage continued communication of your research results in the future.

Dr. Kennerly Digges

I would like to add my welcome to each of you to the Consensus Workshop on Head and Neck Injury. I'm very excited about this workshop and I'm also very excited about the caliber and stature and reputation of the people that are attending. I'm sure that the discussions to come will be both fruitful and challenging and rewarding to all of us.

The purpose of the workshop is to review the data on head and neck injury and to gain a consensus on how to improve head and neck injury criteria. Dr. Ommaya has discussed the format and I'm sure that the opportunity for discussion will be great and I look forward to those discussions.

It has been 3 years since NHTSA sponsored the last Head and Neck Injury Workshop at Ann Arbor, Michigan. The purpose of that workshop was to bring together experts in head and neck trauma research and to develop approaches for improving head and neck injury classification and documentation. At that workshop the limiting feature identified was the inability to observe brain trauma and to relate the seriousness of brain trauma to the outcome to the patient.

An approach suggested for dealing with this problem was the collection of data from practicing physicians, as well as researchers. In order to allow standardized description of the trauma, the workshop developed an anatomical description of the brain and a method of coding injury phenomena and the phenomena's location and the extent of the phenomena.

The second problem was the lack of comparability of head and neck autopsy data due to differences in procedures and differences in emphasis in the autopsy. This problem was particularly acute for neck autopsies. The workshop developed standardized autopsy procedures for the head and neck. In addition, a procedure for categorizing and coding head and neck injuries for statistical processing by computers was developed.

Subsequent to the last workshop, the NHTSA has initiated a program to investigate fatal neck injuries of motorcycle victims with Dr. Harry Hurt of the University of Southern California. The purpose of this study was to determine the nature and extent of head and neck injuries in fatally injured motorcycle riders and that study will be reported on later.

To date, head injury data collection from multiple sources has not been initiated by this agency. However, the agency has sponsored a research program with Dr. Gennarelli at the University of Pennsylvania to explore the hypothesis that the outcome of head injury to a patient can be determined by the trauma which could be observed at the time of injury. Dr. Gennarelli has been conducting clinical studies of brain trauma and has identified those lesions which result in the most serious consequences. The work by Dr. Gennarelli should be beneficial in focusing the investigations and data collection for the researchers.

NHTSA has also sponsored other analytical experimental and data collection research which has added to the knowledge and understanding of head injury during the past 3 years.

For example, NHTSA sponsored research leading to a finite element analysis of the brain. This work was conducted by Dr. Carley Ward while she was at the Naval Civil Engineering Laboratory. The finite element work is useful in defining the relationship between the dosage of the insult to the head and the resulting stresses and strains within the brain.

The sessions to come will provide the opportunity to discuss these and other research worldwide and to collectively evaluate the results.

I'm sorry to say that our biomechanics program at NHTSA during the last 3 years has not been as extensive as I would have hoped. This research was significantly curtailed by a 1977 challenge from Congressman John Moss, who attempted to stop all safety research which involved the use of cadavers. This challenge resulted in the suspension and delay of up to 3 years of some of the critical elements of injury criteria work.

I believe it would be useful at this time to restate the position held by Mr. Moss in this matter. In a letter dated January 6, 1978, to the Secretary of Transportation, Mr. Moss stated his position as follows, and I quote Mr. Moss:

> Let me leave absolutely no confusion about my position in this matter. I believe that the use of human cadavers for vehicle safety research crudely violates fundamental notions of morality and human dignity and, therefore, must permanently be stopped.

Mr. Moss went on:

> I hold this view fully understanding that:
>
> One—The vast majority of the bodies used as cadavers come from the Willed Body Program and that family permission is secured wherever possible to use the cadavers in crash testing.
>
> Two—That NHTSA views the information gained from cadaver testing as critical both to the development of better dummies and to the establishment of meaningful injury criteria.
>
> Three—That good alternatives to cadaver testing are not available to develop this information.
>
> Four—That cadaver testing should no longer be necessary once a suitable dummy is available and acceptable data on human injury tolerance levels are obtained and that;
>
> Five—An acceptance is growing for a researcher's code of ethics governing cadaver use.

Although Mr. Moss's position on cadavers may represent a rather extreme element in our society, it is a position that must be recognized and it must be dealt with.

I might note that an even more vocal constituency exists to prevent trauma research which involves animals.

The nature of trauma research frequently lends itself to sensationalization, particularly when well-known figures such as Congressman Moss decide to attack this type of research. The scientific literature is filled with controversy regarding the deficiencies of both cadavers and animals as human surrogates and it is also easy to find scientists who are willing to make statements to support the extreme views. It is equally difficult to find independent individuals or organizations who are willing to support the need for animal cadaver research in biomechanics, particularly during periods where the potential for sensationalization of the work may exist.

In your discussions and deliberations during the next two days you should keep in mind the sensitivity of some of the alternative research approaches such as those using animals and cadavers. In the event that you find this sensitive work necessary, you should consider ways of dealing with the challenges that may result. It is not inconceivable that an ill-defined research program could cause delay or complete cessation of all research which involves these types of human surrogates.

During the coming year NHTSA plans to initiate a program to develop an improved dummy. This improved dummy is expected to more precisely measure the potential for injury in a variety of crash modes. We expect the development of dummy hardware to continue during the next 4 years. In conjunction with this development, we must develop and we must decide on what types of instrumentation for head and neck injury measurement are necessary and how to relate these measurements to actual injury. We hope that this conference will assist us in answering these difficult questions.

Specifically, I would like to pose to you the following questions to consider during the working session. I have eight of them.

First:
What is the nature of head and neck injury? And as a sub-category of that is: What mechanisms are important and what observations are important?

Second:
What are the important parameters for researchers to measure in the experimental environment?

Third:
What are the benefits and deficiencies of existing injury criteria?

Fourth:
Are there presently available alternatives which are better than the head injury criteria which are currently used?

Fifth:
What are the best available criteria for neck injury?

Sixth:
What additional data needs to be developed to improve head and neck injury criteria?

Seventh, which is the toughest one of all:
What alternative approaches exist for developing the needed data for head and neck injury criteria and

what combination of approaches offers the best way to proceed?

Eighth:

What mechanisms are required to achieve a continuing dialogue and coordination of head and neck injury research?

SESSION 1:

Epidemiology of Head and Neck Injuries in Automotive Accidents

Session 1

Epidemiology of Head and Neck Injuries in Automotive Accidents

Introduction
Robert McLaurin, M.D.

I'm honored to have this opportunity to chair this session. I will note at the beginning that my personal participation in this session will be kept to a minimum which is entirely consistent with my knowledge of the problem. I think that to set the stage for this session it is obvious to everyone epidemiology is important not only because of the considerations of human life and well being that are involved in the problem of head and spinal cord injury, it is also important because of the economic impact that this has both individually and on the nation as a whole. In addition, I would point out that epidemiology becomes important because it assists in defining etiologic relationship of injury and at the same time it helps to define possible means of prevention.

Epidemiology in the past in this field (and in other related fields of the nervous system) has been carried on in a very fragmentary manner, largely on the basis of selected community figures, also on figures engendered by special interest groups, neither of which can be applied to the problem as a whole with any degree of accuracy and, therefore, it is important that we attempt to obtain as accurate figures as possible.

Epidemiology of Head and Neck Trauma in Victims of Motor Vehicle Accidents

William E. Scott

When I was asked by Dr. Ommaya, the chief organizer and man most responsible for this workshop, if I would discuss the epidemiology of head and neck trauma in motor vehicle accident victims, my first response was "Sure, the workshop sounds like a good idea, I'd be happy to address the group." But then I asked myself, what can I tell this group that they don't already know. After all, many of the people in attendance are the medical professionals who see, treat and rehabilitate accident victims—for me to tell them about the problem will be like "hauling coals to Newcastle" or "preaching to the choir." At this point I was about to call the good Dr. Ommaya and gently back out of my commitment. However, short of doing this, I decided that I could contribute something to this workshop if I put the problem in both a historical and national perspective and if I could give you a somewhat abbreviated, but clear picture of the head, neck and spinal cord injury data that we have collected and will continue to collect in our major accident data collection systems.

Unfortunately, people have been killing themselves and others in ever-increasing numbers since cars were first introduced. Ever since we began counting, fatalities have increased in absolute terms each and every year—with two notable exceptions. During World War II, fatalities dropped from 39,000 in 1941 to 24,000 in 1944. Then post World War II, America's love affair with the auto took off in earnest—and deaths increased each year until the major oil shock of 1973–74, which ushered in gas lines, reduced driving and the 55 mph national speed limit. Fatalities dropped from 55,000 in 1973 to 46,000 in 1974.

Throughout this long period of ever-increasing death and injuries from motor vehicle accidents things were clearly getting worse in absolute terms; however, paradoxically, things were getting better in *relative* terms—that is fatality rates were declining.

For example, in 1936, there were 28.38 deaths per 10 thousand population, 12.90 per 10 thousand registered motor vehicles and 14.41 per 100 million vehicle miles. By 1976, these rates had declined to 2.12 per 10 thousand population, 3.17 per 10 thousand registered motor vehicles and 3.25 per 100 million vehicle miles.

Since 1976 some very disturbing things have happened. The long-term historical trend of increasing fatalities has resumed; but the long-term historical trend in declining fatality rates appears to have bottomed out, and in fact, may be on the rise. From a safety point of view even more disturbing things have been happening—indeed these are the facts and events that statistical trends reflect. Safety belt usage has continued to decline steadily since 1976 to a low of about 12 percent in 1980. Speeds and the number of people exceeding the 55 mph speed limit have increased, cars are getting smaller and trucks are getting larger, more numerous and driving more miles, more people are driving motorcycles at a time when 28 states repealed or weakened their helmet laws.

In 1976, 46,000 people died in traffic accidents—last year 51,700 died. Motor vehicle accidents are the leading cause of death up to age 34, and if one looks at all causes of death, up to age 50, motor vehicle accident is the most frequently stated cause. The costs to society are truly staggering. NHTSA has estimated the total cost for all motor vehicle accidents to be in excess of $40 billion annually. Certainly, MVA are a major burden to our health care system and represent a disease of epidemic and growing proportions.

So much for historical and national perspective, now let's look at the overall epidemiology of head, neck and spinal cord injury.

Two accident data files have been analyzed to obtain a greater understanding of the incidence and severity of head, neck and spinal cord trauma resulting from motor vehicle accidents. To describe the overall magnitude of the problem we have analyzed data from our national accident sampling system (NASS).

NASS provides us with a probability sample of the nation's traffic accidents. The NASS design calls for accident data to be collected by trained accident investigation teams in each of 75 sites located across the country. Each team collects a specified set of data on a sample of accidents in its area. Both the sites and the accidents within those sites are chosen using probability sampling techniques. The team obtains medically diagnosed injury data from hospital records or treating physicians.

For a more detailed look at the head, neck and spinal cord injury problem I will present data from our national crash severity study. This study was conducted from January 1977 to March 1979. It is a "purposeful" sample of accidents of towaway severity that was designed to obtain quantitative measures of crash severity that could be linked to quantitative measures of injury severity.

From our analysis of 1979 NASS data we estimate of the 4 million people injured in police-reported accidents, 1,860,000 had at least one injury to the head, neck or back and that for 1.3 million (of the 1.8), the most severe injury was to the brain, skull or spinal column (Figure 1).

7,330,000	Police Traffic Accidents
19,500,000	People
4,026,000	Injured
1,860,000	Injury to Head, Neck, or Back
1,301,000	Most Severe Injury to Brain, Skull, or Spinal Column

Figure 1. NASS National Summary Statistics

From NASS we estimate that 47,000 people died (we know that is about 5 percent low) and that 33,000 had at least one injury to the head, neck or back, while 18,000 (of the 33,000) fatalities had the most serious injury; brain, skull, or spinal column (Figure 2).

47,000	People Killed
33,000	Fatalities with Injury to Head, Neck, or Back
18,000	Fatalities with Most Severe Injury to Brain, Skull, or Spinal Column

Figure 2. NASS National Summary Statistics

The next slide (figure 3) shows the status (vehicle occupant or pedestrian) of those victims having most severe injury to the brain, skull or spinal column. Numerically, passenger car occupants predominate: but, truck occupants and motor cyclists are groups of increasing concern.

Most Severe Injury to Brain, Skull or Spinal Column	
Passenger Car	1,106,000
Light Truck or Van	114,000
Heavy Truck	12,000
Motorcycle	19,000
Pedestrian	19,000

Figure 3. NASS Estimate of Injury Involvement by Vehicle Body Type

Now let's take a look at the estimates of the number of these severe injuries occurring annually by AIS severity measure (figure 4). The next slide (figure 5) is a good indication of the tremendous burden placed on our health care facilities by these accident victims. You will note that 193,000 hospitalized patients required 1,538,000 days of hospital care.

I'd like now to give you a glimpse at more detailed data on head, neck and spinal cord injuries from our national crash study.

Maximum AIS	
Critical - Maximum (AIS 5/6)	18,000
Serious - Severe (AIS 3/4)	46,000
Moderate (AIS 2)	124,000
Minor (AIS 1)	1,106,000
Unknown	80,000

Figure 4. NASS Estimates of AIS Level of Most Severe Injury to Brain, Skull, or Spinal Column

Most Severe Injury to Brain, Skull or Spinal Column	
Fatalities	18,000
Non-Fatalities	1,284,000
No Treatment	447,000
Treated and Released	398,000
Other Treatment	234,00
Hospitalized	193,000*
Unknown Treatment	11,000

*Patients Required Total of 1,538,000 Days of Hospital Care

Figure 5. NASS Estimates of Treatment

The most common injuries, as you would expect, are also the least severe (figure 6). The AIS 1-3 level, they mostly involve pain, muscle strain, headache and minor concussion. At the higher severity levels we are dealing with serious brain damage, neurological deficit, fractured vertebrae and spinal cord damage (figure 7).

Total Injuries	10,453
Most Common AIS 1-3 Injuries	
Neck or Back Pain (AIS-1)	3,902
Neck or Back Muscle Strain (AIS-1)	2,223
Headache (AIS-1)	2,165
Minor Concussion (AIS-2)	1,090

Figure 6. Description of Injuries to NCSS Passenger Car Occupants Involving the Brain, Skull, or Spinal Column

Most Common AIS 4-6 Injuries	
Cerebellur Lesion (AIS-5)	91
Concussion (Unconscious 12 Hours) Neurological Signs (AIS-5)	81
Fractured or Dislocated Vertebrae C-3 and Above, with Cord Damage (AIS-6)	81
Concussion (Unconscious 12 Hours) Neurological Signs (AIS-4)	68

Figure 7. Description of Injuries to NCSS Passenger Car Occupants Involving the Brain, Skull or Spinal Column

The next two slides (figures 8 and 9) show the object most commonly contacted by the seriously injured accident victims. Given the geometry of a vehicle's interior and the kinematics of a crash, you see about what one would expect, people hitting interior pillars and windshield. What was surprising to me is the extent to which people are injured by contacts with objects external to the passenger compartment. These contacts are mostly the result of full and partial ejections and intruding vehicles and poles/trees.

Brain and Skull		
Interior Pillars	47	20%
Exterior to Passenger Compartment	47	20%
Windshield	26	11%
Sunvisors, Fittings and/or Header	25	11%
Roof or Convertible Top	20	9%
Other Miscellanious	69	29%
Total	234	100%

"Exterior to Passenger Compartment" Includes Injuries Associated with Ejection and with Intrusion of Another Vehicle or Object

Figure 8. For Serious Injuries (AIS of 4 or Greater) These Are the Most Common Known Injury Contacts on NCSS:

Spinal Columns		
Impact Force	42	55%
Exterior to Passenger Compartment	13	17%
Other Miscellanous	22	29%
Total	77	100%

"Exterior to Passenger Compartment" Includes Injuries Associated with Ejection and with Intrusion of Another Vehicle or Object.

Figure 9. For Serious Injuries (AIS of 4 or Greater) These Are the Most Common Known Injury Contacts on NCSS:

The next slide (figure 10) shows the relationship between one of the important measures of crash severity Delta V, the change in velocity a person undergoes during a crash, with AIS as the measure of injury severity. The relationship is as you would expect, higher Delta V gives rise to higher injury levels.

Most Severe Injury to Brain, Skull, or Spinal Cord			
AIS	Yes	No	Total
1	14.4	15.9	15.4
2	17.6	19.0	18.4
3	21.0	21.5	21.3
4	24.4	24.7	24.6
5	30.5	31.0	30.7
6	30.5	35.0	31.9

Figure 10. NCSS Average Delta V Associated with Injuries by AIS and Injury Type

Finally, from NCSS we can look at the average length of hospital stay associated with particular AIS injury levels (figure 11). Not surprisingly, we see the average length of hospital stay rising dramatically with injury severity.

Most Severe Injury to Brain, Skull or Spinal Column			
AIS	Yes	No	Total
1	0.41	0.15	0.24
2	3.38	2.52	2.76
3	12.68	9.93	10.26
4	19.44	19.56	19.53
5	52.11	22.04	38.51

Figure 11. NCSS Estimates of Average Days Hospitalization by AIS Level for Non-Fatalities

In summary, with broad brush overview, I have tried to give you a feel for the magnitude and alarming growth and persistence of the motor vehicle accident problem in this country. In briefly describing two of our major accident data collection systems, NASS and NCSS, and in discussing the epidemiology of the head, neck and spinal cord injury problem, I hope I have whetted your appetite for finding out still more about what our data systems can do to help you in your work.

The National Head and Spinal Cord Injury Survey: An Overview of the Study and Selected Findings Relative to Head Injury

Benjamin S. H. Harris III, B.A.
William D. Kalsbeek, M.P.H., Ph. D.
Robert L. McLaurin, M.D.

The National Institute of Neurological and Communicative Disorders and Stroke (NINCDS), one of the National Institutes of Health (NIH), requires accurate information about the magnitude of the head and spinal cord injury problem for purposes of planning, especially for determining research priorities. Therefore, over the period 1974–1977, under contract to the Office of Biometry and Epidemiology of NINCDS (Contracts NO1-NS-4-2334 and 263-78-C-0132), the Research Triangle Institute of Research Triangle Park, NC, conducted a large-scale sample survey of the incidence, prevalence, and costs of head and spinal cord injury (HSCI)—i.e., traumatic injury to the central nervous system (CNS). The survey was designed to provide estimates of the occurrence of new cases, the frequency of existing cases, and the resulting economics costs of HSCI for the United States population. Morbidity and cost estimates for HSCI in 1974 were derived from a probability sample survey of the United States (excluding Alaska and Hawaii). A so-called *casefinding* approach was employed whereby cases of HSCI were located through a search of patient medical records in a sample of hospitals. Medically eligible patients were followed up to determine the status of the HSCI in 1974. Finally, patients in the 1974 prevalence group were interviewed for HSCI costs.

The casefinding survey involved a stratified, three-stage sample of patient medical records. The selection of primary sampling units (PSU's) in the first stage involved three general steps: (1) the total land area of the United States was first divided into PSU's, which are area units consisting of counties or groups of contiguous counties; (2) all PSU's were then stratified according to region of the country and level of urbanization; and finally, (3) 58 PSU's were selected for the national study with probabilities proportional to 1970 population size.

Hospitals were selected in the second stage of the sample design. Within each selected PSU, a list of all hospitals was produced from the 1973 Master Facility

Inventory (MFI) of the National Center for Health Statistics (NCHS), then stratified according to the number of beds, average length of stay for patients, and ownership. A supplementary list of hospitals was developed in each PSU to account for those hospitals which were open during the study period (1970 to 1974) but which were excluded from the original list, primarily hospitals which closed prior to, or opened after, the 1973 MFI. These hospitals were stratified by the date of opening or closing, and a sample was selected with equal probabilities and without replacement in each stratum. Counting both sample lists, 305 hospitals were selected for the survey.

Patient discharges were selected in the third stage of the sample design. Discharges from 1974 and two other years in the interval 1970 to 1973 were surveyed in each selected hospital, allocation of the two non-1974 years determined by a controlled randomization process. For each year allocated to a hospital, a list of all discharged with one or more HSCI diagnoses of interest was constructed from which a scientific sample of discharges was selected for abstraction.

Discharges were selected according to final diagnosis as coded by the *Eighth Revision, International Classification of Diseases, Adapted* (ICDA-8) (1); codes of interest to the HSCI study were grouped by injury location (head or spinal cord) and type of code (included or casefinding). *Included* codes were considered indicative of definitive CNS injury while *casefinding* codes included two groups of diagnoses—CNS conditions which may have resulted from CNS injury, such as epilepsy; and injuries about the head, neck, and trunk, such as fracture of the skull, which may have resulted in uncoded CNS injury. The casefinding codes were intended to assist in the detection of CNS insult resulting from traumatic injury where the final diagnosis and the associated diagnostic code did not establish a definitive relationship between the CNS insult and a traumatic incident. The casefinding codes reduced the problem of missing less obvious HSCI eligibles; the problem of false positives remained, requiring steps taken during the study to review questionable eligibles.

Once records were abstracted, they were converted to machine-readable form and subjected to a computer algorithm in order to determine medical eligibility—i.e., classification as an HSCI and eligibility for further follow-up. All discharges which were found to be medically eligible were designated for follow-up to determine the status of the HSCI in 1974. Furthermore, each person whose record abstract indicated medical eligibility, and whose HSCI prevailed in 1974, was eligible for a personal interview on economic costs.

The list of diagnostic codes of interest and the eligibility algorithm were developed with the assistance of an expert Advisory Committee (2). First the algorithm indicated that the abstracted hospital episode resulted from a traumatic incident and was the patient's first hospitalization for the traumatic incident. Thereafter, all cases exhibiting one or more included codes were considered eligible. Cases of head injury exhibiting casefinding codes only were required to demonstrate the appearance of at least one of the following symptoms of CNS insult within five days of the traumatic incident—unconsciousness, seizures, cerebrospinal rhinorrhea, headache, and/or vomiting.

Overall, approximately 81 percent of sample hospitals participated in the survey; approximately 50 percent of sample patients were successfully followed to determine current HSCI status; and approximately 67 percent of interviews on economic costs were completed for patients determined to be eligible.

The estimate of occurrence of new cases of head injury in 1974, 422,000 cases, was derived from 1,210 cases of head injury obtained in the sample; the corresponding rate of occurrence of head injury per 100,000 population was 200. *Occurrence* refers to the number of cases first treated as inpatients in the nation's hospitals during 1974; persons who were seen in consultation at the hospital but not admitted and persons who were dead on arrival at the hospital were not included in the estimates.

The estimate of frequency of head injury that occurred over the period 1970–74 and still existed in 1974, 926,000 cases, is a function of the 1,726 cases of head injury for 1974 that were included in the sample; the corresponding rate of frequency of head injury per 100,000 population was 439. *Frequency* refers to the number of cases first treated as inpatients in the nation's hospitals during the years 1970 through 1974 that still continued during 1974 (that is, the injury victim was alive in 1974 and received treatment during the last 6 months of 1973 or during 1974). Figures on frequency are probably underestimated (3).

Head injury occurs most often in the 15- to 24-year age group as shown graphically in Figure 1,

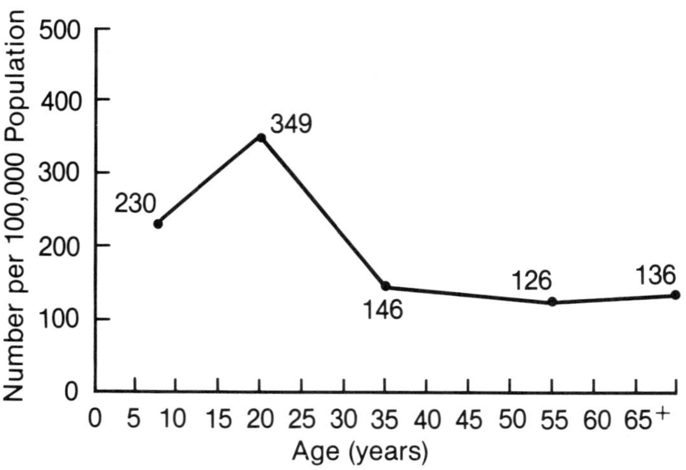

Figure 1. New Cases of Head Injury: Age-Specific Rates, 1974.

which presents 1974 age-specific rates for new cases of head injury. There was no important difference in the occurrence of head injury between white and non-white populations once these had been adjusted for the total numbers. On the other hand, this study showed, as have other local head injury studies (4, 5), that the rate of occurrence of head injury in males is more than twice that for females. The percent distribution by sex of new cases of head injury in 1974 is presented graphically in Figure 2.

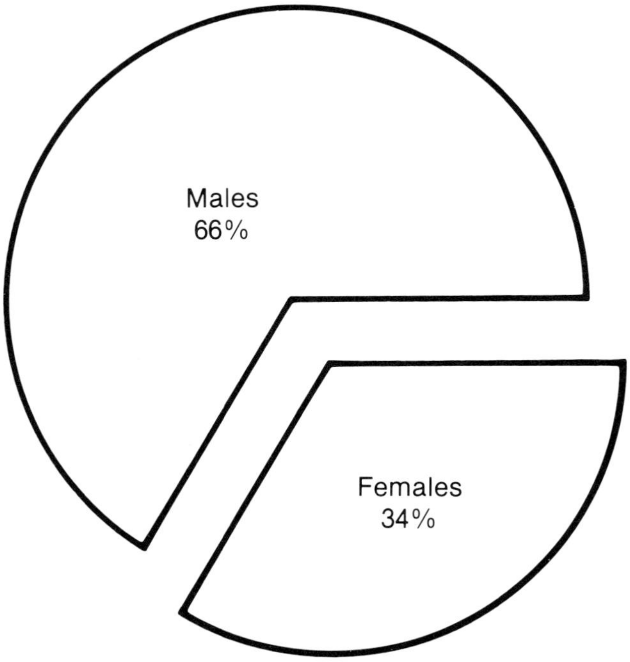

Figure 2. New Cases of Head Injury: Percent Distribution by Sex, 1974.

The rate of occurrence for head injury does not appear to differ significantly from region to region in the United States. Motor vehicle accidents were the most frequent cause of head injury, accounting for 49 percent of all cases occurring during 1974, as shown graphically in Figure 3, which presents the percent distribution by cause of injury of new cases of head injury in 1974. Falls were the second most frequent cause. For motor vehicle accidents, most cases of head injury occurred in the 15- to 24-year age group, whereas most cases of head injury due to falls were seen in the under 15-year-old group; this trend is shown graphically in Figure 4, which presents the percent distribution of new cases of head injury by age group and cause of injury for the study period 1970 through 1974.

Figures 5 and 6 present the monthly and daily occurrence of head injury, respectively. Figure 5 depicts the distribution of cases of head injury for the years 1970 through 1974 by the months in which injury occurred. There was an early peak in occurrence in the month of April, followed by a general increase to the highest monthly percentage in September. Figure 6 indicates that head injuries occur most frequently on Saturdays and Sundays.

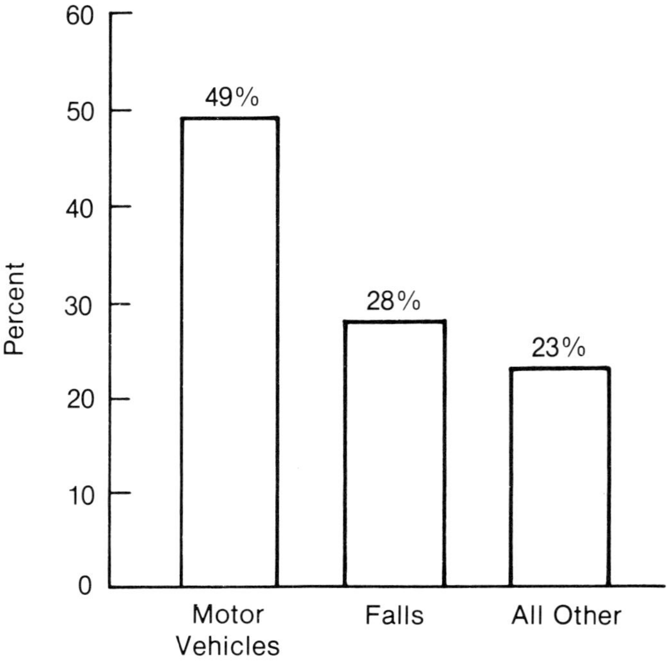

Figure 3. New Cases of Head Injury: Percent Distribution by Cause of Injury, 1974.

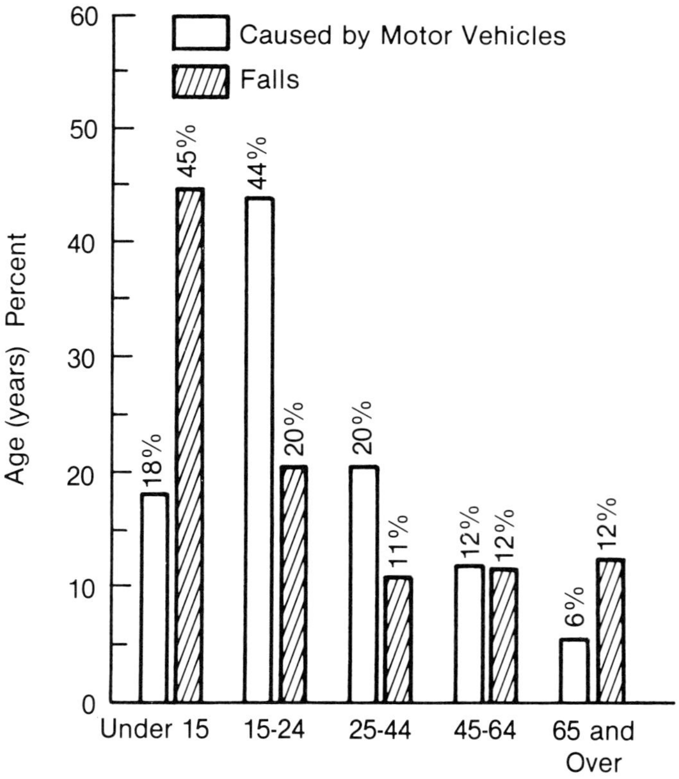

Figure 4. New Cases of Head Injury: Percent Distribution by Age, 1970 Through 1974.

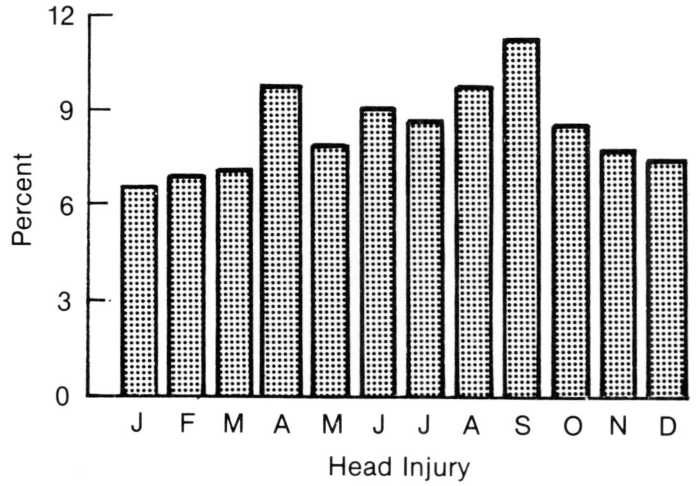

Figure 5. Distribution of Cases of Occurence of Head Injury by the Month in which the Injury Occurred. These Cases Were First Treated in the Nation's Hospitals in the Years 1979 Through 1974. Persons Who Sustained Injury and Died at the Scene of the Injury or Were Dead on Arrival at the Hospital Were Not Included in the Estimates. Data Over a 5-Year Period Have Been Used to Compensate for Small Numbers of Cases.

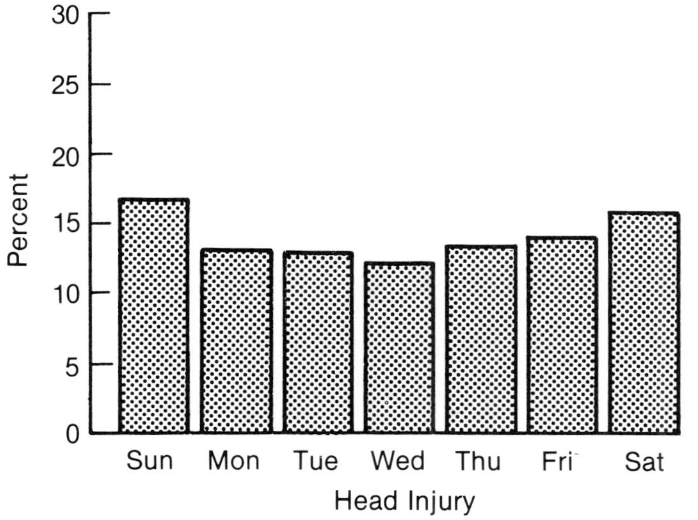

Figure 6. Distribution of Cases of Occurrence of Head Injury by the Day in which the Injury Occurred. These Cases Were First Treated in the Nation's Hospitals in the Years 1970 Through 1974. Persons Who Sustained Injury and Died at the Scene of the Injury or Were Dead on Arrival at the Hospital Were Not Included in the Estimates. Data Over a 5-Year Period Have Been Used to Compensate for Small Numbers of Cases.

The annual occurrence of head injury for the years 1970 through 1974 is presented graphically in Figure 7, separated into principal external causes. It is apparent that there was a significant reduction in head injury cases in the year 1974 when compared to 1973. It is tempting to propose that this drop in occurrence in 1974 was due at least in part to the reduction of the speed limit to 55 miles per hour and the increased use of seatbelts. However, the reduction in the occurrence of head injury in 1974 was a result not only of a reduction in the number of injuries due to motor vehicle accidents, but to an even greater reduction in the number of injuries due to other causes. The present data, therefore, do not support the contention that the reduction in occurrence of head injuries in 1974 can be explained by changes in the regulations governing the operation of motor vehicles.

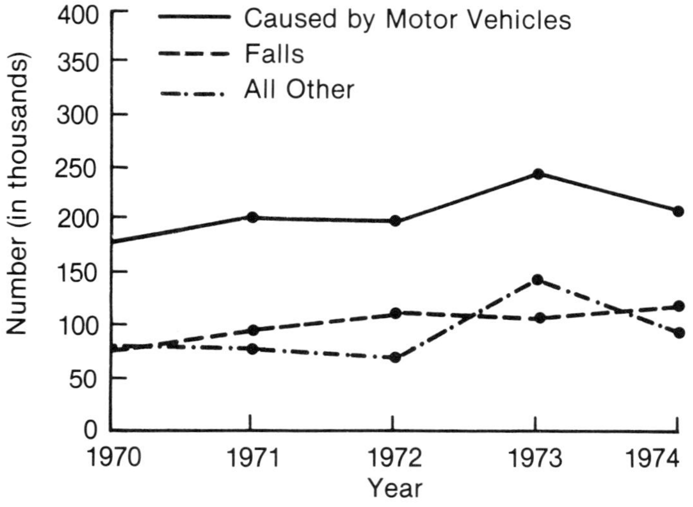

Figure 7. New Cases of Head Injury: Number Occuring Annually, 1970 Through 1974.

The HSCI Survey was an enumerative study. Its chief purpose was to determine the magnitude of the HSCI problem in the United States population. It was the first survey of the U.S. population to focus on measures of morbidity and economic costs specifically associated with head and spinal cord injury. This presentation deals with head injury only. The findings are presented as objective data, but comments directed toward interpretation of the data must be viewed with the understanding that the data are a series of estimates, each with their own level of precision.

Findings from any study must be qualified because of uncertainties, such as bias of selection or errors of measurement, are inevitable. Sources of uncertainty vary with each study. Identification of the chief uncertainties and their effects on conclusions from the data are helpful to the reader. In a special supplement to the *Journal of Neurosurgery* published in November 1980, some uncertainties of the HSCI Survey and their impact on findings are described in more detail (6), as well as additional information on findings of the survey (7).

References

1. National Center for Health Statistics: *Eighth Revision, International Classification of Diseases, Adapted for Use in the United States.* PHS No. 1693. Washington, D.C.: U.S. Government Printing Office, 1967
2. Kalsbeek W.D., Powers C.F., Harwood H.J., et al: *Final Report: Survey of the Incidence, Prevalence and Costs of Head and Spinal Cord Injury.* Research Triangle Park, N.C.: Research Triangle Institute, 1977
3. Anderson D.W., Kalsbeek W.D., Hartwell T.D.: The National Head and Spinal Cord Injury Survey: Design and methodology. *J. Neurosurg 53:*S11-18, 1980
4. Becker D.P., Miller J.D., Ward, J.D., et al: The outcome from severe head injury with early diagnosis and intensive management. *J. Neurosurg 47:*491-502. 1977
5. Jennett B., Teasdale G.,, Braakman R., et al: Prognosis of patients with severe head injury. *Neurosurgery 4:*283-289, 1979
6. Anderson D.W., Kalsbeek W.D.: The National Head and Spinal Cord Injury Survey: Assessment of some uncertainties affecting the findings. *J. Neurosurg 53:*S32-S34, 1980
7. Kalsbeek W.D., McLaurin R.L., Harris B.S.H., et al: The National Head and Spinal Cord Injury Survey: Major Findings. *J Neurosurg 53:*S19-S31, 1980

Head and Neck Injury Involvement in Motorcycle Accidents

Nicholas G. Tsongos

The rapidly increasing popularity of the motorcycle as a relatively inexpensive and economical mode of transportation is evident from the significant increase in registrations. The number of these vehicles being purchased and registered throughout the United States has increased from about two million in 1969 to about five million in 1979. Accompanying the rapid increase in the number of motorcycles is an upward trend in fatal accidents. The number of motorcycle fatalities was 1,870 in 1969, with an increase to 4,893 (1) in 1979.

The motorcycle, with all its excitement and the sense of freedom it provides to the rider, has one serious disadvantage when compared to other transportation modes. Once in an accident, the rider does not have the protective shell of the passenger car. The outcome of the motorcycle accident is well emphasized by its mileage death rate which is estimated (1) to be about 13.8 deaths per one million kilometers of motorcycle travel as compared with the passenger vehicle occupant death rate of 1.5. That makes the probability of an occupant being killed in a motorcycle accident nine times higher than that for passenger car occupants (Figure 1).

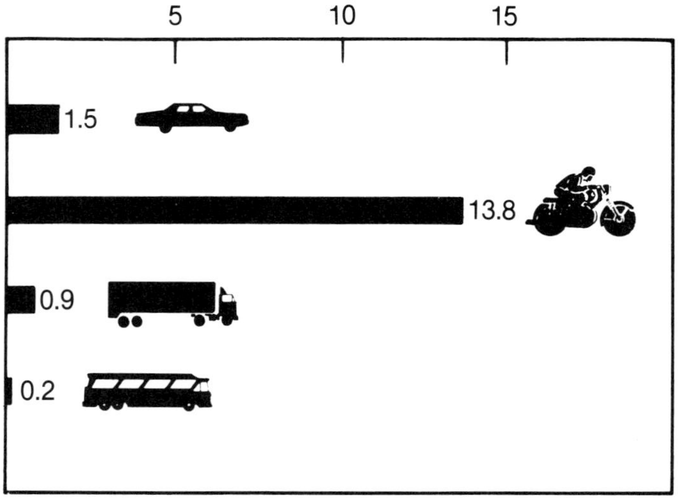

Figure 1. 1979 Fatality Rate per 100 Million Vehicle-Kilometers Travelled

The most common injury to a motorcycle rider involved in an accident is the extremities injury—it comprises about 58 percent of all injuries—(Figure 2) in comparison to the head injury which comprises about one fourth of all injuries (2). Although the extremities injury is the most common in a motorcycle accident, time and care will heal it in most of the cases. This is not the same for a lacerated brain or fractured skull. No matter how minor the accident, there is a good chance that the rider will hit his head, and if it is unprotected, he will suffer serious head injuries. Data collected during the investigation of 900 motorcycle accidents (2) show that the head and neck areas sustained a significant portion of the critical and fatal motorcycle rider injuries, three times higher as compared to all motorcycle rider injuries (Figure 3).

In the same study, 861 discrete injuries to the head and neck regions were identified (Table 1). The distribution of injuries by head-neck region shows the dominance of the forward orientation of the injuries.

The frontal region is very frequently involved in the injuries and could be protected only with the forward structure of a full facial coverage safety helmet.

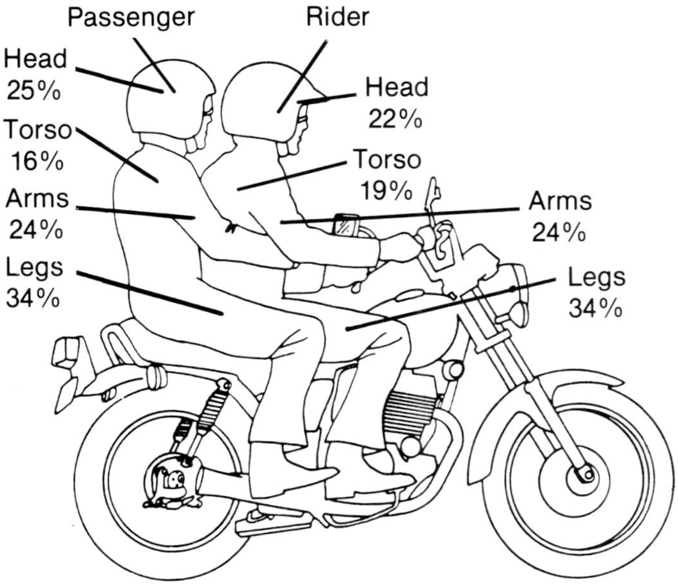

Figure 2. Injury Distribution by Body Area All Riders and Passengers

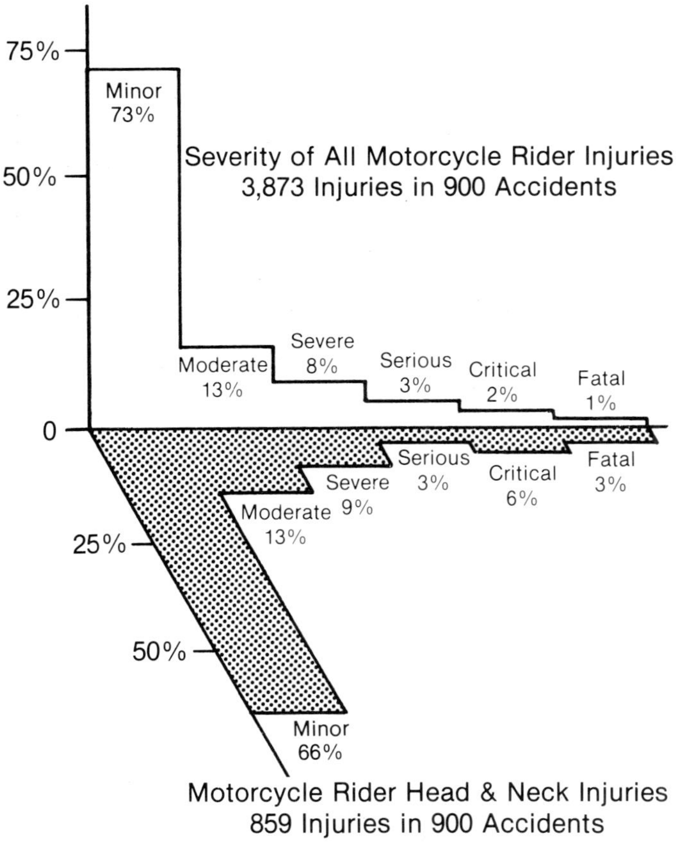

Figure 3. Distribution of Injury Severity

Table 1. Head - Neck Injury Region

Region	Injuries	Percent	Cumulative Frequency
Frontal	119	13.8	13.8
Mandible	99	11.5	25.3
Nasal	49	5.7	31.0
Orbit	48	5.6	36.6
Maxilla	40	4.6	41.2
Zygoma	43	5.0	46.2
Face General	48	5.6	51.8
Basal	39	4.5	56.3
Cervical - General	81	9.4	65.7
Occipital	51	5.9	71.6
Parietal	61	7.1	78.7
Brain - General	103	12.0	90.7
Temporal	44	5.1	95.8
Other	36	4.2	100.0
Total	861	100	

When we examine the head injuries of motorcycle-involved accidents, it is important to segregate the riders who wore helmets and those who did not due to the striking difference of the head injuries between the two groups (2). Figure 4 provides the injury distribution of 900 motorcycle accidents, for riders who wore helmets as compared to those who did not. The head and neck injuries comprised 13 percent of all injuries to helmet users, while for the nonhelmet wearers head and neck injuries comprised 25 percent of all injuries.

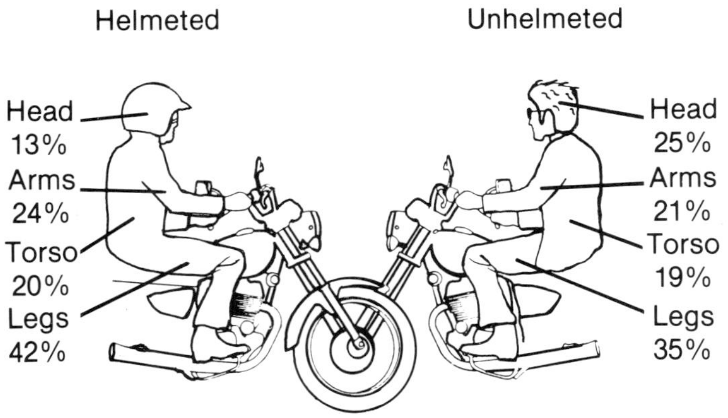

Figure 4. Helmet Use vs. Injury Distribution by Body Area

Table 2 illustrates the distribution of head injuries according to helmet status (3). It will be noted that non-helmeted riders received head injuries which uniformly occurred at a higher rate within *all* AIS Levels, and in each case, the difference is statistically significant. This fact alone is important; however, the distribution of AIS Level 5 injuries is particularly striking. The rate of AIS Level 5 head injuries to helmeted persons was 6.19 injuries for each 1,000 persons involved in accidents. The rate of nonhelmeted individuals who received similar injuries was 431 percent greater, or 32.87 Level 5 injuries for each 1,000 persons involved in accidents. This difference is extremely significant ($X^2 = 11.78$, p .001). None of the information contained in this table relating to injuries to the neck is statistically significant.

Table 2. Number of All Injuries to the Head and Neck with Rates per 1,000 Riders Fatally and Non-Fatally Injured Riders

Injury Location	Injury Severity	Helmet Use: Yes		Helmet Use: No	
		Number	Rate	Number	Rate
Head and Face	AIS = 1	51	78.95	94	162.63
	2	13	20.12	39	67.47
	3	5	7.74	7	12.11
	4	4	6.19	8	13.84
	5	4	6.19	19	32.87
Neck	AIS = 1	16	24.77	20	34.60
	2	0	0.00	0	0.00
	3	2	3.10	1	1.73
	4	1	1.55	1	1.73
	5	0	0.00	1	1.73
Total for Head and Neck Injuries	AIS = 1	67	103.72	114	197.23
	2	13	20.12	39	67.47
	3	7	10.84	8	13.84
	4	5	7.74	9	15.57
	5	4	6.19	20	34.60

Source: University of Kansas Medical School Study

Examining the riders who suffered severe head injuries in motorcycle fatal accidents (2), again we see that the rate of nonhelmeted riders was 2.5 times higher than those of helmeted riders (Table 3).

Within the limitations of this discussion, an attempt was made to emphasize some highlights of the head/neck injuries in motorcycle accidents. The National Highway Traffic Safety Administration has sponsored four motorcycle accident studies which have been completed recently. These studies provide good sources of motorcycle head/neck injury data for further study.

- Motorcycle Accident Factors Study
  (University of Southern California)
- Impact of the Repeal of the Kansas Mandatory M/C Helmet Law
  (University of Kansas Medical Center)
- Impact of M/C Helmet Usage in Colorado
  (Colorado Department of Highways)
- Impact of M/C Helmet Law Repeal in South Dakota
  (University of South Dakota)

In summary, head/neck injuries predominate the severe injuries in motorcycle accidents, with the chest injuries following. Surviving cyclists suffer usually from injury to the extremities. Helmets affect very much the outcome of the injury severity in a motorcycle accident. Helmeted riders have a significant advantage over unhelmeted riders in reducing not only the number, but also the severity of the head injury.

Table 3. Severe Head Injuries (AIS 5 & 6) M/C Riders Involved in Fatal Accidents

Helmet Used	Head Injuries AIS 5 & 6: No	Head Injuries AIS 5 & 6: Yes	Total
No	19 (28.2)*	27 (40.1)	46 (68.3)
Yes	6 (15.8)	6 (15.8)	12 (31.6)
Total	25 (23.7)	33 (31.3)	58 (55.1)

*Numbers in Parenthesis Are Rates/1,000 Riders

References

1. *Fatal Accident Reporting System,* National Highway Traffic Safety Administration, U.S. Department of Transportation, 1979
2. *Motorcycle Accident Cause Factors and Identification of Countermeasures,* University of Southern California, January 1981
3. *Impact of the Repeal of the Kansas Mandatory Motorcycle Helmet Law 1975–1978,* University of Kansas, College of Health Sciences. Final Report October 1980

Risk of Head and Neck Injury if There is No Direct Head Impact

Claude Tarriere

The following data are based on an analysis of frontal, lateral and rear collisions in a series of automotive accidents as shown in Table I.

Results

1. Frontal Collision—In this group, we selected a subsample of 458 cases of front-belted occupants, without rear passengers, who did not sustain direct head impact. In this group, not a single case of significant head injury (AIS=0) was found. Four cases where head contact occurred but location was unknown had no loss of consciousness (AIS=1) (Table II). Regarding risk of neck injuries, in such cases, we found 35 cases of AIS=1 among 458 cases of front-belted occupants (7.6%), who complained only of neck pain and had no other complications.

2. Lateral Collision—In this group, we selected a subsample of pure lateral impacts having impact directions at 8–9 and 10 or 2–3–4 o'clock. None of these occupants suffered head or neck impacts and all were belted (337 occupants involved). Again, as in frontal collisions, we found that, without direct head or neck impact, there was not a single case of head AIS=0 and, there were only 7 cases of neck pain (neck AIS=1) (Table III). In a series of 601 unbelted occu-

Table 1. Peugeot-Renault Accident Investigation Sample

B = Belted Occupants U.B. = Unbelted Occupants

				AIS 6	AIS 3-4-5	AIS 2-1	AIS 0
Frontal	2528 Cars	UB	3461	196	448	2116	688
		B	1398	46	176	669	503
Lateral	684 Cars	UB	964	88	156	506	209
		B	337	17	44	177	100
Roll-Over	489 Cars	UB	710	45	91	430	145
		B	315	4	20	188	102
Rear	461 Cars	UB	631	14	22	376	216
		B	357	5	12	191	148
Others	63 Cars	UB	99	35	20	37	6
		B	36	6	13	15	2
	4225 Cars	UB	5865	378	737	3465	1265
		B	2443	78	265	1240	855
			8308	456	1002	4705	2120
Seat Belt Wearing Unknown			77	2			
			8385	458			

Injury Severity Unknown = 29 Cases (7 B, 22 UB)

Table 2.

No. 228:	Ford Capri: Frontal and Rear Impacts on Motorway. The Right Front Passenger Presents a Head AIS = 1 (Head Trauma Without Unconsciousness) Diagonal Belt Worn with Slack (2 Rib Fractures) Head Impact Probable, but Impact Area Unknown.
No. 1927:	Renault 12: Angled Frontal Impact (10 Hours) and Left Lateral Impact. The Right Front Passenger Presents a Head AIS = a (Head Trauma Without Unconsciousness) 3-Point-Belt-Knee Impact in Radio Set Head Impact Probable, but Impact Area Unknown.
No. 2351:	Ford Escort: Ran Off the Roadway and Frontal Impact Against Tree. The Driver Presented a Head AIS = 1 (Head Trauma without Unconsciousness). 3-Point-Belt Head Impact Probable, but Impact Area Unknown.
No. 2376:	Opel Ascona: Head-On Impact Against a Car (Δ V = 15-25 km/h). Right Front Pasenger Presents a Head AIS = 1 (Head Trauma without Unconsciousness). 3-Point-Belt No Impact Found.

pants who were not ejected by the impact, we were unable to find a single case of head AIS>0. There were only two cases of neck AIS=1 but, in the second case (No. 3657), it is possible that a head impact occurred with an interposition of the arm between head and B-pillar (Table IV). Head impact occurred against the side window in 103 of 1,301 occupants (8%). In this group, the distribution of head injury was as follows: 7 head AIS=0, 73 head AIS=1, 21 head AIS=2, 1 head AIS=3, and 1 AIS=5 (without autopsy); head AIS unknown. Of particular interest are 21 cases where the lateral window was broken, i.e., without effective limitation of lateral flexion of the head on the neck. In this subgroup, 90% of head AIS⩾2. This would suggest a greater degree of brain injury when the window fails to stop lateral head movement. Regarding neck injuries, in such cases, there were 3 neck AIS=1+1 neck AIS=3 (fracture of C3 without neurological symptoms).

3. Rear Collisions (directions 5-6-7 o'clock)—Among 406 occupants, only 3 cases of brain injuries without direct head impact were observed. Of these there were: 2 head AIS=2, 1 head AIS=1, 71 cases of neck AIS=1 (18%), and 1 case of neck AIS=2–3 (Table V).

Conclusion

The risk of head injury is reduced when front-belted occupants are involved in *frontal* collisions *without* head impact, as is also the risk of severe (AIS>3) neck injuries. The same is true of *lateral* collisions. Significant head injuries, but not greater than AIS=2, occurred occasionally in *rear* impacts when no head impact occurred (3 of 406 occupants).

Table 3. Lateral Impacts, Belted Occupants with Head or Neck Injuries but Without Direct Head Impact

337 Belted Occupants in Lateral Impact (All Directions)

234 Belted Occupants in Lateral Impacts (Directions 8-9-10 Hours or 2-3-4 Hours).

— There Is No Case of a Belted Occupant with a Head Injury without Direct Impact of the Head.

— There Are Seven Cases of Neck Injuries without Impact of the Head or the Neck:

No. 1661:	Simca 1100: Δ V 15-25 km/h, 2 Impacts The Driver Was on the Opposite Side to Impact; a Neck Ache Is the Only Injury Observed
No. 3069:	BMW 1602: Δ V = 15-25 km/h, 1 Impact Right Front Passenger, Nearside to Impact, Contusion
No. 908:	Renault 16: Δ V = 25-35 km/h, 1 Impact Right Front Passenger, Opposite Side to Impact, Thorax Ache
No. 3145:	Fiat 124: Δ V < 15 km/h, 2 Impacts Driver, Nearside to Impact, a Neck Contusion Is the Only Lesion Observed
No. 4270:	Renault 16: Δ V = 15-25 km/h, 1 Impact Driver, Nearside to Impact, Contusion
No. 4851:	Simca 1100: Δ V = 15-25 km/h, 1 Impact, Right Front Passenger, Opposite Side to Impact, Not Hospitalized

Table 4. Lateral Impacts: Directions 8-9-10 or 2-3-4 Hours 601 Unbelted Occupants, Not Ejected

No Case of Unbelted Occupant with a Head Injury without Direct Impact	
2 Cases of Minor Neck Injury without Direct Impact of Head or Neck:	
No. 3869:	Citroen 2 CV: Left Lateral Impact, Δ V = 15-25 km/h, 1 Impact Right Front Passenger, Male, Aged 28, Opposite Side to Impact. The Only Lesion Is a Neck Contusion (AIS = 1)
No. 3657:	Renault 16: Right Lateral Impact, Δ V = 25-35 km/h, 2 Impacts Driver, Male, Age Unknown, Opposite Side to Impact, Strain (C3-C4) without Neurological Sign (AIS = 1), (and Also, Left Clavicle Fracture, One Right Rib Fracture, Hip Dislocation, Right Forearm Fracture) No Head Injury but, Perhaps, Impact Against Right B-Pillar with Interposition of Right Forearm.

Table 5. Rear Impact Direction 5-6-7 Hours

406 Occupants Involved in Specific Rear Impacts: 228 Front Occupants and 118 Rear Occupants.	
3 Cases of Head Injuries without Direct Head Impact.	
No. 369:	Volkswagen 1300: ETS < 15 km/h, 1 Impact Right Front Passenger, Female, Aged 33 Head AIS = 2, Unconsciousness 15′ Neck AIS = 1, Contusion C5-C6 No Headrest, Seat Intact, Seat Back Angle: 120, No Head Impact
No. 882:	Open Kadett: ETS < 15 km/h, 1 Impact of Little Violence Driver, Male, Aged 53 Head AIS: 2 Trauma without Unconsciousness, but confused, no Radiological Signs. 3 Days of Hospitalization, 3 Months of Invalidity. No Headrest, Seat Intact, Seat Back Angle 120
No. 1204:	Renault 8: Δ V < 15 km/h, 1 Impact, Driver, Male, Aged 31 Head AIS: 1 Trauma without Unconsciousness No Headres, Seat Intact, Seat Back Angle 130 No Head Impact Note: the Right Passenger Who Had a Headrest Also Suffers from head Trauma without unconsciousness
No. 1581	Renault 4: Impact of Unknown Violence (Against a Lorry) Driver, Female, AGed 32 Head AIS: 1, Head Trauma without Unconsciousness Neck Ache, Hospitalized 10 Days No Headrest, Seat Intact, Seat Back Angle 120 No Impact
No. 89:	Fiat 500, ETS < 15 km/h, 1 Impact Driver, Female, Aged 43 Dislocation C2-C3 without Neurological Sign Strengthening Device (Minerve) During 3 Months (Previous Lumbar Arthrosis) No Headrest, Seat Intact, Seat Back Angle 120 No Impact
71 Cases of Neck AIS = 1: Ache, Contusion or Strain Among Them, One Particular Case No. 1581	

SESSION 2, PART 1:

Physiopathology and Biomechanics of Head Injury

Session 2, Part 1
Physiopathology and Biomechanics of Head Injury

Introduction

A. K. Ommaya, M.D.

This session was chaired by Dr. A. K. Ommaya who briefly reviewed the historical background to current research directions in head injury mechanisms and also described a paradigm for such research as derived from his paper on *Cerebral Concussion and Traumatic Unconsciousness* published in 1974 in the Journal of *Brain* (1). This paradigm and more recent research initiated at NIH and now being continued at the University of Pennsylvania is described in the following paper by Dr. Gennarelli. The following is a brief synopsis of Dr. Ommaya's remarks on methodology arising in the discussion of papers read at this session. Firstly with regard to classification of Head Injuries shown in Table 1 of the paper by Dr. Gennarelli, the subdivision of Diffuse Brain Injuries into 4 categories of increasingly severe nature shown is perhaps better described as numbered grades of the most important brain injury (cerebral concussion) as detailed in Reference 1 mentioned above. This would eliminate the semantic problem of the terms "diffuse injury" and "shearing injury" suggesting a mechanism different from that causing cerebral concussion when all four of the terms in Table 1 are actually only increasingly severe grades of diffuse injury. The advantage of using the classification of Cerebral Concussion diffuse injuries into 6 grades as shown below, apart from semantic clarity, is that the grades also correspond with the AIS levels of increasing severity of brain injury (2).

Diffuse Injuries

Clinical Description	Concussion Grade	AIS
1. Post-traumatic confusion without coma or amnesia	I	I
2. Post-traumatic confusion with post-traumatic amnesia but no coma or retrograde amnesia	II	II
3. Post-traumatic amnesia plus retrograde amnesia but no coma	III	III
4. Post-traumatic coma plus amnesia (classical concussion) with coma <24 hrs.	IV	IV
5. Post-traumatic coma >24 hrs.	V	V
6. Permanent vegetative state or death	VI	V, VI

Secondly, regarding the paper by Nakamura and his colleagues from three Japanese universities and the Japan Automobile Research Institute, the data reported are most interesting in that they conflict with other published data. Thus Thibault et al. have found that under well controlled inertial loading (no contact phenomena allowed) lateral motions of the head on the neck are more injurious than sagittal motions for equivalent accelerations, i.e., completely opposite conclusion to that of the Japanese workers. These differences may well be explained by the markedly different methodologies employed. Thus, the high incidence of skull fractures in the rotational acceleration mode and of clavicular fractures and chest injuries in the translational acceleration mode tend to introduce highly significant head contacts in the rotational mode and of relative chest and neck angulation in the translational mode in the Japanese experiments. The conclusions drawn therefore must be considered very critically in light of these experimental differences. These comments also apply to the conclusions of Ono et al. (3), describing related data from this and previous series of experiments wherein no correlation of concussion with rotational acceleration was reported. Because of the considerable importance of these methodologic issues in data interpretation, the editor will publish a more detailed report which will also include a comprehensive annotated bibliography of head and neck injuries.

References

1. Ommaya, A.K. and Gennarelli, T.A., "Cerebral Concussion and Traumatic Unconsciousness", *Brain,* Vol. 97, 633–654, 1974.

2. *The Abbreviated Injury Scale (AIS), 1976 and 1980,* Revisions. American Association Automotive Medicine, Morton Grove, IL 60053.
3. Ono, K., Kikuchi, A., Nakamura, M., Kobayashi, H., and Nakamura, N., "Human Head Tolerance to Sagittal Impact. Reliable Estimation Deduced from Experimental Head Injury Using Subhuman Primates and Human Cadaver Skulls", Proc. 24th Stapp Car Crash Conference, S.A.E. Penn. 1980.

Mechanistic Approach to the Head Injuries: Clinical and Experimental Studies of the Important Types of Injury

Thomas A. Gennarelli, M.D.

Head injury can no longer be considered as a unitary phenomenon to be discussed as if it were a single entity. Rather, state-of-the-art deliberations must focus on the many individual varieties of pathophysiological disturbance to the skull or its contents which together comprise the head injuries. What, then, are the types of head injury that occur, which types are important causes of death and disability and conversely, which types are more regularly associated with favorable outcome? Since these questions can now be answered with a high degree of confidence, it is possible to relate known or proposed causal mechanisms to each injury type. In this way rational plans can be devised to study these injuries individually and tolerance criteria can be developed for every type of head injury.

Types of Head Injury (Table 1)

In general terms, it is convenient to view head injuries as comprising three distinct varieties.

Skull fracture can occur with or without damage to the brain but is itself not an important cause of neurologic death or disability. Skull fractures can be classified in many ways and are considered open fractures if the dura is torn or closed fractures if it is not. More conventionally fractures are categorized into those of the vault and those of the base. Injuries to the neural substance of the brain are the primary cause of neurological dysfunction and can readily be divided into two categories. **Focal brain injuries** are those in which a lesion large enough to be visualized with the naked eye has occurred and comprise contusions, subdural hematoma, epidural hematoma and intracerebral hematoma. These lesions cause neurological problems not only by virtue of the local brain damage, but, by causing masses within the cranium, they lead to brain shift, herniation and ultimately brainstem compression. These injuries comprise approximately 50 percent of all head injury patients admitted to the hospital and are responsible for two-thirds of head injury deaths. **Diffuse brain injuries,** on the other hand, are associated with more widespread or global disruption of neurologic function and are not usually associated with macroscopically visible brain lesions. Rather they cause widespread disruption of either the function or structure of the brain. Since diffuse brain injuries, for the most part, are not associated with visible microscopic lesions, they have historically been lumped together to mean all injuries not associated with focal lesions. Recently, however, diagnostic information has been gained from computerized tomographic scanning, as well as from neurophysiological and neuropathological studies, which enables us to better define several categories within this broad group of diffuse brain injuries. Four categories of diffuse brain injuries are now recognized:

1. Mild concussion: Several specific concussion syndromes exist which involve temporary disturbance of neurological function without loss of consciousness.

Table 1.

Skull Injuries	Focal Injuries	Diffuse Brain Injuries
Vault Fracture	Epidural Hematoma	Mild Concussion
Linear	Subdural Hematoma	Classical Cerebral Concussion
Depressed	Contusion	Diffuse Injury
Basilar Fracture	ICH	Shearing Injury

2. Classical cerebral concussion: Classical cerebral concussion is a temporary reversible neurological deficiency caused by trauma which results in temporary loss of consciousness (less than 24 hours).

3. Diffuse injury: Diffuse injury is a traumatic brain injury with prolonged loss of consciousness (more than 24 hours). There is usually little or no evidence of brainstem dysfunction but these patients nevertheless may have residual neurological, physchological or personality defects.

4. Diffuse white matter shearing injury (shearing injury or diffuse impact injury): Shearing injuries are an extreme form of diffuse brain injury with considerable anatomical disruption of white matter fibers throughout both hemispheres. This is evidenced by prolonged loss of consciousness (more than 24 hours) and clinical evidence of brainstem dysfunction.

These diffuse brain injuries account for approximately 40 percent of head injured patients admitted to hospitals; and although they comprise only one-third of the deaths, they are the most serious cause of persisting neurological disability in the survivors.

The Importance of Individual Types of Head Injury

In order to determine the importance of individual injuries to death, disability and recovery, injury type and outcome were determined in a series of 434 hospitalized head injury patients. Overall, 1,121 individual lesions were present in these patients (mean 2.58 lesions per patient). Only 26 percent of the patients had a single lesion diagnosis while another 26 percent had two lesions. Twenty-one percent of the patients had three individual head injury lesions, 18 percent had four separate lesions and the remaining 9 percent had five or more lesions. Outcome one month after injury was determined according to the five point Glasgow Outcome Scale. This scale was collapsed into three groups comprising deaths, poor outcome (vegetative and severe disability) and acceptable outcome (good recovery or moderate disability) (Table 2). Over half (54 percent) of the 54 deaths were caused by two lesions, the acute subdural hematoma and the diffuse shearing injury. Conversely, roughly half (48 percent) with acceptable outcome had one of two lesions, cerebral concussion or cortical contusion. These four thus represent the extremes of "bad" and "good" types of head injuries.

Another way of evaluating the importance of these lesions to mortality is to compute the mortality index for each lesion. The mortality index is the product of the individual lesion mortality and its frequency, and thus notes the number of deaths in a head injury series of 10,000 patients attributable to each lesion. Table 3 demonstrates the findings in the overall population studied which comprised all degrees of injury severity. It can be seen that in this series the overall mortality was 1,194 per 10,000 patients (11.94 percent). It is evident that the two most common lesions, cerebral concussion and cortical contusion, are relatively unimportant causes of mortality, whereas the subdural hematoma and shearing injury though infrequent in occurrence together are responsible for over half of all the deaths (57 percent). Thus, the acute subdural hematoma and the shearing injury are the most important causes of death and together are responsible for more deaths than are all other lesions combined.

Table 2. Lesions Associated with Death Best Diagnosis All Patients

1 Month Outcome N = 434

Rank	N	Lesion	% with Lesion Dead
1	18	Acute SDH	47
2	11	Diffuse Shearing	65
3	6	Diffuse Injury	11
4	5	ICH	28
5	4	Cortical Contusion	7
6	3	Pediatric Swelling	12
7	2	Adult Swelling	40
	2	Deep Contusion	67
	2	Brain Step Hemorrhage	100
10	1	Epidural Hematoma	4
	54	Total	12%

Table 3. Importance to Mortality All Hospitalized Patients

	Overall Incidence (%)	Incidence in Non-Survirvors (%)	Mortality Index (Deaths/10,000)
SDH	9	33	423
Shearing Injury	4	20	260
Diffuse Injury	13	11	143
ICH	4	9	112
Cortical Contusion	13	7	91
Cerebral Concussion	24	0	0
Other	33	19	165
Total	100	100	1194

In order to corroborate these findings a multi-center cooperative study was undertaken involving seven head injury centers in the United States. Admission criteria for this study was different than the previously described study of all hospitalized head injury patients and comprised only severely injured patients. This group of severe head injuries was determined by the internationally accepted criteria of the Glasgow Coma Score of 8 or less which persists for a minimum of six hours. Overall focal injuries comprised the 56 percent of the 1,107 patients and had a mortality of 48 percent, whereas the diffuse brain injuries comprised 44 percent of the study population with a mortality of 32 percent. Table 4 ranks the mortality of the individual lesions in this study. In this study coma greater than 24 hours with decerebration is roughly equivalent to the shearing lesion, whereas coma greater than 24 hours not decerebrate corresponds to diffuse injury. It is readily apparent that the subdural hematoma and shearing injury continue to occupy the top of the mortality list and, as in the previous study, are the worst head injury lesions. Computing the mortality index for these two lesions demonstrates that in a similar population of 10,000 severely head injured patients, 1,769 will die from subdural hematoma and 816 from shearing injury. This amounts to 64 percent of the deaths in the severe head injury group.

Table 4. Severe Head Injury Mortality Rank

Lesion	GCS	%
1. SDH	3-5	74
2. Coma V 24 hr-Decerebrate	3-5	57
3. Other Focal	3-5	56
4. Coma V 24 hr-Not Decerebrate	3-5	47
5. EDH	3-5	36
6. SDH	6-8	36
7. Coma 6-24 hr	3-5	30
8. Coma V 24 hr-Decerebrate	6-8	28
9. Other Focal	6-8	18
10. Coma V 24 hr-Not Decerebrate	6-8	11
11. EDH	6-8	9
12. Coma 6-24 hr.	6-8	9

Thus two independent studies of head injury patients both confirm the fact that two lesions are overwhelmingly the most significant causes of death. **In both series the subdural hematoma and the shearing injury are responsible for more deaths than all other causes combined.**

Injury Mechanisms Associated With Individual Types of Head Injury

The types of mechanical injuries to the head are numerous and complex. Figure 1 provides a flow chart analysis of the known and proposed mechanisms of injury. In simplistic terms it is useful to divide commonly occurring types of head injuries into those due to the primary effects of an object striking the head (impacting phenomena) and those effects due to movement of the head (inertial effects).

Contact phenomena are a complex sequence of mechanical events that have been implicated in scalp laceration, fracture of the cranial vault, epidural hematoma and some types of cortical contusions. The magnitude and importance of these phenomena vary with the size of the impacting device and with the magnitude of the force of the impact. Scalp laceration

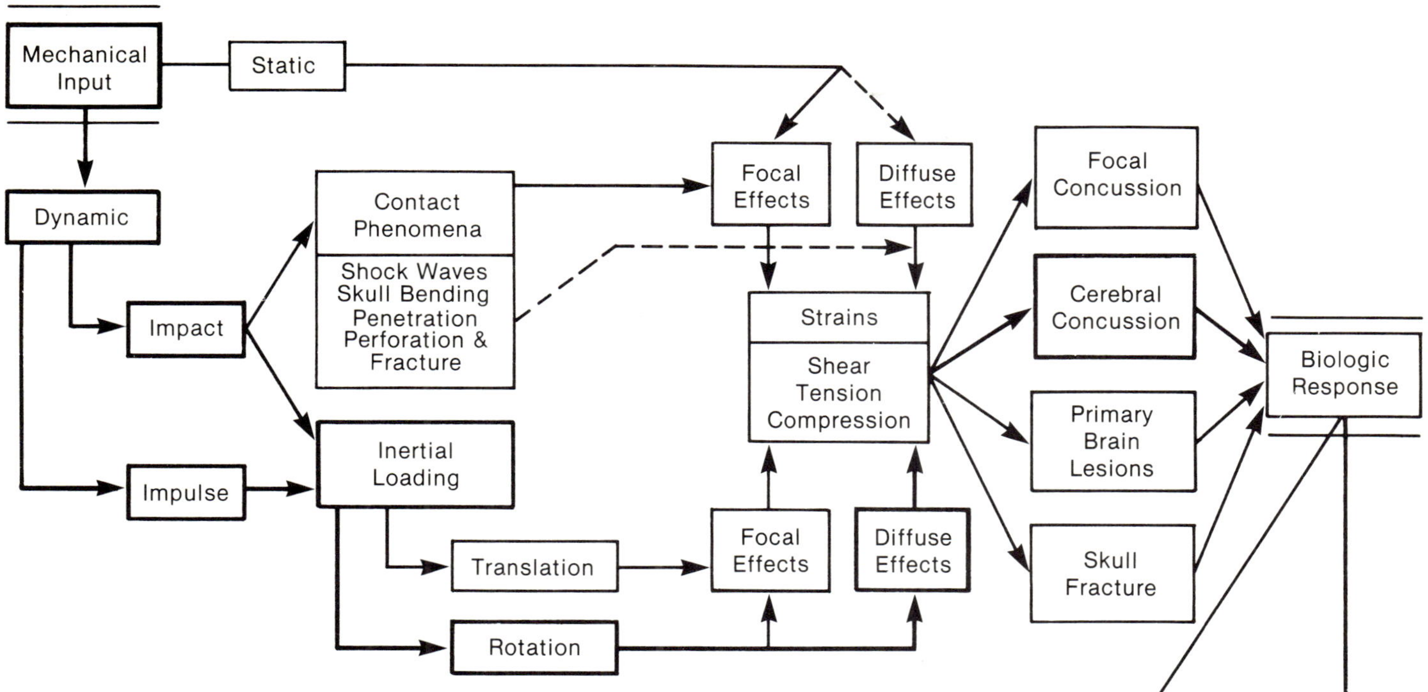
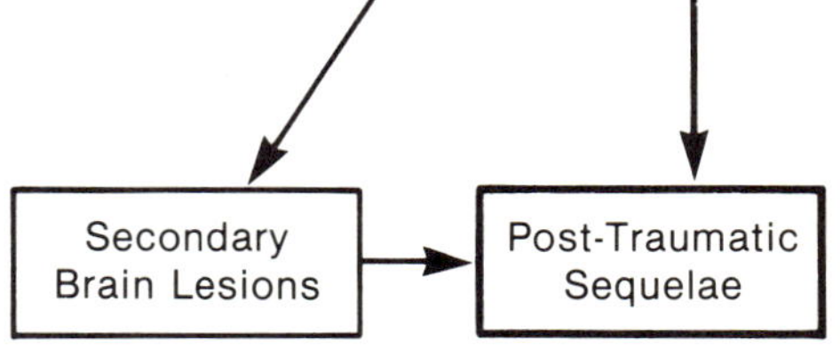

Figure 1.Head Injury Mechanics

and fractures of the cranial vault result almost entirely from local contact phenomena. Epidural (extradural) hematoma involves disruption of vessels (usually arteries) which line the skull or dura and although the hematoma compresses the brain (focally), the injury, mechanistically, is really a form of complicated skull trauma. It, therefore, results from the same types of contact injury that cause skull fracture. Cortical contusions are focal disruptions of the brain surface either beneath (coup contusions) or opposite (contrecoup contusions) the impact site. Considerable work supports the mechanism of the coup contusions, at least, to be due to local contact phenomena beneath the area of impact.

Stress wave propagation and the effects of skull oscillations are other mechanisms resulting from an object striking the skull. These cause skull fracture at a distance from the site of impact and notably basal skull fractures. Additionally, contrecoup contusions are most likely due to remote effects of stress wave propagation or remote skull bending and may result in compressive/tensile strains. Intracerebral hemorrhage/hematoma (ICH) and/or the so-called intermediate contusions are vascular disruptions within the brain substance and also most likely to be caused by concentrated strains caused by stress wave propagation.

Acceleration (inertial) effects of the head whether caused by an impact or by impulsive loading result in the diffuse brain injuries rather than the focal injuries. The one exception to this is the acute subdural hematoma, which results, most often, from physical disruptions of the subdural bridging veins. Ample work documents that translational and rotational components of acceleration, either purely or in combination, are most important for the genesis of concussion and the diffuse brain injuries.

Table 5 reports the data from this series of 434 hospitalized head injury patients and correlates the injury type and its proposed mechanism with the injury importance. It can be seen that the effects of impact to the skull (contact and stress wave injuries) comprise half (54 percent) of all the head injuries but are responsible for only one-fifth (22 percent) of all deaths and a similar number of poor quality survivors (21 percent). On the other hand, injuries which are principally due to acceleration comprise only one-third of all head injuries but are responsible for two-thirds (64 percent) of all deaths and poor quality survivors. Therefore, it is clear that from an overall viewpoint **acceleration is the most important injury mechanism in human head injury with regard to death and disability.**

Methods of Studying the Important Head Injuries and Their Mechanisms

Since acceleration injuries are the most important causes of death and disability, several studies have been undertaken by the author and his colleagues to determine the effects of inertial loading of the head.

Table 5.

Injury and Mechanism	Prevalence (% of All Lesions)	Cause of Death (% of All Deaths)	Cause of Poor Survival (% of All Veg-Sev)
Contact	36	6	12
Scalp Laceration	13	0	0
Vault Fracture	15	0	0
Epidural Hematoma	2	2	8
Cortical Contusion	6	4	4
Stress Wave	18	16	9
Basal Skull Fracture	7	0	0
Contusion - Contre Coup	8	7	4
Intracerebral Hematoma	3	9	5
Acceleration	33	64	62
Concussion	18	0	4
Diffuse Injury	5	11	40
Shearing Injury	2	20	6
Subdural Hematoma	8	33	12
Secondary Injury/Other	13	13	17

Various head injury devices were either modified or constructed in order to provide programmable reproducible inertial loading to the head of the subhuman primate in a fashion which would minimize contact phenomenon and thereby study inertial effects in a more pure fashion. The systems utilized were all characterized by sagittal plane movement, controlled head kinematics and distributed loading. The latter was achieved by encasing the head within a specially constructed helmet system which was rigidly attached to the accelerating apparatus.

In an early series of experiments utilizing the squirrel monkey, the effects of translational and angular acceleration on the brain were directly studied. Two groups of animals were subjected to identical acceleration loading: the first group incurred translational acceleration and the second group utilizing angular acceleration to a 45° arc, the center of rotation being in the cervical spine. The physiological and pathological result of these two groups differed markedly. At the maximum accelerations used, it was impossible to induce a cerebral concussion in monkeys undergoing pure translational acceleration. On the other hand, it was very easy to induce concussion from angular acceleration. It became quite evident therefore that the type of acceleration delivered to the head has a profound influence on the type of resulting neurological dysfunction.

These initial experiments were followed by a series of 100 primate head injuries utilizing just the angular acceleration mechanism. This mechanism was utilized because of the author's interest in cerebral concussion and the diffuse brain injuries. The hypothesis was held that these injuries (cerebral concussion, diffuse injury and shearing injury) form a continuum which results from increasing amounts of shear strain due to increasing angular acceleration (Figure 2). It was hoped that this series of experiments would provide not only a tolerance criteria for cerebral concussion but also for diffuse injury and shearing injury (Figure 3). It was found that utilizing angular acceleration in this series of rhesus monkeys that concussion could be readily produced. However, as acceleration magnitude was increased, prolonged unconsciousness was not achieved; and thus the diffuse injury and shearing lesion were not produced. Instead, as acceleration was increased, subdural bridging veins were torn and large acute subdural hematomas of sufficient size to cause death occurred.

Considering the properties of the subdural bridging veins and their extreme sensitivity to strain rate, it became clear that a tolerance criteria for subdural

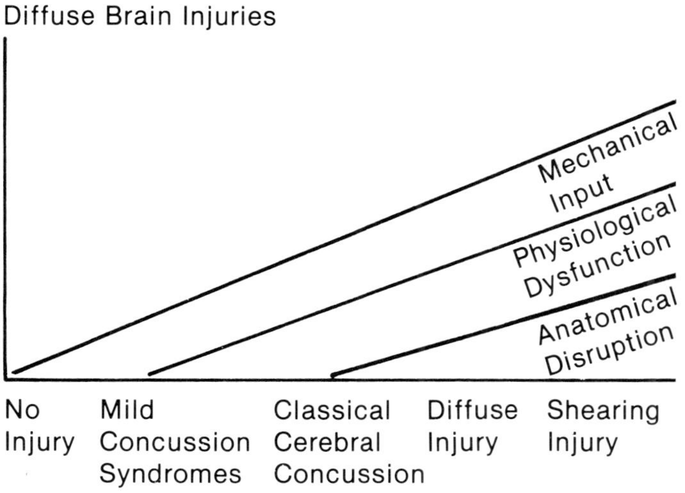

Figure 2.

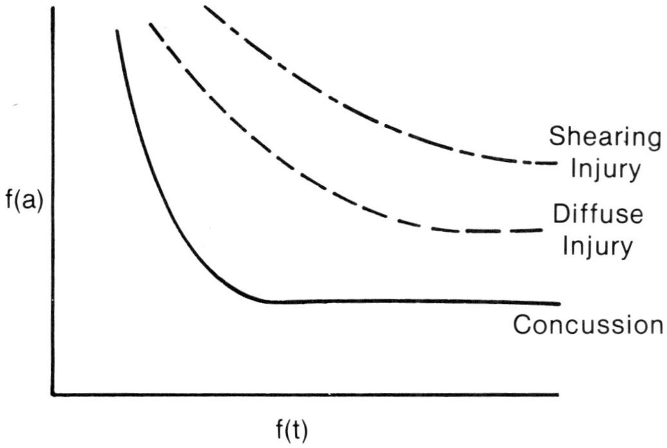

Figure 3.

hematoma was being surpassed. Further it became clear that the tolerance level for creation of subdural hematoma at the short acceleration durations utilized in these experiments was very close to that of cerebral concussion (Figure 4). It is well known from clinical studies, however, that shearing lesions do occur in isolation of subdural hematoma, and further clinical evidence suggested that this might be related to the pulse duration. It was found, for example, that while 71 percent of subdural hematomas were caused by falls, only 10 percent of diffuse injuries and shearing injuries were so caused. Conversely, 24 percent of subdural hematomas were caused by motor vehicle accidents, whereas 90 percent of diffuse and shearing injuries were caused from motor vehicle accidents. This seemed ample evidence that the longer pulse durations characteristically seen in vehicular accidents tend to cause the diffuse and shearing injuries, whereas short duration pulses were more likely to cause subdural hematoma. This hypothesis was confirmed in a subsequent series of animals and suggests the general wave shape of the tolerance curve for subdural hematomas to be that depicted in Figure 4. Subsequent work in the long pulse duration window above concussion to the right of subdural hematoma is showing promising evidence in ongoing work that this hypothesis is valid.

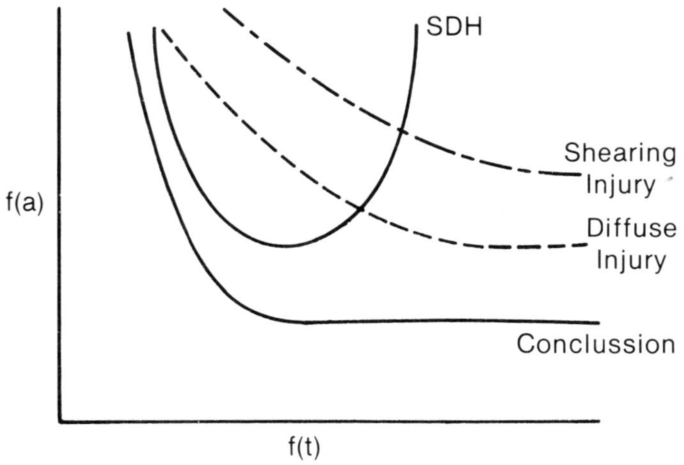

Figure 4.

Summary

It is, therefore, concluded that many of the physiological and pathological consequences of head injury can be produced by a single injury mechanism, namely angular acceleration. At short pulse durations cerebral concussion can be regularly produced with this mechanism along with cortical contusions; but if the acceleration magnitude is increased, a strain rate sensitive subdural bridging vein system tolerance is exceeded, and subdural hematoma results. At longer pulse durations cerebral concussion can be achieved at lower acceleration levels, but it takes considerably more acceleration to cause subdural bridging vein rupture. The incidence of cerebral contusion also appears to decrease as pulse duration is increased. Angular accelerations at relatively high magnitude and long pulse duration are thought to be causal of the diffuse injury and shearing injury. Therefore, **it is concluded that angular acceleration is the proximal cause of the most important causes of death and disability seen in human head injury, namely subdural hematoma and shearing injury.** Further work is anticipated in order to fully substantiate this hypothesis.

Acknowledgement

This work could not have been accomplished without the ideas, stimulation and hard work of numerous co-investigators: Drs. L. Thibault, T. Langfitt and J. Abel at the University of Pennsylvania; Drs. J. H. Adams and D. Graham at the University of Glasgow; Dr. A K. Ommaya at the NIH and NHTSA and the numerous neurosurgical fellows who have participated in the laboratory. Support by NHTSA and NINCDS has allowed those studies to continue.

Head Injury (Neuropathology)

D. I. Graham
J. Hume Adams
T. A. Gennarelli

Introduction

In the previous paper Dr. Gennarelli has shown that in subhuman primates subjected to a controlled 60° sagittal plane of angular acceleration of the head it is possible to induce a wide spectrum of physiological responses that range from no evidence of cerebral disturbance through varying grades of concussion to a rapidly fatal outcome. It has also been established that the magnitude of the input force delivered to the head correlates well with the severity of brain damage. In the present paper we wish to show that this type of experimentally induced head injury produces a wide spectrum of brain damage and is very similar to that observed in man after nonmissile head injury (1) (2) (3) (4).

Materials and Methods

Fifty-three adult monkeys (35 rhesus, 12 cynomolgus, 6 asamensis) were subjected to single sagittal plane acceleration of the head (5). The experimental trauma severity score was assessed for each animal, and the number of animals in each ETS group and their survival are given in Table 1.

There were two categories of animal. The first comprised those animals in which the acceleration produced little or no residual evidence of brain damage. These animals were allowed to survive for varying periods of time and were then electively sacrificed by in vivo perfusion fixation (6). The second category of animal consisted of those that either died instantaneously because of a severe fracture of the skull and physical disruption of the hind brain (the two animals with an ETS score of 6), or very soon after the acceleration impulse because of the rapid development of a large subdural hematoma. Since it was not possible to perfusion fix these animals adequately, fixation was achieved essentially by immersion. There was therefore inevitably histological artefact in these brains.

Table 1. Experimental Head Injury in 53 Subhuman Primates

Experimental Trauma Severity Score	1	2	3	4	5	6
Number of Animals	2	2	13	20	14	2
Survival	48h-14d	5-6h	22h-14d	2h-8d	10m-9h	nil
Fracture	—	—	2	3	7	2
SDH	—	—	6	14	13	—
ICH	—	—	—	4	—	—
Contusions	2	1	8	16	12	—
Mean Total Contusion Index	2.0	1.0	2.0	5.8	5.4	—
Hypoxic Brain Damage						
1. Neocortex	—	—	—	2	2	—
2. Ammons Horn	—	—	3	11	4	—
Brain Shift	—	—	—	2	4	—
Necrosis in PHG	—	—	—	2	4	—
Central Chromatolysis						
1. Motor Cortex	—	—	4	6	—	—
2. Brain Stem	—	—	1	5	—	—

m = minute, h = hour, d = day
SDH = Subdural Haematoma, ICH = Intracerebral Haematoma, PHG = Parahippocampal Gyrus

Neuropathology

After a variable survival the fully heparinsed animals were perfusion fixed using a technique similar to that described by Brierly et al. (1969). Briefly, a cannula with a short lip and filled to the tip with isotonic saline was introduced into the ascending aorta, the descending thoracic aorta was clamped, and the right atrium incised. Physiological saline was then infused for about 20 seconds (150–300 ml at pressure of 150 mmHg). The perfusate was then switched to FAM (a mixture of 40 percent formaldehyde, glacial acetic acid and absolute methanol 1:1:8 by volume) which was delivered for about 20 minutes (3,000 ml at a pressure of 150 mmHg). After perfusion the animals were decapitated and the head immersed in FAM at 4° C for a minimum of 4 hours. The brains were then carefully dissected from the skull, re-immersed in FAM at 4° C for an additional 24 hours and transferred to a mixture of 70 percent methanol and 30 percent water. The specimens wrapped in cotton wool moistened with 70 percent spirit and sealed in polythene bags were then sent by air-mail to the Institute of Neurological Sciences, Glasgow.

After photographing all surfaces of the brain and transecting the brain stem at the level of the midbrain, the cerebral hemispheres were cut into coronal slices 5 to 6 mm. thick. The cerebellum was detached from the brain stem and the cerebellar hemispheres cut at right angles to the folia. The brain stem was cut into horizontal slices. A composite photograph was taken of all the slices for future reference. Three to four (depending on the size of the brain) of the slices of the cerebral hemispheres and two or three of the sections of the brain stem were embedded in celloidin. Sections were cut at 30μ and stained by Nissl's method using Cresyl violet and by Heidenhain's modification of the Woelke technique for myelin. Representative blocks of the remaining slices of the cerebral hemispheres, a block from each cerebellar hemisphere, and the remaining slices of the brain stem were embedded in paraffin wax. Sections 6 to 7μ thick were stained with haemalum and eosin and by the method that combines Luxol fast blue and Cresyl violet. The great majority of the sections were also stained by the Palmgren technique for axons and by Nauomenko and Feigin technique for microglia. With experience it was found that sections 20μ thick and stained with Cresyl violet were particularly informative.

The sections were examined using a Watson Zoom stereo-microscope with transmitted light at a magnification of between $\times$ 10 and $\times$ 50. Using this system it was particularly easy to recognize contusions and recent infarction, and in the longer surviving animals the loss of nerve cells and any associated reactive changes. Conventional light microscopy was used routinely in the animals of short survival since any suspected recent hypoxic lesions were accepted as genuine only if the ischaemic cell process (ischaemic cell change with or without encrustations) as defined by Brierly et al. (1969) in FAM perfusion fixed material was present. All abnormalities identified in the brains of the animals were charted on a series of line diagrams of the cerebral hemispheres, cerebellum and brain stem.

Results

These are summarized in Table 1.

Fracture of the skull. This occurred in 15 percent of the head injured primates with an ETS score of 3 or 4. The incidence rose to 50 percent in animals with an ETS score of 5 and, as already noted was present in both of the animals that died instantaneously after the acceleration impulse.

Subdural hematoma. Subdural hematomas (SDH) were identified in 33 animals. Whereas some 46 percent of the animals with an ETS score of 3 had an SDH, the incidence rose to 70 percent in animals with an ETS score of 4 and 93 percent in animals with an ETS score of 5. The highest incidence of SDH therefore occurred in animals with the highest ETS score. The subdural hematomas were graded as small,

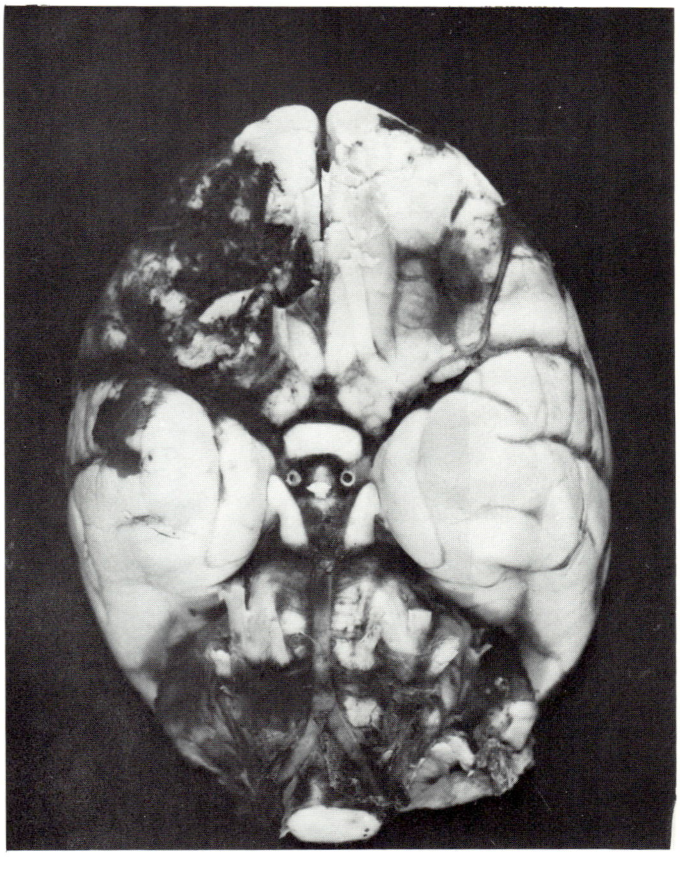

Figure 1.

medium or large in relation to their volume, all of the large SDHs occurring in the animals with an ETS score of 5. If an attempt was made to evacuate an SDH in an animal with an ETS score of 5, an external hernia cerebri developed very rapidly.

Intracerebral hematoma. An isolated intracerebral hematoma in the frontal or the temporal lobes was an uncommon finding occurring in only four animals, all with an ETS score of 4.

Contusions. An isolated intracerebral hematoma in the frontal or the temporal lobes was an uncommon finding occurring in only four animals, all with an ETS score of 4.

These are the hallmark of a head injury and occur as haemorrhagic lesions particularly at the crests of gyri. Contusions affecting principally the undersurfaces of the frontal and temporal lobes were observed in 39 animals (Figure 1). In an attempt to assess contusions more precisely we have developed a contusion index which has allowed the depth and extent of contusions in various regions of the brain to be expressed quantitatively (7). The regions chosen, i.e., the anatomical locators, in the present investigation were the frontal, temporal, parietal and occipital lobes and the cerebellum. Contusions not extending through the full thickness of the cortex received a depth grading of 1, those affecting the full thickness of the cortex 2, and those extending into the white matter 3 (Figure 2). Contusions restricted to the crest of one gyrus or to two contiguous gyri were given an extent grading of 1, more extensive contusions on one surface of the locator 2, and contusions affecting more than one surface 3. The contusion index (CI) for any one locator was obtained by multiplying the depth grading by the extent grading and could therefore range from 0 ($0 \times 0 =$ contusions absent) to 9 ($3 \times 3 =$ deep and extensive contusions). Using these figures it was therefore possible to obtain mean contusion indices (MCI) for the entire brain. The CI's for the various anatomical locators used are given in Table 2 where it is seen that contusions are most severe in the frontal and temporal lobes (5). The MTCI's are given in Table 1 where it can be seen that contusions were most severe in animals with an ETS score of 4 or 5.

Table 2. Experimental Head Injury in 53 Subhuman Primates

Mean Contusion Index	(n = 39)
Frontal Lobes	2.0
Temporal Lobes	1.1
Occipital Lobes	0.5
Parietal Lobes	0.04
Cerebellum	0.6

Hypoxic brain damage. In four animals, two with an ETS score of 4 and two with an ETS score of 5, there were multiple well-defined foci of neuronal necrosis throughout the neocortex. There was, however, a much higher incidence of hypoxic damage in the Ammon's horns particularly in animals with an ETS score of 4 where it was seen in 55 percent of cases. In general the lesions were restricted to the Sommer sector.

The histological appearances of the Ammon's horns varied with the length of survival. Classical ischaemic cell change with encrustations were seen in the hippocampus of one animal two hours after the acceleration injury. In animals surviving for a few days

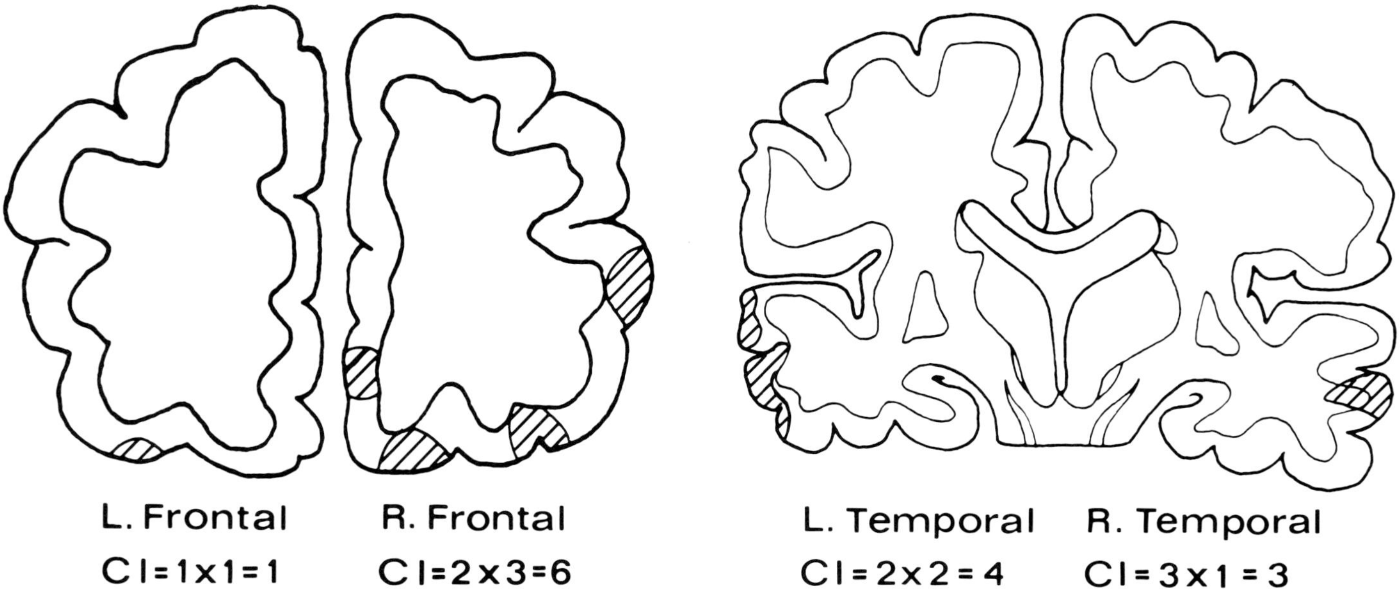

Figure 2.

there was characteristically loss of nerve cells and early reactive changes in the form of microglial hyperplasia and enlarged astrocytes.

Internal herniation and raised intracranial pressure. In six animals with SDH (two with an ETS score of 4 and four with an ETS score of 5) there was a shift of the midline structures of the brain and in six (two with an ETS score of 4 and four with an ETS score of 5) there was pressure necrosis in the parahippocampal gyrus of the type associated with a high intracranial pressure (8).

Central chromatolysis. A further fairly common abnormality was the occurrence of central chromatolysis in the Betz cells or enlarged motor neurons in the brain stem. It was seen in the former cells in ten animals and in the latter in six animals, all of which had an ETS score of 3 or 4, and which had survived for between 2 and 8 days after injury.

Other abnormalities. Other histological abnormalities identified were single tiny foci of haemorrhage in the brain stem in two animals with an ETS score of 5, both of which survived for 10 minutes after injury, and the occurrence of very occasional axonal retraction balls in the white matter of one animal with an ETS score of 4 that was sacrificed some 8 days after injury.

Discussion

One of the difficulties in assessing the incidence and type of brain damage in the present series was the length of survival (ranging from instantaneous death to elective sacrifice at two weeks) after injury, nevertheless Table 1 shows a definite tendency for brain damage to be more severe in the animals with higher ETS scores. There therefore appears to be a relationship between the energy input and the brain damage as well as between the energy input and the ETS score. It is also clear that most of the types of brain damage that are encountered in nonmissile head injury in man can be produced in varying degrees by this model.

The most important factor governing the outcome in any patient with a head injury is the damage sustained by the brain, and it is well recognized that in many patients not all the brain damage has occurred at impact. Some impact damage is immediate while some of it is delayed, i.e., brain damage brought about by processes (primary complications) initiated at the moment of impact but which do not become clinically apparent for some hours or even a day or more after injury. Other types of brain damage are not directly attributable to impact but are sequelae to other processes (secondary complications). Based on a comprehensive neuropathological study of a consecutive series of fatal cases and as a result of these studies our current approach (9) to the pathology of brain damage in nonmissile head injury is as follows:

1. Immediate impact injury.
   a) Contusion and lacerations.
   b) Diffuse damage to white matter.
   c) Other types of diffuse brain injury.
2. Primary complications.
   a) Intracranial haemorrhage.
   b) Brain swelling.
3. Secondary complications.
   a) Brain damage secondary to raised intracranial pressure.
   b) Hypoxic brain damage.
   c) Infection.

Contusions were common in the experiments described in this paper and their distribution was similar to that observed in man (5) (7). As has been already noted there is a tendency for the mean total contusion index to increase with the ETS score. Furthermore it has been shown as mechanical input increased, frontal contusions occurred before temporal contusions and that the threshold for frontal contusions was less than that for temporal contusions (5). It was therefore possible to show that if there was sufficient input to cause a temporal contusion, then a frontal contusion was also present. That this in fact was true was shown by the observation that only once did a temporal contusion occur in the absence of frontal contusion. Furthermore the frontal contusions in general were statistically more intensive than the temporal contusions. The data therefore supports the hypothesis that in an angular acceleration the threshold for frontal contusions is less than the threshold for temporal contusions. Classical diffuse damage to white matter was not found in the present experiment—this is not surprising since the animals that survived for more than a few hours returned to a normal or near normal clinical state soon after the impact, i.e., prolonged coma or even severe irreversible brain damage compatible with survival was not produced in this study. The occurrence of central chromatolysis in some of the animals with an ETS score of 3 and 4 and the very occasional finding of axonal retraction balls are however at least suggestive of minimal direct damage to axons. With regard to other types of immediate impact damage, there were two animals of short survival with an ETS score of 5 that had petechial haemorrhage in the brain stem. It is not suggested that such haemorrhages were responsible for death: they merely indicate a damage of a type that was incompatible with life (10).

Of the primary complications, intracranial hematoma is particularly common in man, and in this series of experiments there were numerous examples of subdural hematoma and four instances of intracerebral hematoma in the frontal and temporal lobes. Brain swelling was also a prominent feature in the severely injured animals with acute subdural hematoma as was shown by the rapid appearance of an external hernia cerebri when a craniectomy/craniotomy was undertaken.

Secondary haemorrhage in the brain stem as a result of an intracranial expanding lesion (9) is probably the most common terminal event in a fatal nonmissile head injury in man. This was not observed in the present series presumably because so many of the animals with acute intracranial expanding lesions died so soon after the acceleration impulse. There were, however, occasional examples of brain shift and of necrosis in the parahippocampal gyrus of a type associated with a conventional tentorial hernia and a high intracranial pressure (8).

A major problem in assessing the incidence and type of brain damage in the present series was the fact that many of the more severely injured animals (ETS score of 5) died very soon after injury. As already noted perfusion fixation in these animals was not satisfactory with the result that in those animals sacrificed within one or two hours of acceleration impulse it was not possible to differentiate histologically between "dark cell artefact" (11) and ischaemic cell process (6) (12). It is therefore inevitable that hypoxic brain damage was less common in the ETS score 5 animals. In spite of the limitations it was, however, possible to identify hypoxic brain damage in the neocortex of four animals and in the Ammon's horn of 18 animals with an ETS score of 3 and 4. The pathogenesis of this hypoxic brain damage is uncertain, particularly as it was not associated with either a prolonged elevation of intracranial pressure or with a greatly reduced cerebral perfusion pressure (13). This was in contradistinction to the ETS score 5 animals which developed massive intracranial hypertension such that the cerebral perfusion pressure fell to ischaemic levels and the animals died from lack of cerebral perfusion.

There were no cases of posttraumatic infection in the present series.

Conclusion

Most types of brain damage that are commonly found in patients' dying as a result of a nonmissile head injury can be induced by single sagittal plane acceleration of the head. The findings suggest that it should be possible to correlate the biomechanics of the model with the broad spectrum of ETS and brain damage, to identify brain damage attributable to immediate impact and to monitor the pathophysiology of any sequelae.

Acknowledgments

It is a pleasure to thank the Department of Medical Illustration of the Southern General Hospital for help in preparing the illustrations and Mrs. K. McCallum for typing the manuscript.

References

1. Gennarelli TA, Adams JH and Graham DI: Acceleration induced head injury in the monkey. 1. The model its mechanical and physiological correlates. *Experimental Clinical Neuropathology;* eds. K. Jellinger, F. Gullotta, M. Mossakowski. *Acta Neuropathol* (Berl) Suppl vii, 23–25, Berlin Springer-Verlag. 1981
2. Gennarelli TA, Segawa H, Wald V, Marsh K and Thompson C: Physiological response to angular acceleration of the head. *Seminars in Neurological Surgery—Proceedings of the Fourth Chicago Conference on Neural Trauma.* Raven Press (NY)—in press. 1981
3. Adams JH, Graham DI and Gennarelli TA: Acceleration induced head injury in the monkey 11. Neuropathology. *Experimental Clinical Neuropathology;* eds. K. Jellinger, F. Gullotta, M. Mossakowski. *Acta Neuropathol* (Berl) Suppl vii, 26–28. 1981
4. Adams JH, Graham DI and Gennarelli TA: Neuropathology of acceleration-induced head injury in the subhuman primate. *Seminars in Neurological Surgery—Proceedings of the Fourth Chicago Conference on Neural Trauma.* Raven Press (NY)—in press. 1981
5. Gennarelli TA, Abel JM, Adams JH and Graham DI: Differential tolerance of frontal and temporal lobes to contusion induced by angular acceleration. *Proceedings of 23rd Stapp Car Crash Conference,* pp 561–586. Society of Automotive Engineers (NY). 1979
6. Brierly JB, Brown AW, Excell BJ and Medrum BS: Brain damage in the rhesus monkey resulting from profound arterial hypotension. 1. Its nature, distribution and general physiological correlates. *Brain Res.* 13, 68–100. 1969
7. Adams JH, Scott G, Parker LS, Graham DI and Doyle D: The contusion index: a quantitative approach to cerebral contusions in head injury. *Neuropathol Appl Neurobiol* 6, 319–324. 1980
8. Adams JH, and Graham DI: The relationship between ventricular fluid pressure and the neuropathology of raised intracranial pressure. *Neuropathol Appl Neurobiol* 2. 323–332. 1976

9. Adams JH, Graham DI, Scott G, Parker LS and Doyle D: Brain damage in fatal non-missile head injury. *J Clin Pathol* 33, 1132–1145. 1980

10. Tomilson BE: Brain-stem lesions after head injury. *The Pathology of Trauma* eds. S. Sevitt and HB Stoner. *J Clin Pathol* 23, Suppl (Roy Coll Path) 4, 154–165. 1970

11. Cammermeyer J: The importance of avoiding "dark" neurons in experimental neuropathology. *Acta Neuropathol* (Berl), 245–270. 1961

12. Brown AW: Structural abnormalities in neurones. Hypoxia and Ischaemia ed. BC Morson. *J Clin Pathol* 30 Suppl (Roy Coll Path) 11, 170–180. 1977

13. Gennarelli TA, Czernicki Z, Segawa H, Wiser R, Marsh K, Wald V, Adams JH and Graham DI: ICP in experimental head injury. *Intracranial Pressure IV,* eds. K Shulman, A Marmacou, JD Miller, DP Becker, GM Hochwald and M Brock, pp 28–32. Berlin Springer-Verlag. 1980.

Impact Responses of the Protected and Unprotected Head

Alan M. Nahum, M.D.
Frank Raasch, M.D.
Carley Ward, Ph. D.

A series of impact experiments were conducted with cadavers to explore the potential of the cadaver as a model for some aspects of head injury stimulation. Seated stationary cadaver subjects were impacted by a rigid mass travelling at a constant velocity. Various padding materials were interposed between the skull and impactor to vary the duration of the applied load. The input force and the biaxial acceleration-time histories of the skull were recorded during the impact event. Static fluid pressurization of the cranial vascular network and cerebral spinal fluid space to in vivo pressure levels at impact also was performed. Follow-

Impact Conditions								
Experiment	36	37	38	41	42	43	44	54
Impactor Mass (kg)	5.36	5.59	5.32	23.09	5.23	5.23	5.23	5.23
Impactor Velocity (m/s)	8.75	9.94	9.60	12.83	12.95	12.95	4.36	8.41

Figure 1. Impact Parameters for Frontal Series

Results of Coding							
Experiment	Peak Input Force ($N \times 10^3$)	Peak Head Acceleration ($m/s^2 \times 10^3$)	GSI	HIC	t_1 (ms)	t_2 (ms)	Injury Code
36	7.78	2.30	1068	923	2.4	4.4	1
37	7.90	2.00	861	744	3.1	5.5	0
38	10.80	2.42	1153	980	1.1	2.9	2
41	14.84	3.90	4756	3765	5.9	8.6	2
42	5.20	1.59	842	703	2.0	7.1	0
43	10.59	2.23	1008	804	3.7	6.1	0
44	6.53	1.52	675	551	2.8	7.0	2
54	10.84	2.34	1061	820	2.8	4.5	0

Figure 2. Results of Frontal Impact Series

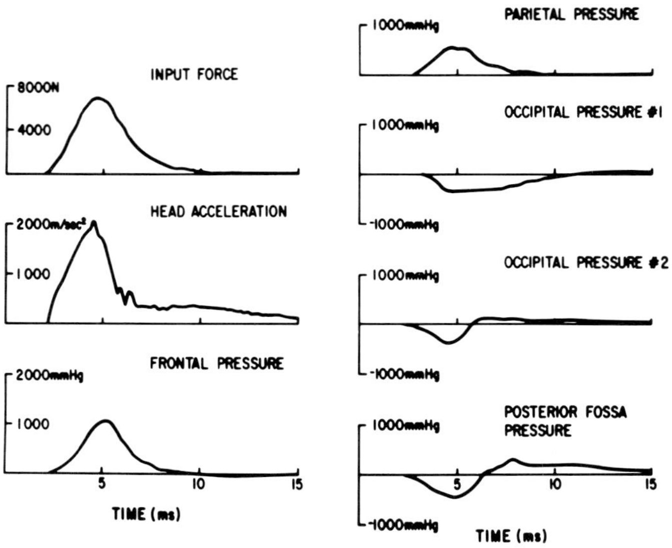

Figure 3. Intracranial Pressure Responses from Sample Experiment

ing the impact, the brain was perfused with a 10-percent formalin and carbon particle solution. The brain and cervical spine were subsequently evaluated by pathologic exam. In addition to dynamic measurements of input force and head acceleration, a series of intracranial pressure-time histories was recorded by the insertion of intracranial pressure transducers.

Series I consisted of eight frontal impact experiments using individual unembalmed anatomic specimens. The impactor mass range was 5.23 to 23.09 Kg and the impactor velocity from 8.41 to 12.95 m/s (Figure 1). Peak input forces varied from 5.20 to 14.84 kN with resulting peak head accelerations of 1.52 to 3.90 $m/s^2 \times 10^3$ (Figure 2). The resulting intracranial pressure reponses (Figure 3) showed a pattern of highest positive levels beneath the impact site in the frontal area with a gradual decrease in pressure from anterior to posterior and finally negative pressures in the opposite or occipital area of the intracranial cavity. The maximum negative pressures were recovered in the area of the foramen magnum. Both injury severity indices and injury pathology were calculated (Figure 4) for these experiments. A plot of head rotation versus pressure for one of the experiments (Figure 5) revealed that pressures had virtually returned to normal before significant head rotation commenced. A second (Series II) set of graded experiments was conducted sequentially on a single specimen (Figure 6). The impactor mass remained constant while the velocity varied between 4.42 and 8.69 m/s.

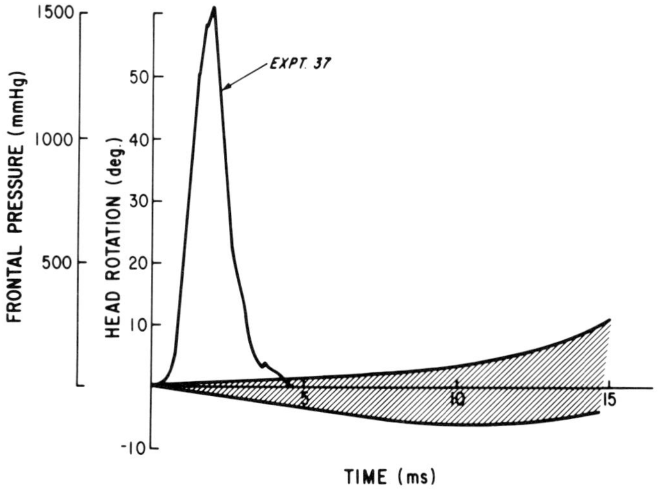

Figure 5. Head Rotation vs. Intracranial Pressure

Table III.
Series I Pressures

Experiment	Peak Input Force (N × 10³)	Peak Head Acceleration (m/s² × 10³)	Frontal (mm Hg	Parietal	Occipital #1	Occipital #2	Posterior Fossa	Carotid Siphon (mm Hg)
36	7.78	2.30	1022	594	−205	−78*	−480	—
37	7.90	2.00	1059	552	−341	−363	−452	—
38	10.80	2.42	1041	494	−205	—	−485	—
41	14.84	3.90	3207	1414	857	—	−426	352
42	5.20	1.59	—	70	—	—	−329	550
43	10.59	2.23	2031	1664	482	—	−136	811
44	6.53	1.52	764	150	109	—	− 19	860
54	10.84	2.34	2059	1354	248	—	−483	356

*Epidural

Figure 4. Severity Indices for Frontal Impact Series

Impact Conditons							
Experiment	46	47	48	49	50	51	52
Impactor Mass (kg)	5.23	5.23	5.23	5.23	5.23	5.23	5.23
Impactor Velocity (m/s)	4.42	4.42	4.21	8.35	8.35	8.29	8.69

Figure 6. Impact Conditions for Sequential Impact Series

			Series II Pressures					
Experiment	Peak Input Force (N × 10^3)	Peak Head Acceleration (m/s × 10^3)	Frontal (mm Hg	Parietal	Occipital	Posterior #1	Fossa #2	Carotid Siphon (mm Hg)
46	1.50	0.31	174	127	24	−44	−38	158
47	1.22	0.29	194	122	42	−24	−23	148
48	4.27	1.28	929	397	64	−282	−229	362
49	9.35	3.42	1969	1261	311	−405	−433	517
50	6.28	1.49	1173	628	122	−252	−233	1344
51	16.60	5.39	3785	2371	995	−609	−620	2619
52	13.34	4.29	3506	1883	533	−652	−662	2222

Figure 7. Impact Results for Sequential Impact Series

Peak input force (Figure 7) ranged from 1.22–16.60 kN with resulting peak head accelerations of 0.31–5.39 m/s × 10^3. A plot of peak pressure versus head acceleration (Figure 8) showed a linear relationship. Severity indices (Figure 9) were also calculated. A linear relationship between average frontal pressure and average head acceleration was also observed and thus peak pressure (Figure 10) is nonlinear with respect to the severity indices GSI and HIC. In these indices, the 2.5 power of the acceleration term produces an exponential curve.

Series III consisted of seven sequential frontal impacts to a single embalmed helmeted specimen with impactor masses in the range of 5.3–14.82 Kg and velocities of 6.4–12.7 m/s (Figure 11). Peak head accelerations (Figure 12) ranged from 1.13 to 1.98 m/s² × 10^3. A comparison table from an unhelmeted series at the bottom of the table suggests the reduction in injury severity for comparable kinetic energies.

Series IV consisted of individual helmeted specimen impacts (Figure 13) with a mass of 14.8 Kg and impactor velocities of 5.8–9.8 m/s. A comparison with a prior unhelmeted series (Figure 14A) shows a reduction in severity indices for helmeted heads. A comparison of pressures for the helmeted and unhelmeted series (Figure 14B) shows that the pressures are lower but that the HIC values are higher because the acceleration pulses are longer in duration. However, pulse

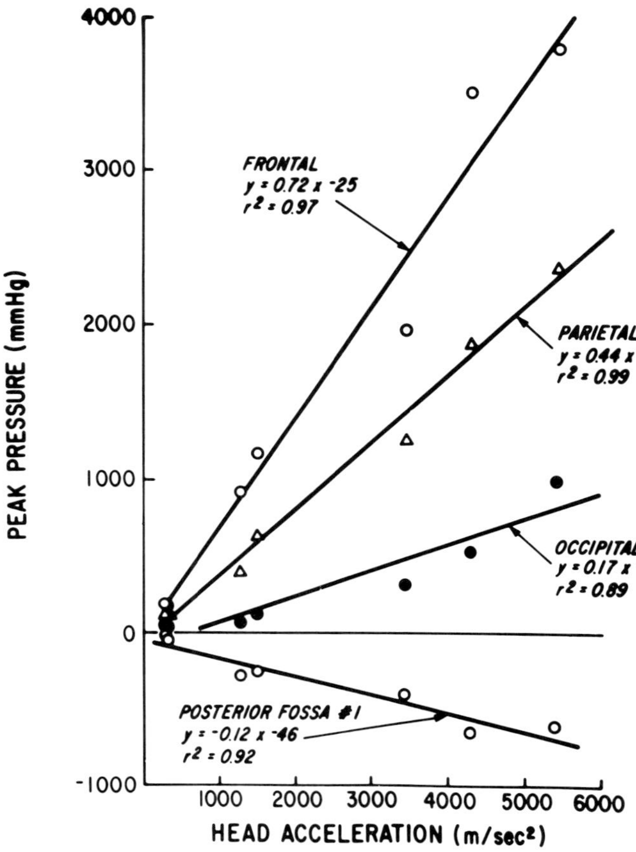

Figure 8. Head Acceleration vs. Peak Pressure

Experiment	Peak Input Force (N × 10^3)	Peak Head Acceleration (m/s^2 × 10^3)	GSI	HIC	t_1 (ms)	t_2 (ms)
		Impact Severity Rating				
46	1.50	0.31	36	32	2.7	13.0
47	1.22	0.29	24	21	4.5	12.7
48	4.27	1.28	342	297	2.2	4.8
49	9.35	3.42	1153	1008	1.3	2.2
50	6.28	1.49	675	539	4.4	9.5
51	16.60	5.39	4394	3895	3.6	4.4
52	13.34	4.29	3687	3182	1.9	3.2

Figure 9. Severity Indices for Sequential Impacts

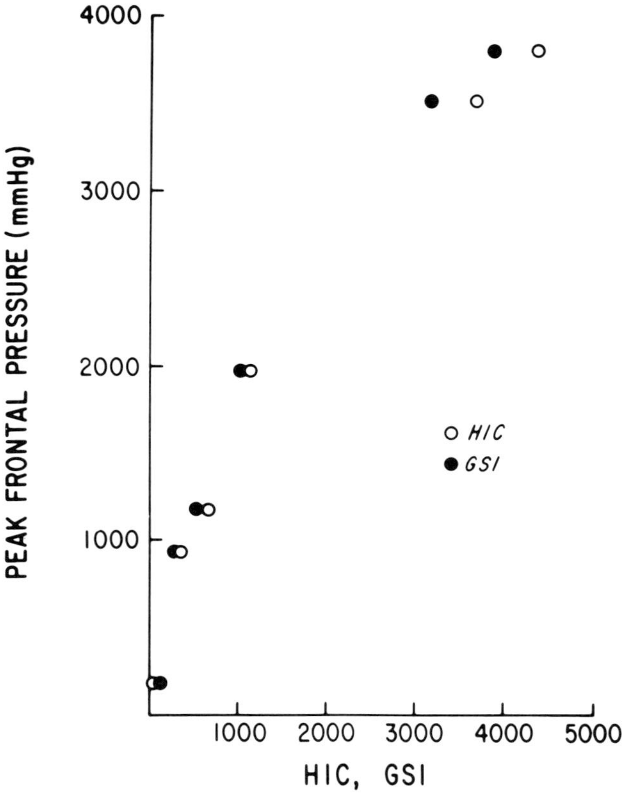

Figure 10. Peak Frontal Pressure vs. Severity Indices

duration has little or no effect upon peak intracranial pressure and influences only the pressure pulse durations. Helmeted head accelerations (show comparison here) do not have the high frequency components and fast rise times of unprotected heads. The helmet prevents high magnitude short duration intracranial pressures.

In Series V, four sequential impacts were performed against the temporo-parietal area of a single embalmed specimen. The velocities (Figure 15) ranged from 6.6 to 7.5 m/s, and the impactor mass was 4.17 Kg. Peak head accelerations (Figure 16) ranged from 0.92 to 2.1 $m/s^2 \times 10^3$.

In the second set of experiments, side impacts (Series VI) were performed on individual unembalmed cadavers. Impact velocities (Figure 17) ranged from 7 to 10.1 m/s with a 4.2 Kg impactor mass. Resulting peak head accelerations ranged from 3.2 to 6.9 $m/s^2 \times 10^3$ (Figure 18). The intracranial pressure measurements (Figure 19) indicate positive pressures (right frontal) close to the impact site and negative pressures opposite the impact (left frontal, left parietal, left occipital, left posterior fossa).

A plot (Figure 20) of frontal pressure versus head acceleration shows a good correlation while head acceleration versus HIC (Figure 21) also shows a satisfactory correlation.

Experiment	055W	056W	057W	058W	059W	060W	063W
			Helmeted Multiple				
Velocity (M/Sec)	7.51	10.30	12.70	6.44	7.38	9.97	9.95
Impactor Mass (KG)	5.30	5.30	5.30	14.92	14.92	14.92	14.82

Figure 11. Helmeted Sequential Impacts

Experiment	KE (kg.M²/sec.²)	Peak Head Accelerations ($m/s^2 \times 10^3$)	GSI	HIC	t_1	t_2
		Helmeted Multiple.				
055W	149	1.65	668.6	563	3.3	6.3
056W	281	1.13	251.5	221	3.8	6.8
057W	427	1.43	420.8	367	3.9	6.6
058W	303	1.19	350.7	298	5.1	10.0
059W	406	1.51	640.8	546	4.8	8.7
060W	741	1.67	1091.5	1010	2.9	7.6
063W	733	1.98	1087.1	1000	5.5	9.9
		Unhelmeted Multiple.				
46	51	0.31	36	32	2.7	13.0
47	51	0.29	24	21	4.5	12.7
48	46	1.28	342	297	2.2	4.8
49	182	3.42	1153	1008	1.3	2.2
50	182	1.42	675	539	4.4	9.5
51	179	5.39	4394	3895	3.6	4.4
52	179	4.29	3687	3182	1.9	3.2

Figure 12. Comparison of Helmeted and Unhelmeted Impact Results

		Helmeted Single.			
Experiment	64W	65W	66W	67W	68W
Impactor Velocity (M/sec)	9.85	8.47	5.81	7.24	7.86
Impact Mass	14.83 (KG)				

Figure 13. Helmeted Single Impacts

Experiment	KE (kg.M²/sec.²)	Peak Head Accelerations (m/s² × 10³)	GSI	HIC	t_1	t_2
		Helmeted Single.				
64W	719	2.69	2819.6	2684.9	2.5	6.7
65W	532	1.97	1626.8	1542.1	2.6	7.4
66W	250	1.26	543.9	465.3	4.1	9.3
67W	388	1.96	1584.8	1581.1	3.4	8.0
68W	458	1.43	857.2	806.6	3.1	8.9
		Unhelmeted Single.				
36	205	2.30	1068	923	2.4	4.4
37	276	2.00	861	744	3.1	5.5
38	245	2.42	1153	980	1.1	2.9
41	1900	3.90	4756	3765	5.9	8.6
42	438	1.59	842	703	2.0	7.1
43	438	2.23	1008	804	3.7	6.1
44	50	1.52	675	551	2.8	7.0
54	184	2.34	1061	820	2.8	4.5

Figure 14A. Comparison of Helmeted and Unhelmeted Impacts

Experiment	KE (kg.M²/sec.²)	Peak Head Acceleration (M/sec² × 10³)	Parietal	Occipital	Posterior Fossa	Carotid Siphon	Foramen Magnum
			Helmeted Single.				
64W	719	2.69	887	−487	−201	5185	—
65W	532	1.97	436	−157	−536	2676	¢
66W	250	1.26	398	− 79	−139	1365	—
67W	388	1.96	479	− 45	−184	6749	—
68W	458	1.43	365	−268	−332	1518	1193
			Unhelmeted Single.				
36	205	2.30	594	−205	−480	—	—
37	276	2.00	552	−341	−452	—	—
38	245	2.42	494	−205	−485	—	—
41	1900	3.90	1414	857	−426	352	—
42	438	1.59	70	—	−329	550	—
43	438	2.23	1664	482	−136	811	—
44	50	1.52	150	109	− 19	860	—
54	184	2.34	1354	248	−483	356	—

Figure 14B. Comparison of Helmeted and Unhelmeted Impacts

Lateral Multiple Impact - Series I				
Experiment	70W	71W	72W	73W
Velocity (M/sec)	6.55	7.54	7.54	6.55
Impactor Interface Material Thickness (cm)	Ensolite (3)	Ensolite (3)	Polystyrene (3.1)	Polystyrene (3.1)
Impactor Mass	4.17 (KG)			

Figure 15. Parameters of Lateral Impacts

Lateral Multiple Impact - Series I						
Experiment No.	KE (KgM^2/sec^2)	Peak Head Accelerations ($M/s^2 \times 10^3$)	GSI	HIC	t_1 (Msec)	t_2
70W	89	1.39	744	639	5.9	11.2
71W	119	2.10	1671	1466	7.6	11.8
72W	119	1.36	880	752	5.7	11.2
73W	89	.92	388	333	5.9	13.7

Figure 16. Results of Lateral Multiple Impact Series

Lateral Single Impact - Series II					
Experiment	74W	75W	76W	77W	78W
Impactor Veolicty (M/sec)	8.05	7.03	8.83	9.68	10.16
Impactor Interface Material Thickness (cm)	Ensolite (3)	Ensolite (3)	Ensolite (3)	Polystyrene (3.1)	Polystyrene (3.1)
Impactor Mass	4.17 (KG)				

Figure 17. Parameters for Single Lateral Impacts

Lateral Single Impact - Series II						
Experiment No.	KE (KgM^2/sec^2)	Peak Head Accelerations ($M/s^2 \times 10^3$)	GSI	HIC	t_1 (Msec)	t_2
74W	135	3.55	2678	1973	7.8	11.3
75W	103	3.20	1848	1340	6.2	7.9
76W	163	6.90	6797	5246	5.7	6.5
77W	195	3.51	3553	2844	8.9	12.1
78W	215	5.80	4653	3249	9.1	10.1

Figure 18. Results of Lateral Single Impacts

Experiment	KE (KgM²/sec²)	Peak Head Accelerations (M/sec² × 10³)	Right Frontal	Left Frontal	Pressures (MM-Hg) Left Parietal	Left Occipital	Left Posterior Fossa
					Lateral Single Impact - Series II		
74W	135	3.55	454	−207	−900	−156	—
75W	103	3.20	372	−143	−718	—	−330
76W	163	6.90	1800	−155	−711	—	—
77W	195	3.51	—	−410	(−176)[1] (−18)[2]	—	—
78W	215	5.80	1432	−507	−806	−335	—

[1] Anterior Parietal
[2] Posterior Parietal

Figure 19. Pressures from Lateral Single Impacts

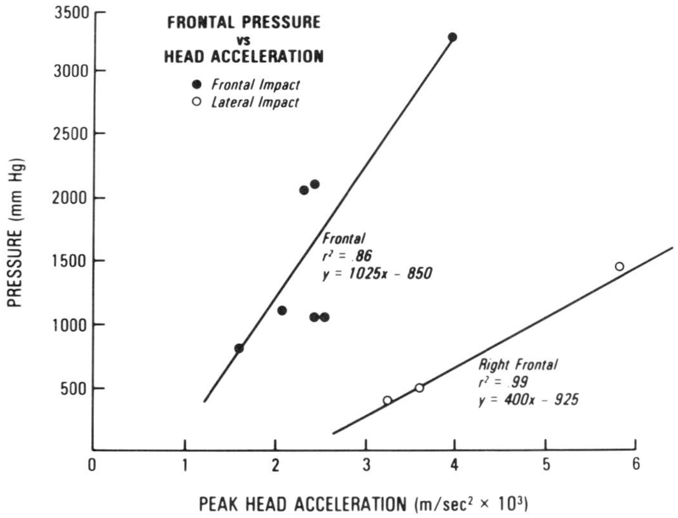

Figure 20. Frontal Intracranial Pressure vs. Head Acceleration

Conclusions

In a series of frontal and lateral head impacts intracranial pressures were recorded at varying locations. The measurements appeared to be reproducible. In the experiments head accelerations correlated well with the HIC, and at least several of the pressure patterns correlated with peak head acceleration. Pressures showed a pattern of positivity at the area of impact and negativity at the opposite side of the cranial cavity.

The potential of the human cadaver as a model for head injury has yet to be fully explored. Future research using cadavers should emphasize the following areas:

1) *cadaver characterization:* prior to the use of any cadaver complete information should be obtained regarding diseases, prior treatment and cause of death; standard geometric and anthropometric measurements should be obtained. Then standardized tests of bone and soft tissue tolerances should be conducted upon representative samples of bone and soft tissue.

2) *investigation of cadaver brain:* a full study of the biomechanical and pathophysiologic properties of the cadaver brain should be undertaken; this would provide well-defined physical properties and would answer such questions as the properties of the vessels (and their response to trauma) and indicate potential methods of assessing posttraumatic injury, e.g., damage to cortical areas or long tracts.

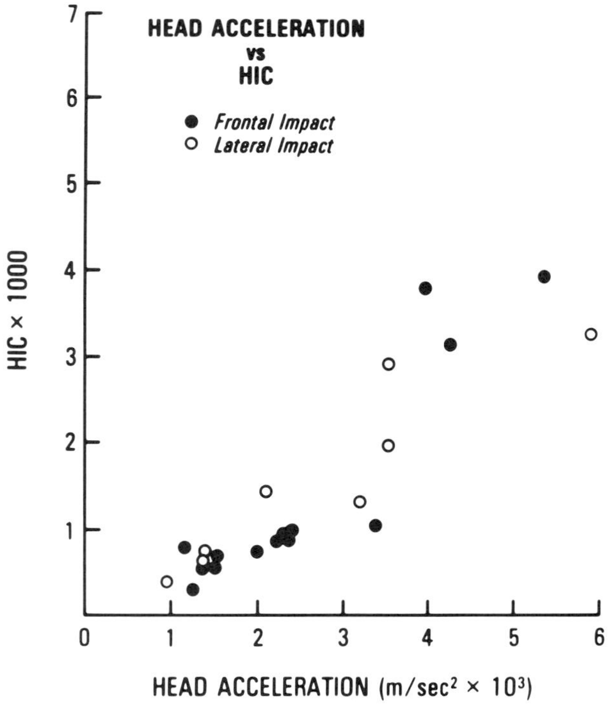

Figure 21. Head Acceleration vs. HIC

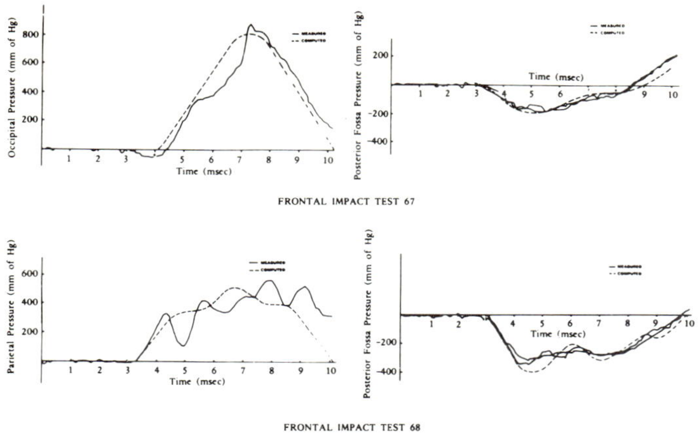

Comparison of computed and measured pressures.

Figure 22. Comparison of Computed and Measured Pressures

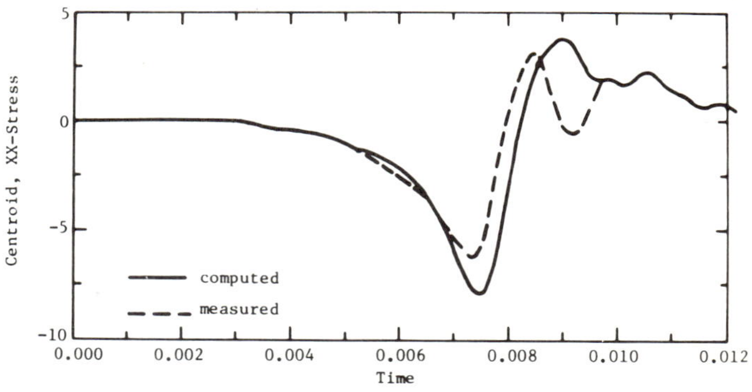

Figure 23. Comparison of Measured and Computed Pressures in Right Frontal Lobe

Pressures computed by a brain model showed good correlation with measured pressures in frontal impacts (Figure 22) and for many of the side impact studies (Figures 23A and 24). Pathologic studies of impacted pressurized brain specimens showed ruptures of small veins with resulting epidural and subdural bleeding, and these data were used as indices of the most minimal detectable injury. Peak pressures can be used as a measure of the intracranial response to head acceleration following head impact. Simulations suggest that serious brain injuries occur when the peak intracranial pressure exceeds 34 psi. Tolerance curves have been prepared and compared with other existing head injury severity indices.

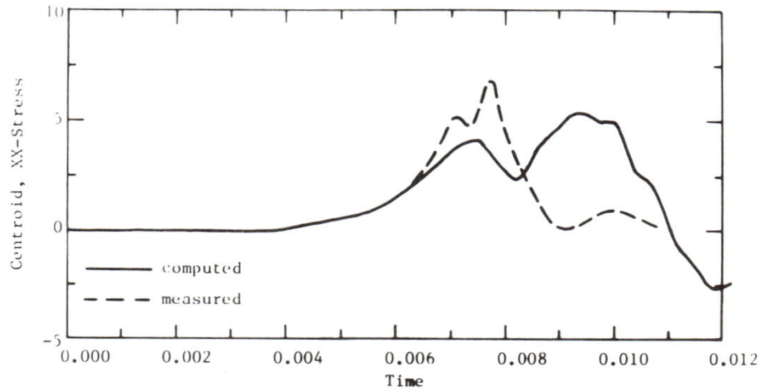

Figure 24. Comparison of Measured and Computed Pressure in Posterior Fossa

Investigation of Brain Injuries Using the C.T. Scanner

Claude Tarriere

Work in progress for:

E.E.C. Research Programme on the Biomechanics of Impacts with Relation of Future Vehicle Safety Regulations

Introduction

In this study of 133 cases of head injury produced by a variety of causes, the etiological circumstances were noted whenever these data were available, although they are not actually the subject of this study. For that matter, these data were frequently inaccurate. Only seven cases of pedestrians who had been struck by cars (No. 13, 19, 29, 30, 77, 78 and 100) were the subject of a complete accident analysis. They were considered to be usable as a basis for establishing the link between the experimental data in cadavers and the real-world physical circumstances, if the scanner pictures can be considered to be comparable.

In addition to records of age and sex, two clinical data base impressions were recorded:

(a) The initial examination, upon admission to emergency care at the initiating hospital center, was the reason for transfer to a neurosurgical department. When patients had been brought directly to a neurosurgical department, we used the emergency team's records.

(b) The status upon arrival at a neurosurgical department. Since this clinical picture had been established by neurologists, it was chosen for the AIS ratings, as it was clearly more accurate, even when there were differences in the extent of gravity shown in the two pictures, as frequently occurred. These differences in extent of gravity can be in both directions; i.e., increasing or decreasing the AIS!

The following were also noted: associated lesions, concomitant problems that could interfere in the evolution of the organic disturbance, length of stay in neurosurgery department and methods employed by the latter, as well as the patient's final condition at time of discharge from the hospital.

C.T. Scanner Study

The scanner study was performed using a CGR[x] device in accordance with routine procedures established for this apparatus as provided by the Compagnie Generale de Radio-électricité.

Data from Accident Victims

(1) Etiological circumstances

Figures 1, 2 and 3 show the distribution of cases. The type of accident was specified in 131 out of 133 observations.

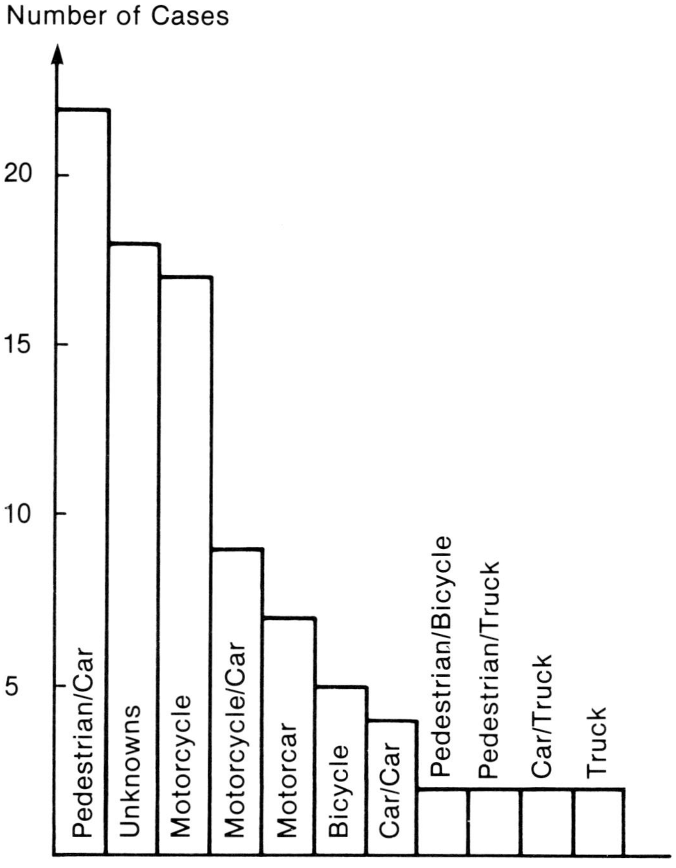

Figure 1. Distribution of Recorded Cases by Type of Traffic Accident

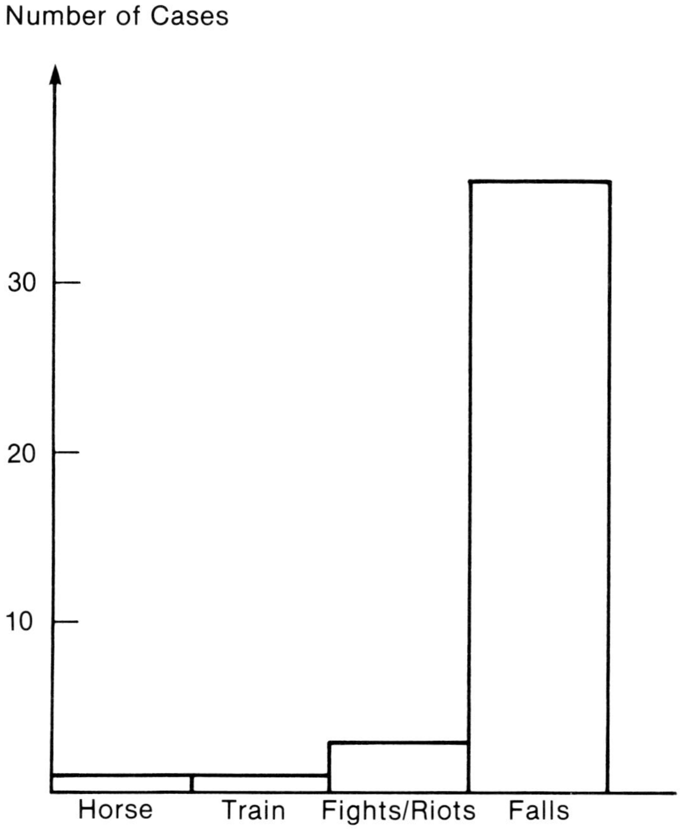

Figure 2. Other Recorded Cases than Traffic Accidents

(2) Age and sex

These data are summarized in Figures 3 and 4. The distribution between the sexes shown in Figure 3 and for age in Figure 4 is in agreement with standard accident data.

(3) Time of scanner use

Note was taken of the hour and date on which the scanner was used in relation to the time of occurrence of the accident. This emerges as highly important. We thus have 101 cases for which the time of use was specified:

—34 of the scanner pictures were made within six hours after the accident.

—41 of the scanner pictures were made from six to twenty-four hours after the accident.

Thus, 75 out of 101 of the C.T. scans (74%) were made on the same day as the accident (less than 24 hours afterwards). The 26 others ranged in time from over 24 hours to one week subsequent to accident occurrence.

This study is hence based on a majority of early scanner images. The advantage of this feature is that it eliminated secondary lesions and perhaps supplies more accurate injury-related data. In fact, through the performing of successive scanner studies, we know that certain kinds of lesions are rapidly reversible. However, there is one disadvantage, in that this method fails to properly recognize certain lesions that emerge later when the initial scanner image was normal, as previously reported (2). This theoretical drawback was eliminated in our study, by successive scanner pictures made, in most cases, if the clinical status continued to display the same level of gravity in spite of an initially normal C.T. scan.

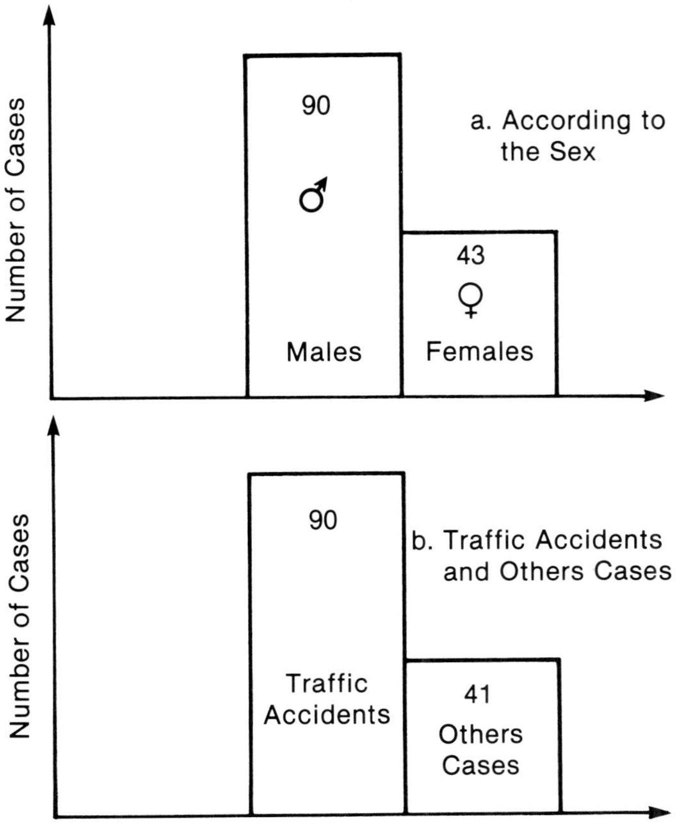

Figure 3. Distribution of Recorded Cases:

(4) Clinical data

The distribution of the AIS according to AIS–80 criteria was as follows:

3	AIS 1	2%	
12	AIS 2	9%	
24	AIS 3	18%	29%
31	AIS 4	23%	
29	AIS 5	21%	
34	AIS 6	25%	69%
Total 133	Cases		

29% of the AIS were 3, which corresponds to injuries of the head.

69% of the cases were serious head injuries, with AIS levels between 4 and 6, as shown above.

(5) C.T. Scan data

Various injury images were found with the scanner, both in isolated occurrence and in associated occurrence.

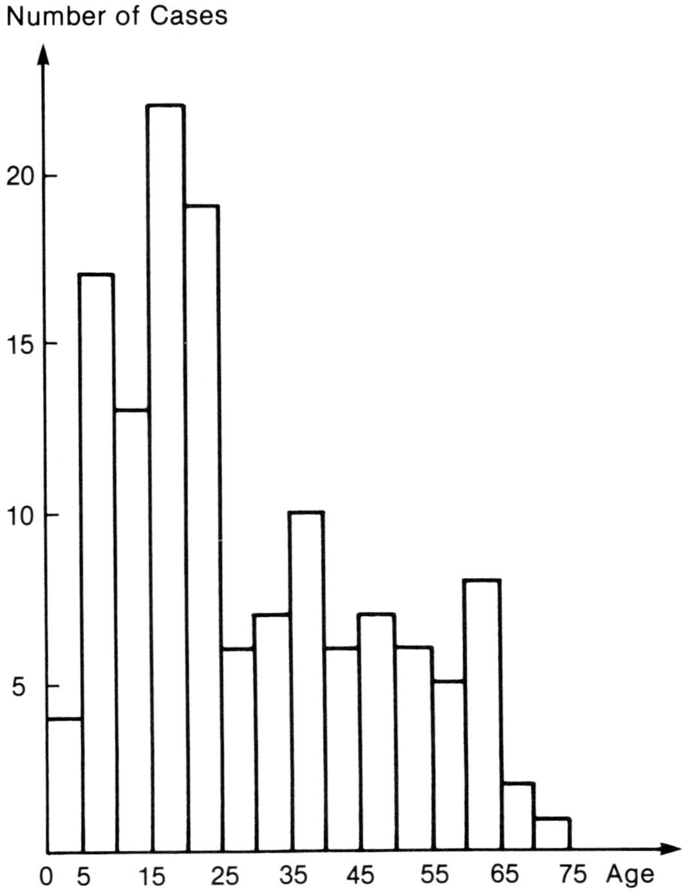

Figure 4. Ages of the Victims

With respect to intracranial contents, we found the following:

—Juxtadural hematoma (extra and subdural)
—Hemorrhagic contusion occurring in the form of hyperdensity and cerebral edema, both localized or diffused.

The distribution of these lesions was investigated with each type of image.

Certain scanner images were normal, i.e., with no injury image. This fact was noted 15 times out of 133, or in 11.2% of the cases. From the AIS standpoint, these normal scanner findings correspond to the following:

—Cerebral concussion

Number	AIS grade	Number of cases	
3	1	34, 80, 82	
4	2	17, 18, 21, 22	60%
3	3	10, 25, 79	
3	4	13, 37, 78	
2	5	57, 74	
0	6	....	

It emerges that, out of these 15 normal scanner images, in 10 cases out of 15, i.e., 60%, the AIS grade was 3.

The concussion picture (brief unconsciousness with no neurological sign, AIS=2) had no proven anatomical substratum. It is hence normal to have a C.T. scan record which is negative in such cases. In contrast, out of five remaining cases, with grades of AIS 4 or 5, if we eliminate the two scanner pictures (No. 37 and 57) taken after a seven-day interval, three of them are beyond argument. Three out of five, or 20%, show a normal scanner image and 1 AIS 4 or 5 (Nos. 13, 74 and 78). These three victims were aged under 10 years (4, 6 and 9 years).

— **Cerebral edema**

This term should perhaps be avoided: it may be better to use the term "cerebral intumescence" which does not prejudge its mechanism. We found this kind of image in the three following forms:

- Bi-hemispheric edema
- Bi-hemispheric edema + edema of the brain stem
- Hemispheric or even more specifically located edema

These three types were found in 38 of the 133 cases, either occurring alone or in association with sub-arachnoidal blood, i.e., in 28% of the cases.

The AIS distribution of these cases was in the >3 range and the associated lesions were of two types:

(a) An image of an edema associated with a grave injury that is invisible to the scanner because of its size. This injury is presumably located in the brain stem and is invisible because of its size or because the conditions attendant upon the taking of the scanner image; it is presumably accompanied by an edema that follows a favorable development pattern.

This hypothesis is supported by the presence, in a few cases, of clinical signs peculiar to the brain stem alone, despite the absence of any engagement or intumescence.

(b) The edema image is presumably linked to numerous, diffuse petechiae, a finding that has been reported by certain authors. In this case, it is hard to understand the different development patterns that can exist between two images of edemas with different AIS.

— **Extradural hematoma occurring alone**

This image was found occurring alone in 7 cases out of 133: 5.2%.

Number of cases	AIS	Case no.
1	2	85
2	3	2, 84
1	4	101
3	5	19, 89, 91

The extradural hematomas of AIS 3 were of either small volume (84, 85) or of slow development (2).

However, the extradural hematomas of AIS 4 or 5 were larger than, or equal to, 3 centimeters in thickness at the time of the intervention.

—**Contusions occurring alone**

Under this heading, we found hemorrhagic contusions, which hence mean hyperdensity whatever their locations (hemisphere, cerebellum, brainstem).

42 contusions, or 31%.

Distribution by AIS grades:

Number of cases	AIS	Case No.
0	1	....
2	2	1, 130
7	3	27, 31, 32, 92, 105, 115, 116
13	4	3, 8, 9, 20, 46, 94, 95, 96, 107, 126, 128, 129, 133
8	5	24, 68, 93, 108, 110, 127, 131, 132
12	6	14, 43, 54, 97, 98, 102, 106, 113, 118, 119, 120, 121

Whatever its size, the presence of a hemorrhagic contusion is hence most frequently synonymous with seriousness of injury: e.g.,

9 out of 42, or 21% had an AIS <3
33 out of 42, or 78% had an AIS=4 to 6

We tried to correlate the injury location and the AIS. Unfortunately, the number of cases was still too small. Thus:

- Frontal contusion, 7 cases:

2 AIS 2, 2 AIS 3, and 3 AIS 4.

- Temporal contusion occurring alone, 4 cases:

2 AIS 3, 1 AIS 5, and 1 AIS 6.

- Occipital contusion, 1 case:
  1 AIS 6.
- Contusion of two adjacent lobes, 10 cases:
  3 AIS 4 and 1 AIS 5.
- Contusion of 3 adjacent lobes or of 2 or several separate lobes, 16 cases:
  2 AIS 3, 6 AIS 4, 4 AIS 5; and 4 AIS 6.
- Contusion of brain-stem, 2 cases:
  1 AIS 3, and 1 AIS 5.
- Contusion of brainstem+hemispheric edema, 4 cases (N): 56, 60, 73, 41:
  1 AIS 6, 1 AIS 6, 1 AIS 6, and 1 AIS 6.

In the light of this distribution, it is clear that the number of cases is too small to yield a meaningful correlation. The latter must exist, as is shown in the following:

Study of the seven frontal contusions occurring alone, four of which have an AIS <3.

Increased AIS in the case of the occurrence of multiple contusions: 14 cases out of 16 with an AIS >4.

—Multiple injuries

Under this heading, we include the association of several types of images. It is possible to have all the variants that associate the four preceding types of lesions discussed. We deem it unwise to draw conclusions therefrom before having an accurate correlation for every type of image. If one has this data available, it may be expedient to proceed as in the calculation of a regional AIS.

Discussion

Correlation between C.T. scan images and clinical status is possible, but it is necessary to have extremely extensive series. Late model C.T. scanners are very reliable and negative examinations seldom occur.

As concerns correlation between scanner images and clinical pictures, this clearly must be dependent on age, sex and other factors likely to influence the development pattern; e.g., pre-existing physical defects, polytraumatisms, etc. It can be considered that the acquisition of a large number of data will result in the equation "type of image = gravity"; in fact, the only problem still remaining is the development pattern of the scanner images, due to mechanisms of edema and/or of engorgement. The problem is solvable by including early and serial C.T. scan evaluations.

The second part of the investigation is devoted to experimental cadaver lesions: by definition, these are not evolutive, but this difficulty vanishes if we assume that these lesions represent the initial capillary rupture; hence the lesions' initial mechanism may permit the prediction of the extent of the lesion (hemorrhagic contusion) from the observed density of the capillary lesions in the cadaver.

At the completion of this investigation, it will be possible to classify the experimental lesions into AIS grades that are slightly different from the ones which might be assigned by pathological anatomy.

Example: Case no. 105/131, in which the brainstem lesion proven by the scanner image undergoes a favorable development pattern. The AIS provided by the initial clinical picture could be weighted by the patient's condition at the time of hospital discharge, since certain development patterns are too different, with a single initial AIS.

However this may be, these experimental lesions will yield an appreciation of gravity that can, in turn, be placed in parallel with the physical conditions of the lesions observed. These physical conditions are various known parameters (acceleration, or derivatives of acceleration), and they will then yield a threshold of injury and/or of tolerance.

The other methods using C.T. scan data correlation

A—Autopsy: Out of 101 cases, after drafting an autopsy request for, we were able to get only one autopsy for 22 fatalities.

In view of the current manner in which this matter is administered, we feel that it is impossible to solve this problem. However, the correlation between pathological anatomy and scanner image has been described by other teams whose members readily obtain authorization to perform autopsies. The scanner examination is the equivalent of a macroscopic anatomo-pathological examination of a live subject. Its resolution power is 7 mm, but C.T. scans may fail to show all petechial hemorrhage, especially in the brain stem.

B—Two other methods:

1—We did not note any other cases of non-neurosurgical death and this means that we should extend our contacts to include other traumatological teams.

2—The interpretations of four instrument-fitted cadavers proved meaningless. It appears that this method cannot be applied to C.T. scan data.

In view of these difficulties—either of an administrative nature or inherent in the technique employed (power of resolution of the scanner at 7 mm)—we decided to employ only the method of correlation between scanner image and clinical picture of the neurosurgical patients.

Experimental Data from Human Cadavers

Origin of data

Fresh cadavers were prepared with vascular pressurization and instrumented with nine accelerometers screwed on the skull.

Test conditions:

- Frontal impact:
  - a) free falls; different jerks for the same mean acceleration
  - b) sled tests
  - c) reconstructions of frontal collisions
- Facial impacts:
  - a) free falls
  - b) reconstructions of pedestrian collisions (not available)
- Lateral impacts:
  - a) free falls
  - b) reconstructions of lateral collisions

Validity of the vascular pressurization technic as a means for detecting brain injuries

An attempt of validation of the interpretation of cerebral injuries observed by autopsy upon fresh cadavers was done a few years ago. A comparative study of cerebral lesions induced by impacting dead and living animals was carried out. The animal selected was the rabbit and for the tests with dead animals, the method of preparation used was the same as that developed for humans.

One of the experimental methods used to define human cerebral tolerance involved performing head impacts on human cadavers whose average arterial pressure had been reestablished by injecting an appropriate liquid. In order to be able to detect these cerebral lesions (even a moderate one such as the rupture of a capillary), the liquid injected contains particles of carbon, the diffusion of which, outside a vessel, indicates the rupture of the latter. This "hemorrhage" is visible to the naked eye only when it is major; a microscope research is necessary when it is of a lesser severity.

This original experimental approach had to be validated in order to ensure that the preparation of the cadavers was not likely to produce artifical lesions and, conversely, that it did not minimize the risk of lesion attributable to a given impact severity. It was only the comparison of dead animals (prepared in the same way as human cadavers) with living animals subjected to the same head impact, which enabled certain validation elements to be obtained for our pressurization technique.

The study was carried out in two phases:

—1st phase: production of moderately severe cranial trauma without cerebral lesion on 20 animals

—2nd phase: production of sufficiently violent cranial trauma to produce cerebral lesions on 52 animals

Conclusions of this attempt of validation

The results are of interest in that they support the hypothesis that this method for detecting cerebral lesions can be used with human cadavers. During the first phase, the results allowed us to establish that, in the absence of lesions on living rabbits, there were no lesions on the dead ones. In the second phase, it was shown that, when lesions are observed on the living rabbits, they are also observed on the dead ones, with a trend to be more severe on the dead. This observation is rather favorable in that the method cannot be criticized for minimizing the risk of lesions in relation to the real-life accident. Some differences in nature and location of lesions have been observed between living and dead rabbits. This is a subsidiary conclusion of this study, the purpose of which was the validation of a method for evaluating the cerebral risk on the cadaver in the case of hemorrhage (vascular pressurization and diffusion of carbon particles in the case of vascular lesions). Obviously, this study is only an indication. It is difficult to draw, from the rabbit, a general conclusion valid for the human being.

The problem of edema

In cadaver experiments, a limitation exists in the prediction of brain injuries. Although we can bring to light the smallest capillary rupture by a "hemorrhage" of carbon particles, brain edema cannot be simulated. We have to accept this limitation and to estimate the magnitude of the missing information in our brain injury risk evaluation. Table 1 gives the distribution of brain injuries for a sample of 133 head-injured people who have undergone a C.T. scan examination.

In 28 cases (21%), an edema alone would be the origin of the brain injuries:

3 AIS=2
7 AIS=3
9 AIS=4
5 AIS=5
4 AIS=6

However, the "hemorrhage" is the most common injury. Alone or in association with another brain injury, it accounts for about 80% of cases.

Table 1. Brain Injuries Distribution Among 133 Scanned Patients

Type of Brain Injury	No. of Cases		(%)
Contusion Alone	42		31
Contusion Alone or Associated	72		55
Edema Alone	28		21
Edema Alone or Associated with Sub-Arachnoidal Blood	38		28
Edema Alone or Associated with All Types of Brain Injuries	53		40
Brain Stem	12 or 13		10
Brain Stem Contusion Alone	2	(105, 131)	
Brain Stem Edema Alone	2	(73, 76)	
Brain Stem Contusion + Edema Elsewhere	1	(59)	
Brain Stem Contusion + Constusion Elsewhere	1	(108)	
Brain Stem Contusion and in Different Brain Areas	3	(12,60, 53)	
Brain Stem Edema and in Different Brain Areas	3	(42,67,69)	
Brain Stem Injury Not Certain	1	(14)	
Extra-Dural Hematoma Alone	5		4
Extra-Dural Hematoma Alone or Associated	15		11
Sub-Dural Hematoma Alone	5		4
Sub-Dural Hematoma Alone or Associated	13		10

Nature and Mechanisms of the Experimental Brain Injuries Observed

(1) Free falls

First experimental series (head frontal and lateral padded impacts)

Table 2 provides some details for frontal, lateral and facial head impacts. The brain stem injuries are the most frequent and severe ones. All information is given in C. Got et al.

Table 2. Summary of Cerebral Lesions

Type of Impact	No. of Subjects	No. of Serviceable Subjects	Injured	Brain Stem Lesions	Corpus Callosum	Peripherical Impact Area	Peripherical Opposite Area	Others
Side Temporal	22/20	17/16	9/9	7/6	1/0	1	1	1
Face and Forehead	7/5	7/5	5/5	4/3	1/1			
Forehad (3 m of Free Fall)	13/13	7/7	6/6	4/4	2/2			

Note: First Figure: All Subjects
Second Figure: Helmeted Subjects, or Equivalent Cases, i.e., Padded Head Impact

From SAE Paper 780 887

New series (head frontal padded impacts)

Cases 159 to 177.
13 cases could be used: 4 with a brain stem contusion, 1 case with contusions on "posterior quadrigeminal tuberculum" and on "hypocampus."

(2) Brain injuries without direct head impact in lateral collisions (Driver on the impacted side)

(a) Lateral collision Peugeot 504/Citroen LN

Out of a series of 14 tests of actual lateral collisions reconstructed with cadavers (where the head AIS for the seven actual victims was 2), there is only one severe injury observed on cadavers (Table 3). It is a case where the belt was missing for the driver. Because of this experimental mistake, the head and shoulders of the driver were partially ejected through the lateral window broken by the shoulder impact. The amplitude of the sideways bending of the head exceeds 75 as compared with 10 for the two other cadaver tests where the amplitude is limited by the window glass. The head hit the hood of the striking car very slightly (HIC value=100).

It is interesting to note that the body motion observed in this case is associated with severe and very unusual injuries.

There are no cortical injuries, but very scattered peripheral hemorrhages on the right temporo-parietal area (superficial hematomas in parietal and "frontale-ascendante" areas, reaching F2 and P2, with some "suffusions" under the piemer) and two small injuries measuring 1 mm in diameter and located symmetrically in the brain stem, at the cerebral pedunculus, with a slight hemorrhage in the "faisceau longitudinal median droit et gauche" area. These injuries, very similar to some findings of Ommaya and Gennarelli in animal experimentation, suggest a brainstem elongation due to extensive sideways bending of the head.

(b) Lateral collision Renault 12/Renault 12

The two cars were running at 50 km/h in this experimental collision.

The driver in the struck car is a man 53 years old, 1.74 m height, 75 kg weight.

There is no direct head impact but a complex kinematic with a lateral flexion and, in a second step, the laterally flexed head rotates forward. This complex head movement has a very large amplitude. As in the Citroen LN case, there are no cortical lesions but multiple injuries on the brain stem at protuberance and cerebral pedunculum levels, and also at spinal bulb level where the hemorrhages are very small.

(3) Injury mechanisms

a) First free-fall series

- Frontal padded impacts

  Table 4 suggests that head-torso hyperextension angle could have a noticeable influence on the brain injury generation.

- Lateral impact

  In the whole series, the head lateral bending is important. Consequently, it is impossible to separate the influence of the different kinematic parameters.

b) New series (frontal padded impact)

Several parameters have to be considered:

—Impact speed

—Head/thorax angle during the "rebound" phase (Figure 5)

—The linear and angular resultant accelerations

Table 3. Lateral Collision—Peugeot 504 Against Citroen LN

Test No.	Head/Thorax Flexion Angle (Degree)	Angular Velocity (rad/s)	Angular Acceleration (rd/s2)	Linear Acceleration (9) Max.	Linear Acceleration (9) 3ms	HIC	Cerebral AIS	Observations
Citroen LN Series								
195	75	40	3000	105	25	100	4	No Head Impact
191	10	67	16000	145	50	198	0	Head Impact
194	10	38	18000	175	95	495	0	Head Impact
Renault 15 Series								
158	80	58	16500	205	150	1980	0	Head Impact

Table 4. Head Frontal Padded Impacts (First Series: Cases No. 102 to 144)

	Head/Torso Angle (Degrees)	Max. Acceleration (9)	3 ms Acceleration (9)	Jerk 10^5 g/s	HIC
AIS = 0	56 to 65	145 to 500	135 to 185	0,16 to 2,49	900 to 2500
AIS = 2	66 to 80	130 to 384	118 to 150	0,17 to 0,87	1000 to 2200

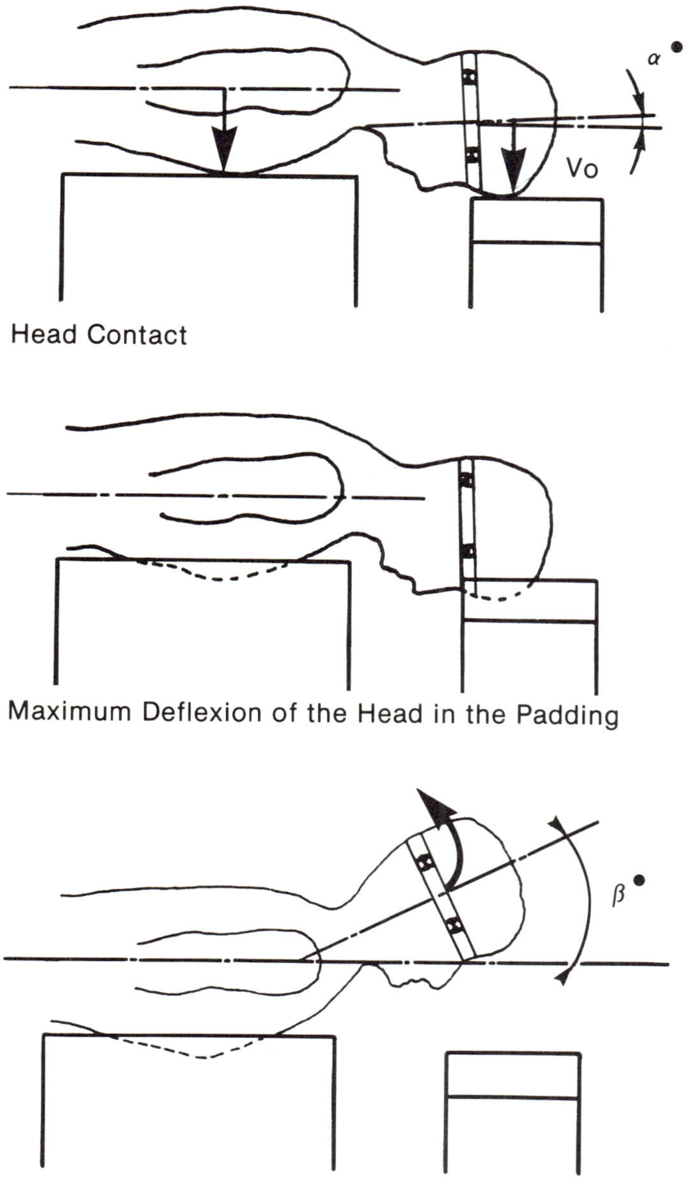

Head Contact

Maximum Deflexion of the Head in the Padding

Head Rebound

Figure 5. Head Kinematic

—The rate of onset of the linear acceleration (jerk)

The brainstem contusions observed in this series have to be associated with a combination of high linear acceleration and a high jerk (Table 5).

As one can see on Figure 6, for the same class of HIC or acceleration, above a level of 10^5 g/s, the jerk has an influence on the injury severity level (half of the subjects are injured). But this influence is not heavy if we consider the relatively low severity of the injuries observed.

Figure 7 clarifies the influence of the head/thorax angle.

For the same acceleration (or HIC) range and jerk, the susceptibility to brain injuries could be low (cases 159, 160, 162) or high (cases 107, 108, 110). The amount of neck hyperextensions during the "rebound" phase makes the difference.

c) Brain injury mechanism for head bending (Citroen case)

In lateral collision, the Citroen LN test was carried out three times: the results are assembled in Table 3.

On the basis of these results, it seems that the brain injuries (case 195) are due to the large magnitude of the head/thorax flexion because of the relatively low linear and angular velocity and deceleration (this cadaver, the only one injured, was also the only one without head impact).

However, in another test with a Renault 15, we also found a large magnitude of head/thorax lateral flexion (80) without brain injury: in this last test, the cadaver head flexion was stopped by the B-pillar impact.

Table 5. Head Frontal Padded Impacts (New Series: Cases No. 159 to 177)

	Head/Torso Angle (Degrees)	Max. Acceleration (9)	3 ms Acceleration (9)	Jerk 10^5 g/s	HIC	Force (daN)
AIS = 0	19 to 56	105 to 240	90 to 165	0,17 to 1,52	450 to 1960	780 to 950
AIS = 2	0 to 50	150 to 246	102 to 170	0,99 to 1,58	750 to 1770	450 to 1060

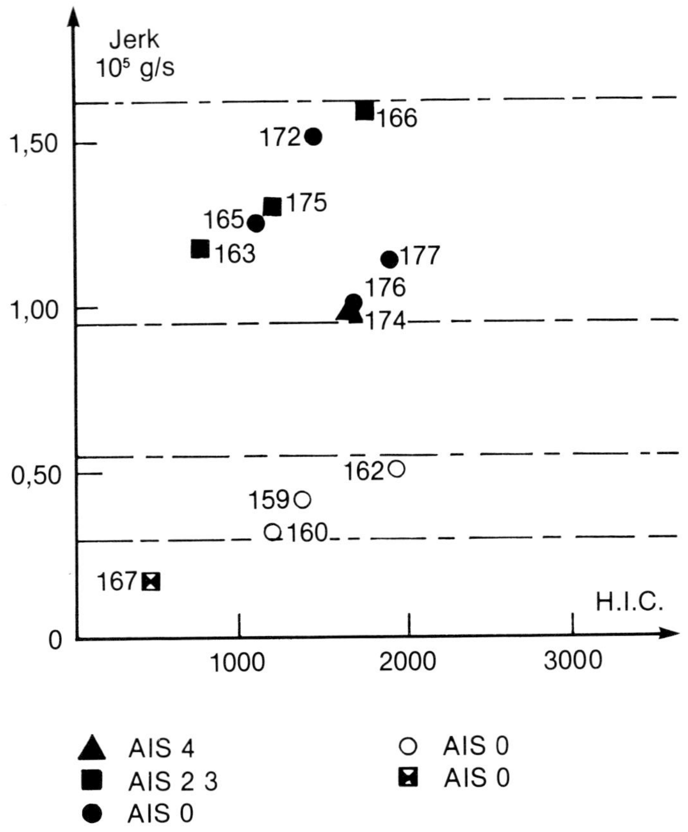

Figure 6. Linear Rate of Onset Jerk Versus H.I.C. Cadaver Test Results

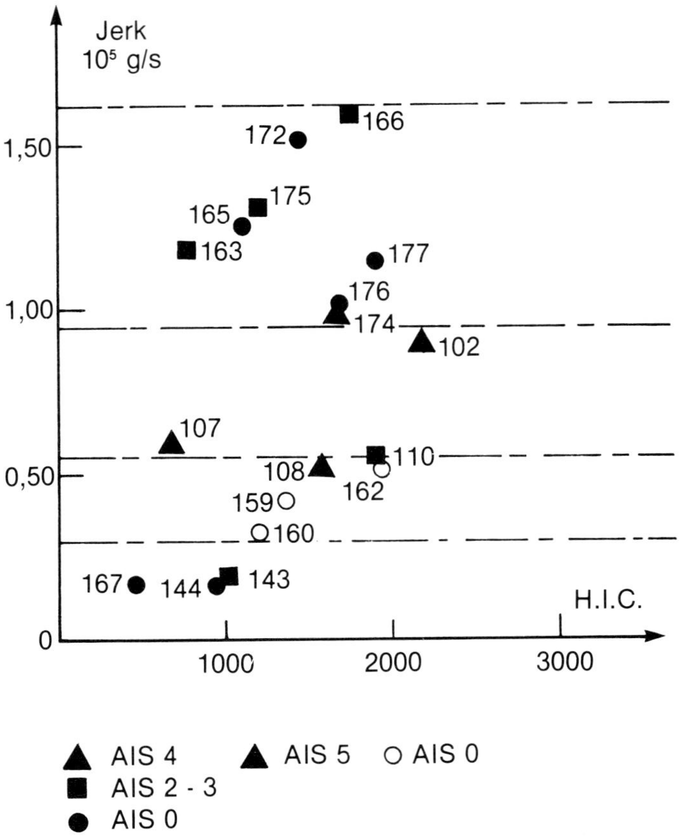

Figure 7. Linear Rate of Onset Versus H.I.C. Head Cadaver Test Results

Could we say that the same lateral bending induces head-neck compression when there is an impact, head-neck extension when there is no impact? Without injury in the first case, with a severe injury in the second one?

Interpretation of experimental cerebral injuries on cadavers

The autopsies for the actual-accidents' victims and the scanner investigations for nonfatal accidents' victims constitute the references for the interpretation of experimental cerebral injuries in cadavers. From our validation studies, it appears that, very often, the actual injuries are more extensive than the experimental ones. A too short duration of "bleeding" after experiment could be one explanation. It is recommended, in future work, to avoid stopping vascular pressurization before 5 or 10 minutes after impact. It is interesting to note that 22% of scanner images correspond to an AIS<3 and that 43% correspond to AIS 4. This means that references may be available for interpreting experimental brain injuries in the middle-range of the severity scale.

References

Bousigne's thesis, Toulouse, 1980.

Computed Tomography in Head Injuries, by W. Lanksch, T. Grumme and E. Kazner; published by Springer.

C. Got et al, 1978, SAE Paper 780, 887.

Ommaya, A.K. and Gennarelli, T.A. Comparison of Translational and Rotational Head Motions in Experimental Cerebral Concussion, Proceedings of 15th Stapp Car Crash Conference, Coronado, California, 1971.

Mechanical and Clinical Approaches to Head Injury Criteria

Sten Lindgren

Anatomy

The dynamic anatomy of the skull can be regarded as a combination of hemisphere and sphere, as in this drawing published 1964 (1) (Figure 1). This is one reason why the intracranial mechanics must be regarded differently due to impact site, type of impact and impact direction (Figure 2) (2).

The hemispherical anatomy of the skull may influence the deformations of the skull with local brain tissue reaction as well as the so-called steady acceleration pressure pattern, modified by impact direction and impact site. The different tangential forces related to the radial distance to the rotational axis may produce rotational centers also related to the intracranial compartmental anatomical characteristics. This will be discussed later during this symposium (3) and has been the subject for calculations by Ward and Thompson (4).

Mechanics—Tolerance

It is quite obvious that the different types of mechanical changes (Figure 3) after impact to the head may cause various types of injuries at different locations. Attempts to investigate such relationships, here called "Biomechanical research pattern" may be presented as a series of events worthwhile studying. Some decades ago even the impacting object (including mass, shape, contact surface) and type of impact had to be directly related to the resulting injuries. Even if the impact direction is axisymmetric, angular movements of the skull may occur before, during or after the impact. The location of a rotational axis may also change (Figure 4).

The physical and mathematical basis for one of the s.c. cerebral concussion tolerance curves and Head Injury Criterion has recently been reviewed by J. Newman (5). The experimental procedures used for the short duration part of the curve with often less

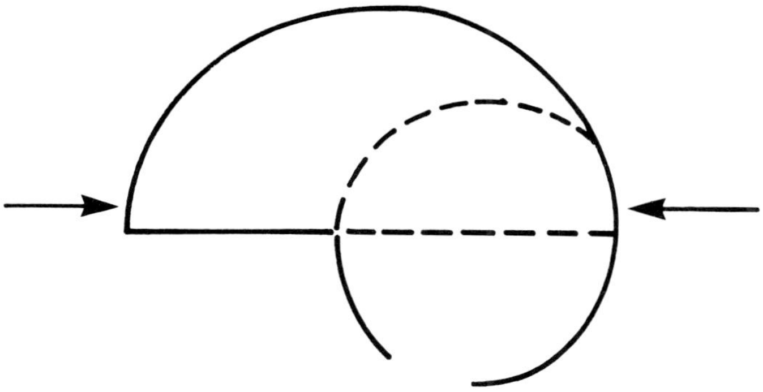

Figure 1. Schematic Drawing of the Dynamic Anatomy of the Skull

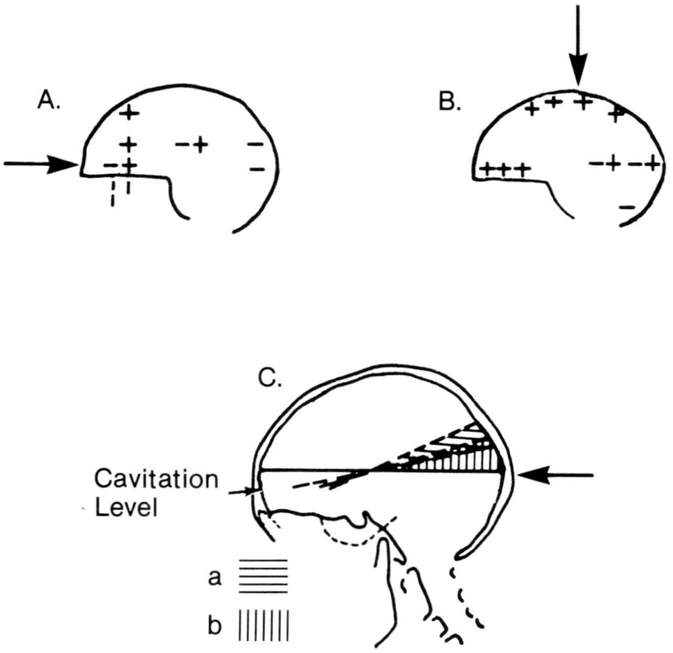

A. Frontal impact (cf. Fig. 24). Downward acceleration of the anterior skull base gives the partly negative "coup"-pressure.
B. Vertex impact (cf. Fig. 27). The pressures at the anterior skull base do not represent contre-coup (180°) or equatorial (90°) pressures.
In A and B the anterior fossa seems to represent part of a hemisphere.
C. Pressure and deformation within the skull contents
a: Pressure transients due to the deformations of the shell resulting in local acceleration differences between shell and content, directed perpendicularly to the shell.
b: Pressure pattern occurring in an ideally stiff shell (impacted on by a big comparatively soft object), in this case probably representing acceleration and velocity differences between the whole skull and its contents.
Displacement of contents: related to **a**, to possible flow between the intracranial and extracranial intraspinal cavities and modified by the properties of the contents including the occurrence of cavitation.
Rate of displacement: related to the just mentioned factors and **b.**

Figure 2. Schematic Drawings

Head Injuries

Biomechanical Research Pattern

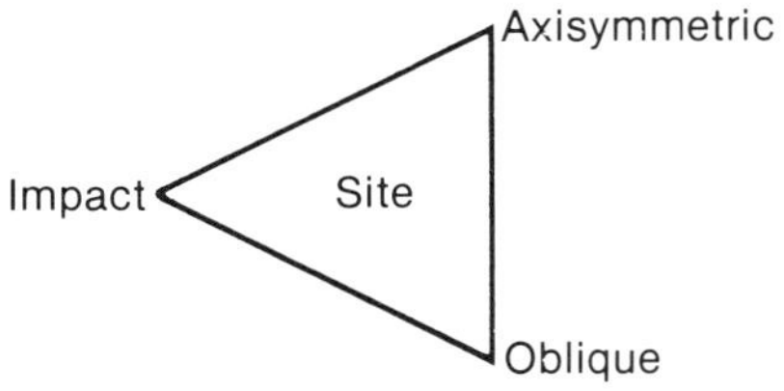

Direction	Skull Response	Intracranial Response	Injury
	Tolerance Curves? "Injury Criteria"??	(Compartmental) Forces, Pressures, Deformations	Site, Nature Grading (AIS, EIS)
	Deformational, -Skull Contact - Local Propagated - Local Total Volume Change	Local Tissue Displacement at Skull Deform, Fracture, Modified by Anatomy (Hemisph. etc.) Cavitation?	+ Surface Hemorrhages: Extra - Intradural Focal Brain Lesions ? Damge
	Translational, Accel., Veloc.	Accel, Pressure Pattern - ("Steady") - Impact Directional (Caviation - Supporting?) Transversal Displacement?: in Ant. Post. Imp. - at For. Magn. in Vertex Imp.- at Tentorium	0? +? (Magnitude?) +? Axial (Coma?)
	Angular, Accel., Veloc. - Before, During, After Impact	Different Tangential (and Radial) Forces Related to Rot. Axis. Compartmental Movements - Rot. Centers, CSF Modifications	+ Brain Surface, Veins - Lesions, Hemorrhage + Axial (Coma?)
	Cranio-Spinal Movem.	Brain Axis - Deformation?	?

Impact: Mass, Shape, Contact Surface and Other Characteristics of the Impacting Object Are Not Particularly Considered Here.

Skull Response: Axisymmetric Impact May Produce Effects of Angular Movements - Accelerations, Velocity - Due to Motions Before (Fall, Whiplash), During or After (Influence of Head-Neck Junction) the Impact.

Intracran. Resp.: Deformation Is Perhaps the Most Important Direct Mechanical Cause of Injury. Its Pathophysiological and Pathoanatomical Criteria May Be Related to Stress - Strain Conditions, at Various Locations. Laboratory Tests of Samples of the Various Materials Have Not Been Included.
S.C. Cavitation Includes Phenomena of Implosion, Turbulence, Etc.

Injury: AIS - EIS See Text and Fig. Coma Is Denoted for "Concussion". Axial: Diencephalon -Medulla.

Figure 3.

well-defined sites of impact and relations of the direction of impact to that of the big acceleration used to produce cadaver skull fractures should predict acceleration unconsciousness in living human beings. Even if unconsciousness occurs without skull fracture, severe skull fractures more often occur with severe coma. However, if the fracture occurs at the site of impact, particularly to the side of the skull, its peak acceleration is decreased and "contact time" increased more than if a linear meridional fracture is produced (the effect may be similar to intracranial fluid volume pulses). In a recent study of AIS skull injury versus AIS brain injury Gennarelli (6) found very little relationship.

Increased magnitude of the same type of impact may not produce only the same types of injuries, but more severe. Resonance frequencies of the skull and skull bone material properties, particularly at the site of impact, may suddenly modify the response. Of other nonlinear events such as mechanical failures, a specific problem is the cavitation phenomenon, perhaps occurring in the contrecoup region and at other sites, also influenced by local skull bone deformations (7) (Figure 2c). The last conclusion is supported by Stalhammers experiments (8) where the mere production of a negative intracranial pressure as part of a "steady acceleration pressure pattern" in living rabbits did not elicit any cerebral morphological changes.

The intermediate time duration portion of the tolerance curve has been related to animal experiments from 1954 (9). With the use of intracranially directed gas (10) and later on fluid (11) volume pressure pulses the "experimental animal brain concussion" symptoms may be regarded as pathophysiological indicators of functional brain material properties (Figure 5). It has, however, been shown that the symptoms produced in this way could be prevented by an anterior skull decompression, indicating the significance of the brain axial dislocations in the tentorial opening—fora-

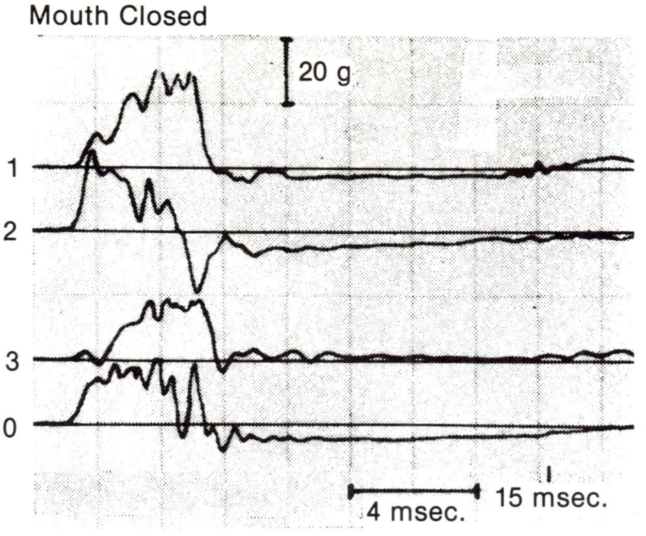

Figure 4a. Impact to the Chin (Ref. 12). Direction of Forces (Modified by Anatomy) and of Accelerometers (Fixed to the Skull by Metal Screws). Acceleration Curves.

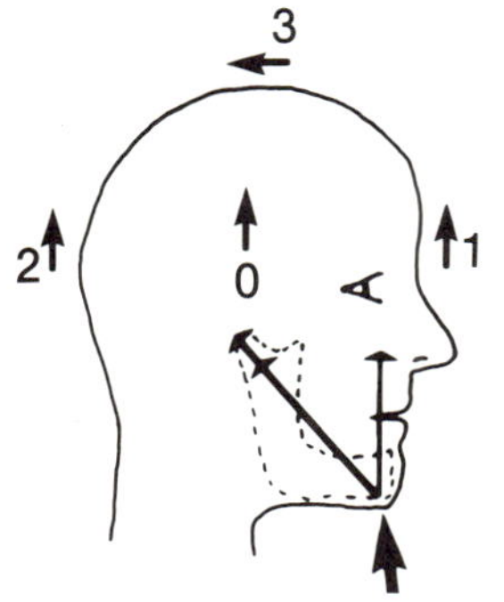

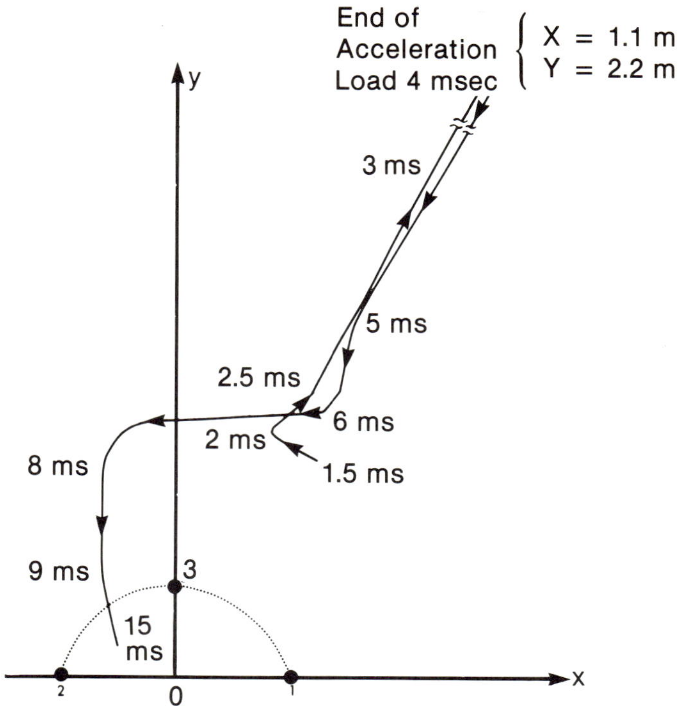

Figure 4b. Locaton of Rotational Axis Calculated from Acceleration Data. The Instantaneous Rotational Axis Is Moving Away from the Head in Anterior - Superior Direction During the Acceleration Load, Turning Point at 4 msec. Then the Posterior Rotation Dominates with Rotational Axis Moving into the Head - Further Accentuated at 15 msec.

men magnum area (12) (Figure 6). Stress-strain tissue relations and physiological parameters may be combined.

Among other types of tolerance studies in this connection may be mentioned the rotational concussion studies of Ommaya and Hirsch (13) and tests of tissue tolerance such as those of Lowenheilm (14).

Neurophysiology

Neurophysiological as well as neurosurgical experience of other kind related to similar symptomatology also points to the significance of the central parts of the brain and brain stem, but is more difficult to apply to head injuries. However, in some series of animal experiments the concussion symptoms are attributed to severe disturbances of the reticular activating systems (15) and less significance was given to the changes in cortical activity (16). Only the former conclusion was supported by Ommaya and Gennarelli (17) with rotational impact experiments and studies of the transmission of the somatosensory evoked responses of the cortex. It has also been suggested that the duration of the changes of the CNS-reactivity is not only related to varying severity of lesions at a similar location in the brain axis but also to different sites of such lesions (16). Greenberg et al. (18) found in patients that duration of coma more than 30 days had a stronger correlation with dysfunction of cerebral hemispheres than with brainstem dysfunction. They do not comment on the group with shorter duration of coma, which "could not be related to either hemispheric or brainstem dysfunction," nor on the hypothesis of a centripetal sequence of events from cerebral cortex to medulla.

Pathoanatomy

Pathoanatomical findings of presumably "immediate impact damage" to the brain have more often been related to specific mechanical events in the literature:

a) The brain surface lesions, including bridging veins and subcortical structures, are probably due to intracranial difference of the tangential forces at angular movements—except for the orbital surface of the frontal lobes, where deformation of the skull base may be a contributory factor in anterior impacts (Figure 2).

Gurdjian et. al. 1954-1955
Relationship Between Pressure-Time and Degree of Cerebral Concussion

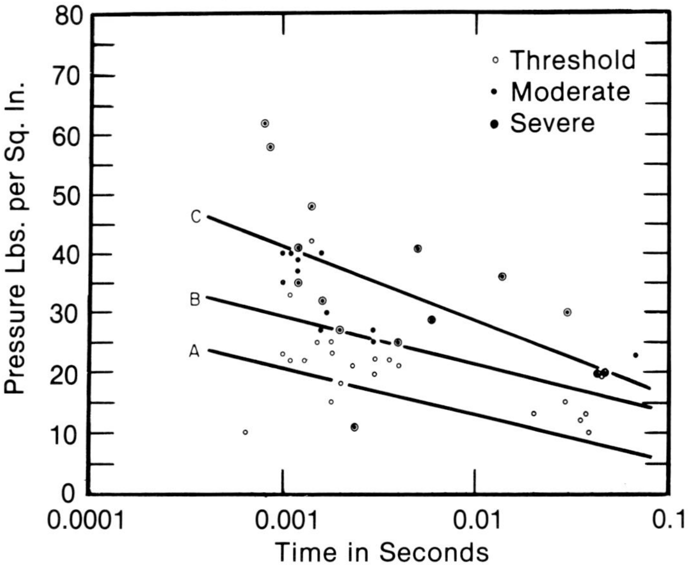

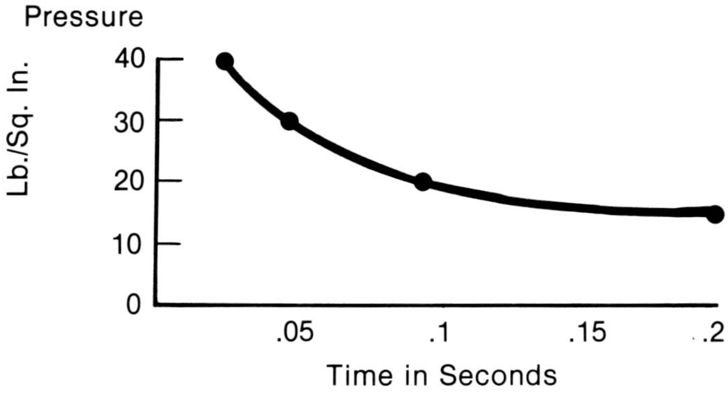

Pressure and time correlation in cases with severe concussive effects. The higher the level of the pressure used the lower the time duration in order to effect a severe result.

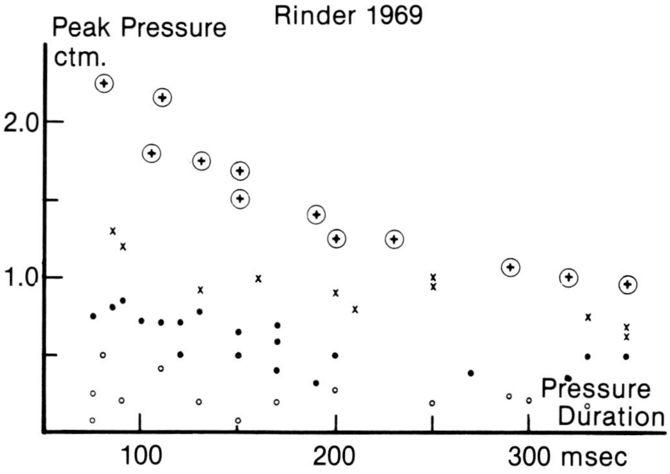

Results of experiments with induction of pressure pulses of 25—300 msec duration, showing relations between "severity" of the concussive response and peak amplitude and duration of the pressure pulse.

The piston was displaced 1—5 mm at a mean velocity of 0.05—0.2 m/sec. ○ = no effects; ● = "light" effect; X = "moderate" effect; + = "severe" effect (criteria are stated in "Results", p. 6, line 6 from bottom).

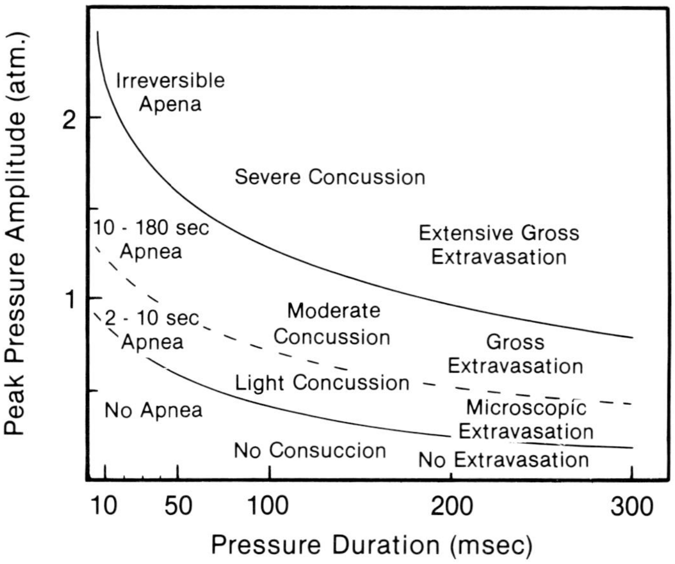

Diagram showing approximate relations between peak amplitude of intracranial presure increase at load-input to the skull cavity, and "severity" of concussive response and extent of extravasation of labelled albumin at induction of pressure pulses of varying duration.

Severe concussion: irreversible apnea, rise in blood pressure, tachy- or bradycardia.

Moderate concussion: 10—180 sec apnea, rise in blood pressure, bradycardia.

Light concussion: 2—10 sec apnea, fall inblood presure, bradycardia.

No concussion: no effect on recorded physiological parameters.

For further explanation, see Results.

Figure 5

However, that part of the skullbase, including the tentorial area underneath the hippocampal gyri, may also form a border for compartmental tissue rotational movements and deformations. With lateral impacts such a compartmental effect of the falx may be evident from the findings of Shatsky et al. (19)—occurring with a pronounced skull and brain deformation. This means that discussion about mechanisms of "cortical damage" always has to be related to its location and its depth.

b) The brain surface linear lesions along linear, meridional fractures are probably due to widening of the fracture and simultaneous negative focal pressure at the time of fracturing (2).

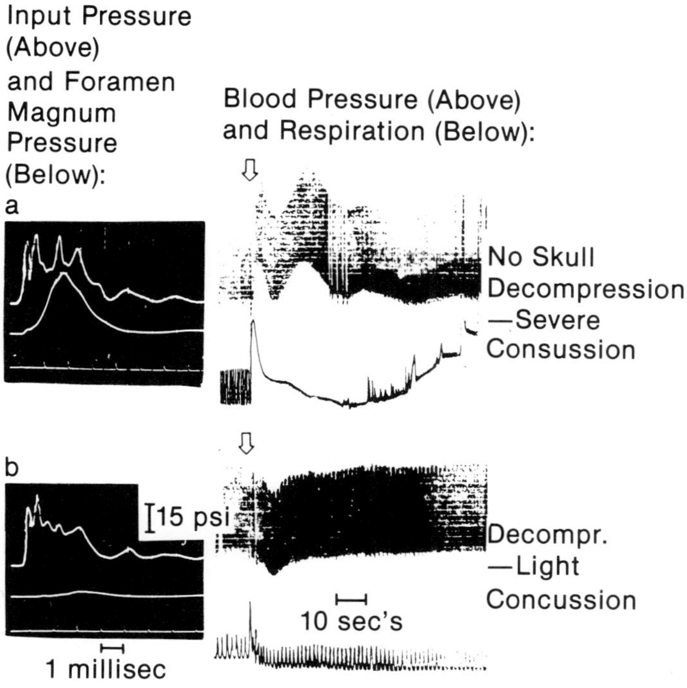

Percussion-concussion, pressure at input (parietal) and foramen magnum level, with simultaneous recording of blood pressure and respiration.

Figure 6.

c) The s.c. contrecoup-lesions which have a comparatively late clinical appearance, 1-2 days after trauma, and become ischemic, necrotic or hemorrhagic in nature, often subcortical, are sometimes related to s.c. cavitation phenomena or to local oscillatory skull movements. Gennarelli et al. (20) found that "as mechanical input increases, frontal lobe contusions occur before temporal contusions" and this was thought to be evidence of the importance of the angular movements and the tangential displacements; the same findings have by other investigators been taken as evidence of the importance of the more marked negative part of the acceleration pressure pattern in the frontal area with occipital impacts. The rarity of occipital contusions with frontal impacts is still somewhat confusing; there is still too little evidence for explanations such as the damping effect of the facial bone structures and the anterior skullbase influencing the acceleration characteristics as well as of the smooth, deformable tentorium posteriorly facilitating tissue movements.

d) The cerebral subcortical white matter ("diffuse" or may be disseminated) injuries are often attributable to angular movements of the skull—but still the suggested intracranial mechanics are less well defined—"shear strain" is not a complete mechanical description. The part of the white matter primarily involved must always be considered.

e) The periventricular and the corpus callosum hemorrhages have sometimes been attributed to the assumed total volume changes of the skull during and after impact. A combination of the technique in the promising studies of Shatsky et al. (19) and Hodgson and Thomas (21) with the newer techniques in pressurized cadavers could be valuable. S.c. resonance cavitation is here probably only of theoretical interest. With vertex impact directions the pressures in a transverse direction are different in the anterior and posterior parts—which in this connection may be regarded as a pressure gradient and of hypothetical interest (Figure 2)?

f) The axial mechanical disturbances from the diencephalon down to the medulla through the tentorial opening and the foramen magnum are attributed sometimes to the angular movements of the skull with radial and differential tangential forces in the brain as a whole—sometimes also within the respective compartments resulting in different tissue movements and deformations close to the "separating" planes—sometimes, at anteroposterior impacts, to the transversal pressure gradient from the skull contents down to the cervical medulla and—sometimes explained as caused by the movements in the head-neck junction.

The proponents of the angular movement of the skull as a mechanical cause of lesions similar in the cerebral subcortical white matter as well as in the white matter in the brain axis, have assumed that the location of such disturbances are parallel to an increasing mechanical input in a centripetal sequence from the cerebral hemisphere down to the medulla. This was supported by the findings in squirrel monkeys by Ommaya and Gennarelli (17) of intracerebral petechial hemorrhages disseminated in the supratentorial subcortical regions but rarely in the "brainstem." It may be possible that different magnitude of impacts elicits other types of intracranial mechanical events, particularly along the base of the hemispherical compartment including the tentorial opening.

Hume Adams et al. (22) in fact found an interesting pattern of focal lesions in the rostral brainstem area and in the corpus callosum at an autopsy in cases of relatively short survival time. (In those cases they point out that the damage occurring in the midbrain and the pons seems to be related to the axonal fibre direction!) However, in the intermediate survival cases signs of diffuse damage to the white matter of the cerebral hemisphere were also revealed. This difference is not easily explained with the hypothesis of a similar mechanical cause along cortex-brain-stem direction and most marked in the cerebral cortical-subcortical region. Information concerning possible relationship between assumed magnitude of impact, severity of clinical condition at admittance and various length of survival should be valuable in these otherwise very well-selected and pathoanatomically examined cases.

They also described another pattern of injury in two patients dying within 12 hours with "a fracture of the skull and innumerable petechial hemorrhages in the cortex and white matter of the cerebral hemispheres," midbrain, rostral pons, around the aqueduct and in the tegmentum without the above mentioned focal pattern. He also mentions (23) the findings of other neuropathologists that patients with very short survival time have marked "primary brain stem injury."

The importance of craniospinal movements is still under debate regarding evidence of medullary functional and anatomical disturbances.

C.T.-Scanning

Computerized tomography of the brain is the clinical possibility of pathoanatomical investigation of particularly focal lesions and dislocations. We have sometimes seen hemorrhages in the hypothalamic-pendun-cular region and in the rostral part of the brain stem explaining deviation of the later course of patients with similar early AIS level. The C.T. scanning is very informative also in revealing multiple contusions, edema, etc. It may add to the pathoanatomical investigations by giving a morphological picture also of the more slight disturbances, particularly in children, such as hyperemia or edema of the brain and other conditions of relatively short duration. Supplementary information from intracranial pressure recordings must so far often be used to explain cerebral dysfunction as C.T. findings still can only indirectly indicate the presence or absence of high intracranial pressure. The main cornerstone will always be the clinical picture, sometimes with support of neurophysiological laboratory findings.

Clinical Picture

Even if the clinical severity of one type of symptoms does not describe the severity of the whole spectrum of injuries, usually the degree and duration of unconsciousness and associated signs have been used. Even if such disturbances of consciousness sometimes may be continuous, there are a number of practical reasons to define certain time durations of importance for medical judgment—diagnostic and prognostic.

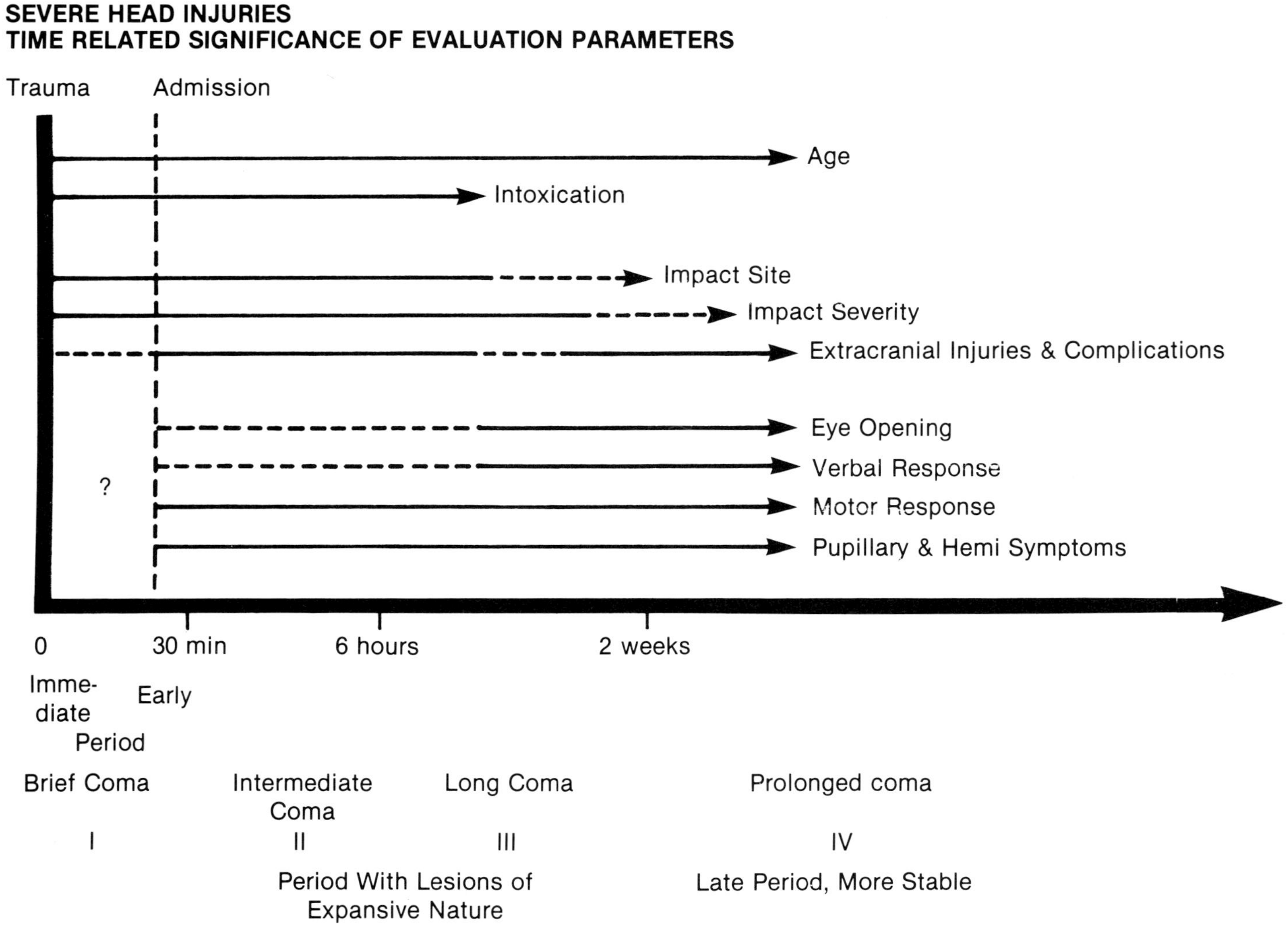

Figure 7.

The posttraumatic severity of a condition and the resulting outcome often depends on factors of partly time-related significance such as age, intoxication, extracranial injuries or complications, etc. The grading of the damage is, for the clinician, facilitated by observation of the response to external stimuli usually verbal or painful. Some time-related factors are shown in Figure 7.

In the immediate posttraumatic period the well-known pathophysiological disturbances in "animal experimental brain concussion" have been classified by Abel et al. (24) in a similar way as the AIS numbering. For clinical purposes it is necessary with a basis for judgment of the clinical condition, the diagnosis and the prognosis throughout the whole posttraumatic period. We have very little clinical knowledge of the **immediate** human posttraumatic reaction and a little more of the early findings, except in "sports" events such as boxing. The immediate posttraumatic reaction in such events has sometimes also been described as specific for a certain type of violence. Moreover, with most injuries medical evaluation of the significance of various symptoms can hardly be started earlier than 30 minutes after trauma. Conditions with unconsciousness disappearing within 30 minutes have been called **Brief coma** (Figure 8).

During the following two weeks disturbances of consciousness may not be directly caused by the trauma but added, s.c. secondary complications such as intracranial hematoma. However, during this long period the acute management often is most critical during the first 6 hours, which has been defined as an **Intermediate coma** period. Judgment of neurosurgical groups of patients and their comparison in terms of "acute" diagnosis and treatment this may be enough (Figure 11). However, the long-term recording of other functions than consciousness, with regard to wakefulness or awareness, is a matter for psychopathological or neurological scoring, partly for the requirements of ADL and employment.

Summary

Traumatic and posttraumatic events reported from mechanical, physiological, pathoanatomical and clinical studies of head injuries are discussed. The relationship between mechanical parameters and the appearance and duration of coma is of particular interest for the studies of cerebral concussion tolerance curves. Some still relevant research is reviewed and discussed.

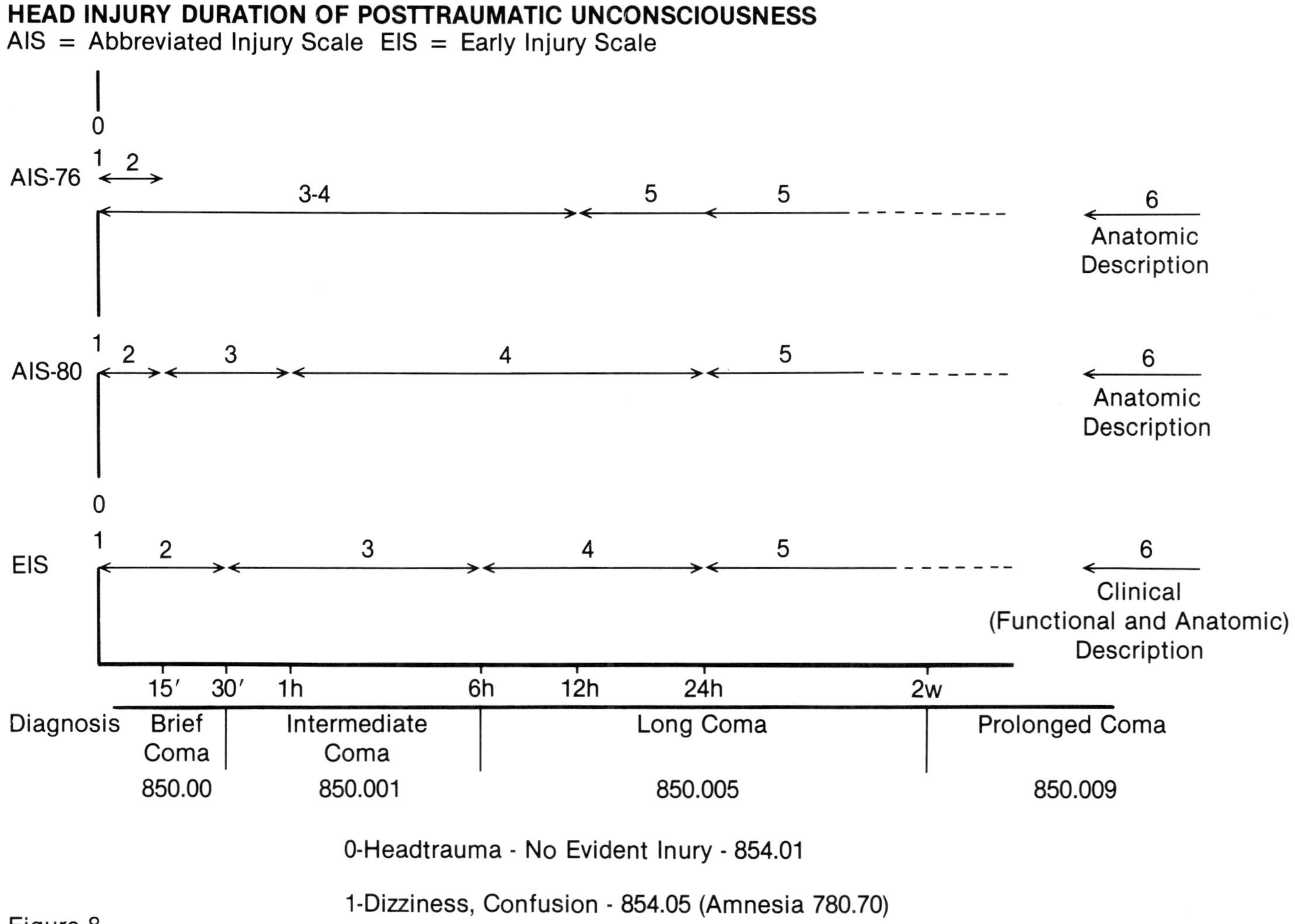

Figure 8.

Record: Head Injuries

Inst, Clinic, Ward, OPD

Pt ID

Accident Date Time

Place of Acc.

☐ Home ☐ Work ☐ Other ____________

Age

☐ Male ☐ Female

Accident Type

Information From:

Fall
☐ On the Level
☐ From Height
☐ Steps
☐ After Fainting

☐ No Information

☐ Other ________

Collision
☐ Pedestrian
☐ Cyclist
☐ Moped Or Mc
☐ Car Driver
☐ Passenger Front
☐ Passenger Back
☐ Safety Belt Used
☐ Helmet

Head Impact By
☐ Floor, Wood, Concrete
☐ Ground, Road Surface
☐ Windshield
☐ Dashboard
☐ Steering-Wheel
☐ Blow?

Unconscious Transport: _______

☐ At Accident ☐ Later ☐ Answers ☐ Moves ☐ Vomits

☐ Intoxication? . . . ☐ Airway; Free ☐ Resp Support: . .

Examination Date Time ☐ 1st Hospital ☐ 2nd Hospital

Head Injuries / Site of Impact: ☐ Face ☐ Frontal ☐ Occip. ☐ Right Side ☐ Left Side ☐ Vertex

Reaction Level

On Request	On Pain-Movem	Opens Eyes
0☐ Alert	0☐ Normal	0☐ Spontaneous
1☐ Simple Answers Obeys Command ☐ Amnesia PTA RA Duration: . . . . ☐ Disoriented ☐ Restless, Confused	1☐ Agitated Movements	1☐ To Speech
2☐ Drowsy, Answers Slowly	2☐ Irritated Coordin	2☐ On Command
3☐ Irrelevant Sounds	3☐ Withdrawal	3☐ To Pain
4☐ Nil	4☐ Flexion	4☐ Nil
5☐ Nil	5☐ Extension	5☐ Nil
6☐ Nil	6☐ Nil	6☐ Nil

General Condition

Airway Intub ☐

Respir ☐ Normal . . . . rate/min
☐ Shallow ☐ Deep ☐ Irreg

BP Pulse Rate

Shock Temp

Other Injuries

Previous Neurol Dis

Focal Symptoms Dysphasia ☐

Note Side Differences:
Ability to Move Impaired In

	Right	Left
Arm	☐	☐
Leg	☐	☐
Face	☐	☐
Tonus Reduced In		
Arm	☐	☐
Leg	☐	☐
Plantar Resp - Ext	☐	☐
Neck Stiffness (Caution!)	☐	

Eye Movements ☐ Follows

☐ Fixed Forward ☐ Deviat ☐ Undul

Pupils	Right	Left
Large	☐	☐
Small	☐	☐
Equal	☐	
Reaction to Light		
Direct	☐	☐
Indirect	☐	☐

Figure 9.

1. All Ages: - Head Trauma, Slight (Direct Or Indirect). Wounds. Slight Non-Localized Pain In Head Or Neck. Facial Fractures. No Unconsciusness. Dizzy. Confused

2. All Ages: - Head Trauma, Moderate. Frontal Impact. Wounds. Localized Pain In Head Or Neck. Facial Displaced Fracture. Eye Ball Damage.
Unconsciousness V 30 Min. PTA Brief. Vomiting. Drowsy, Eyes Open Or Answers On Request.
- Spine: Dorsal and Lumbar Damage, No Neurological Symptoms.

3. All Ages: - Head Trauma, Moderate. Frontal Or Vertex IMpacts. Skull Fracture (Vault + Temporal Bone). Severe Maxillar Fractures. Unconscious V 6 Hrs. Amnesia. - If Still Unconscious: Purposeful Motor Pattern With Or Without Pain Stimuli.
- Spine: Cervical Damage, No Neurological Symptoms. - Dorsal and Lumbar Damage With Neurological Symptoms.

4. V 50 Years Old (- and Also Nr 5 If V 20 Years): Head Trauma: Particularly Temporal Or Occipital Impacts. Skull Fracture (Open Or Base). Airway Obstruction.
Unconscious V 24 Hrs. Flexor Motor Pattern. Hyperthermia.

   Intracranial Expansive Lesion ("Secondary" Complication) Indicated By Deeper Unconsciousness, Hemisymptoms, Unequal Pupils.
- Spine: Lower Cervical Damage With Neurological Symptoms.

5. V 50 Years Old - Findings As In Grade No 4 — Or All Ages V 20 Years: - Head Trauma, Moderate to Severe, All Sites Particularly Occipital.
Unconscious V 24 Hrs. Respiratory Abnormlities. Extensor Motor Pattern. Pupils Fixed.
Symptoms Indicating Intracranial Expansive Lesion.
- Spine: Upper Cervical Damage With Neurological Symptoms.

6. All Ages: - Head Trauma, Severe.
Unconscious. Respiratory Insufficiency - Or Lasting Apnea.
On Pain No Reaction Or Extensor Motor Pattern. Dilated Fixed Pupils. Anatomic Lesions, Related to This Functional Deficit.

   All Head Injury Degrees May Develop Secondary Complications Indicating - Intracranial Expansive Lesion. Intrathoracic and Intraabdominal Injuies Etc. May Add to the Degree of Injury. - This "Final" Result May Be Graded According to Neurological Scales.

Figure 10a. Early Injury Scale (Degree of "Threat to Life") (V 30 min. After Accident)

AIS (Code) (Abbreviated Injury Scale) (Threat to Life)	Early Injury Scale (Degree of "Threat to Life") (>30 Min. After Accident)	ICD (Who) (International Classification of Diseases) (Worst Diagnosis in Each Group) Observation (>30 Min. - 2 d.)		Diagnosis (V 2 Days) (Additional Coma)
0. No Injury Evident		0. Head Trauma, Alert (Trauma Capitis NUD)	854,01	0. See Observation
1. Minor	1. All Ages: - Head Trauma, Slight (Direct or Indirect). Wounds. Slight Non-Localized Pain in Head or Neck. Facial Fractures. No Unconsciousness. Dizzy. Confused.	1. Confused - Amnesia Wounds (Head, Neck, Face) Facial Fractures	854,05 - 780,70 873, 874, 879 804,00	1. See Observation
2. Moderate	2. All Ages: - Head Trauma, Moderate. Frontal Impact. Wounds. Localized Pain in Head or Neck. Facial Displaced Fracture. Eye Ball Damage. Unconsciousness < 30 Min. PTA Brief. Vomiting, Drowsy, Eyes Open or Answers on Request. - Spine: Dorsal and Lumbar Damage, No Neurological Symptoms.	2. Brief Posttr. Coma <30 Min. (Coma Breve Posttr. - Commotio Cerebri). Drowsy, Slow Answers, Opens Eyes Spine: Damage of Dorsal or Lumbar Spine.	850,00 805,21	2. See Observations
3. Severe (Not Life-Threatening)	3. All Ages: - Head Trauma, Moderate. Frontal or Vertex Impacts. Skull Fracture (Vault + Temporal Bone). Severe Maxillar Fractures. Unconscious < 6 Hrs. Amnesia. - If Still Unconscious: Purposeful Motor Pattern with or without Pain Stimuli. - Spine: Cervical Damage, No Neurological Symptoms. - Dorsal and Lumbar Damage with Neurological Symptoms.	3. Intermediate Ptr. Coma < 6 Hrs. Verbal Response Only to Pain, Coordinated Movements, With-drawal Spine: Damage of Verv. Spine. Damage of Dorsal and Lumbar Spine with Neurol. Symptoms	850,001 805,00 806,21	3. See Observation
4. Serious (Lifethreatening - Survival Probable)	4. <50 Years Old (- and Also Nr 5 if <20 Years): Head Trauma: Particularly Temporal or Occipital Impacts. Skull Fracture (Open or Base). Airway Obstruction. Unconscious < 24 Hrs. Flexor Motor Pattern. Hyperthermia. Intracranial Expansive Lesion ("Secondary" Complication) Indicated by Deeper Unconsciousness, Hemisymptoms, Unequal Pupils. - Spine: Lower Cervical Damage with Neurological Symptoms.	4. Posttr. Coma < 24 Hrs. Nonpurposeful Flexion. Focal Expansive Contusion Spine: Lower Cerv. Damage with Neurol. Symptoms	850,005 851,001 806,00	4. Long Posstraum. (<2 Weeks) 850,005
5. Critical (Survival Uncertain)	5. >50 Years Old - Findings as in Grade No 4 - - - or All Ages >20 Years: - Head Trauma, Moderate to Severe, All Sites Particularly Occipital. Unconscious > 24 Hrs. Respiratory Abnormlities. Extensor Motor Pattern. Pupils Fixed. Symptoms Indicating Intracranial Expansive Lesion. - Spine: Upper Cervical Damage with Neurological Symptoms.	5. Posttr. Coma >24 Hrs Extension Movements (on Pain) Expansive Lesions as Above Spine: Upper Cerv. Damage with Neurol. Symptoms	850,005 806,005	5. Long Prt. Coma (or Prolonged Posstr. Coma (>2 Weeks) 850,09
6. Fatal (Maximum - Currently Untreatable)	6. All Ages: - Head Trauma, Severe. Unconscious. Respiratory Insufficiency - or Lasting Apnea. On Pain No Reaction or Extensor Motor Pattern. Dilated Fixed Pupils. Anatomic Lesions, Related to this Functional Deficit. All Head Injury Degrees May Develop Secondary Complications INdicating - Intracranial Expansive Lesion. Intrathoracic and Intraabdominal Injuries etc. May Add to the Degree of Injury. - The "Final" Result May Be Graded According to Neurological Scales.	6. As Above Under "5".		6. As Above Under "5".

Figure 10b. Continuous Injury Scaling - Neurotraumatology (Gothenburg)

Trauma Capitis (Head Trauma)		854.01		
Vulnus Capitis (Scalp-Wound)		873.00		
Vulnus Colli (Neck-Wound)		874.00		
Vulnera Faciei (Face-Wound)		879.00		
		Non Compl.	Compl	Sequele
Fractural Cranii (Skull Fracture)		800.00	800.10	800.90
Fractura Cranii Baseos (Skull Base Fracture)		801.00	801.10	
Fractura Cranii Cum Impressione		803.00	803.10	803.90
Fractura Cranii Sive Oss. Facei Mult		804.00	804.10	
Fractura Cranii (?) Cum Liquorrhea			801.10	
Amnesia - Confusion, Vertigo Etc (Without Coma) Traumat		854.05		
Coma Breve Posttraumaticum (Commotio Cerebri) (Brief Posstr. Coma, Concussion <30 Min)		850.00		
Coma Intermedium Posstraumaticum (Intermediate Posstr. Coma 30 Min - 6 Hrs.)		850.001		
Coma Longum Posstraumaticum (Long Posstraumatic Coma 6 Hrs - 2 W)		850.005		
Coma Prolongatum Posttraumaticum (Prolonged Posstr. Coma, Vegetating State Etc >2 W)		850.009		
Encephalopathia Posttraumatica				850.90
Hydrocephalus Posttraumatica				854.90
Laesio Cerebri Focalis Non Expansiva (- Symptomatological Diagnosis) (Focal Nonexp. Cer. Lesion-)		851.00	851.10	851.90
Contusion Cerebri Focalis s. Hemat. Intracerebr. Expansiva (Focal Expansive Cer. Contusion or Hematoma)		851.001	851.101	
Pneumocephalus			851.102	
Varia - Al. Defin (Contus. Mult., Oedema Malign Etc)		854.00	854.10	(c. corp. alie)
Fat Embolism		995.10		
Hematoma Extradurale		852.00		
Hematoma Subdurale ac. (Hydrom-Hygrom)		853.00		
Hematoma Subdurale Subacuta		853.001		
Hematoma Subdurale Chron. Taum.				853.90
Hematoma Subdurale Non Traum. (431.91)				
Aneurysma (Art. Ven.) Traum.		995.30		
Laesio Nervus Cranialis	II	950.00		
Laesio Nervus Cranialis	III, IV, VI	951.00		
Laesio Nervus Cranialis	Others	951.01		
Laesio Nervus Perifer.		959.22	959.32	959.92
Defectus Cranii Posttraum.			800.10	800.90
Osteitis Cranii Posttraum.			800.10	800.90
Abscessus Cerebri Posstraum.			800.10	800.90
Fractura et Luxatio Vert. (Without Spinal Cord Symptoms)	cerv thor lumb	805.00 805.21 805.21	805.10 805.31 805.31	
Fractura et Luxatio Vert. (With Spinal Cord Damage Incl. Hematoma)	cerv thor lumb	806.00 806.21 806.22	806.10 806.31 806.32	
Myelopathia Traum ac. (Spinal Cord Damage - - Acute - Incl. Hematoma)	cerv thor lumb	958.00 958.21 958.22		
Myelopathia Traum Chron. (Spinal Cord Damage - Chronic)	cerv thor lumb		958.90 958.91 958.92	

Figure 11. ICD Traumatology

Some of the failures may be related to:

1. The dynamic anatomy of the skull and of the intracranial compartments have been paid too little interest. It will influence the cranial and intracranial response to impacts in terms of skull deformations of intracranial pressure and tissue deformation pattern.

2. Some basic experimental mechanical procedures have to be repeated with the modern technique available. Electrophysiology has been successful but may be supplemented with new techniques for analysing the location of lesions.

3. The reports regarding a relationship between impact magnitude and the involvement of the cortex and of the central parts of the brain and brain stem have been controversial. Some experimental and postmortem findings point to the possibility of a compartmental influence on the location of the lesions.

4. The lesions in the white matter as well as those in the cortical and subcortical tissues have often been less well described with regard to location, which is sometimes the case also with the lesions along the axis of the brain, the "brainstem."

The understanding of the mechanisms of such lesions will be facilitated with better cooperation between pathologists, roentgenologists (tomographic scanning) and clinicians.

5. The clinical definition of head injury levels and their posttraumatic time-related factors have to be even more considered than in the present AIS scale. The severity of the disturbances of functions and the nature of the lesions expressed in terms of a modified "International Classification of Diseases" can be the basis for international comparison of head injury: epidemiology, prevention, diagnosis and results of treatment.

A physical criterion on "Head Injury" may be based on for instance *one* type of mechanical response of the skull or/and of the brain and its vascular and nervous supply, provided this is related to *the* injury investigated; grading may then be possible.

References

1. Lindgren, S., "Studies in Head Injuries: Intracranial Pressure Pattern During Impact." *Lancet i,* 1251–1253, 1964.
2. Lindgren, S., "Experimental Studies of Mechanical Effects in Head Injury." *Acta. Chir. Scand. Suppl,* 360, 100 pp. 1966.
3. Aldman, B., Ljung, C., and Thorngren, L., Unpublished Observations, 1981.
4. Ward, C.C., and Thompson, R.B., "The Development of a Detailed Finite Element Brain Model," Proc. of the 19th Stapp Car Crash Conference, 641–674, 1975.
5. Newman, J.A., "Automobile Occupant Injury Criteria, Part 1: Head Injury." *Autom. Safety Eng.,* February 1980.
6. Gennarelli, T.A., "Analysis of Head Injury Severity by AIS–80," Proc. Am. Ass. Automot. Med., 1980.
7. Lubock, P., and Goldsmith, W., "Experimental Cavitation in a Model Head-Neck System," *J. Biomechanics* 13, 1041–1052, 1980.
8. Stalhammer, D., "Experimental Brain Damage from Fluid Pressures due to Impact Acceleration," Thesis, Goteborg, 1974.
9. Newman, J.A., "On the Use of the Head Injury Criterion (HIC) in Protective Headgear Evaluation," Proc. of the 19th Stapp Car Crash Conference, 615–640, 1975.
10. Gurdjian, E.S., Lissner, H.R., Webster, J.E., Latimer, F.R., and Haddad, B.F., "Studies on Experimental Concussion. Relation of Physiologic Effect to Time Duration of Intracranial Pressure Increase at Impact," *Neurology* 4, 674–681, 1954.
11. Rinder, L., "Experimental Brain Concussion by Sudden Intracranial Input of Fluid," Thesis, Goteborg, 1969.
12. Lindgren, S., and Rinder, L., "Decompression in Precussion Concussion: Effects on 'Concussive Response' in Rabbits," *J. Trauma* 7, 493–499, 1967.
13. Ommaya, A.K., and Hirsch, A.E., "Tolerances for Cerebral Concussion from Head Impact and Whiplash in Primates," *J. Biomechanics* 4, 13–21, 1971.
14. Lowenheilm, C.G.P., "On Bridging Vein Disruption and Rotational Cerebral Injuries Due to Head Impact," Thesis, Lund, 1977.
15. Foltz, E.L., and Schmidt, R.P., "The Role of the Reticular Formation in the Coma of Head Injury," *J. Neurosurgery* 13, 145–154, 1956.
16. Ward, A.A., *The Physiology of Concussion,* In Head Injury, Conference Proceedings, J.G. Lippincott Co., Philadelphia, 1966, pp. 203-208.
17. Ommaya, A.K., and Gennarelli, T.A., "A Physiopathologic Basis for Non-invasive Diagnosis and Prognosis of Head Injury Severity. Head Injuries," Proc. Second Chicago Symposium of Neural Trauma, 1976, pp. 49–75.
18. Greenberg, R.P., Miller, J.D., and Becker, D.P., "Clinical Findings Associated with Brainstem Dysfunction: an Electrophysiological Study in Severe Human Head Trauma," Seminars in Neurological Surgery, Neural Trauma, Raven Press, New York, 229–236, 1979.
19. Shatsky, S.A., Alter III, W.A., Evans, D.E., Armbrustmacher, V., and Clark, G., "Traumatic Dis-

tortions of the Primate Head and Chest: Correlation of Biomechanical, Radiological and Pathological Data," Proc. of the 18th Stapp Car Crash Conference, 351–381, 1974.

20. Gennarelli, T.A., Abel, J.M., Adams, H., and Graham, D., "Differential Tolerance of Frontal and Temporal Lobes to Contusion Induced by Angular Acceleration," Proc. of the 25th Stapp Car Crash Conference, 563–586, 1979.
21. Hodgson, V.R., and Thomas, L.M., "Acceleration Induced Shear Strains in a Monkey Brain Hemisection," Proc. of the 25th Stapp Car Crash Conference, 1979.
22. Adams, J.H., Mitchell, D.E., Graham, D.I., and Doyle, D., "Diffuse Brain Damage of Immediate Impact Type," *Brain* 100, 489–502, 1977.
23. Adams, J.H., "The Neuropathology of Head Injuries," In Vinken, Bruyn: Handbook of Clinical Neurology 23, part I, 1975.
24. Abel, J.M., Gennarelli, T.A., and Segawa, H., "Incidence and Severity of Cerebral Concussion in the Rhesus Monkey Following Sagittal Plane Angular Acceleration," Proc. of the 25th Stapp Car Crash Conference, 35–53, 1978.
25. Lindgren, S., "Acute Severe Head Injuries," *Acta Clin. Scand.* Suppl., 254, 1960.

Which is the More Severe Impact on the Head: Sagittal or Lateral?

Preliminary Report

Norio Nakamura
Hideaki Masuzawa
Hiroaki Sekino
Hiroshi Kono
Atsumi Kikuchi
Koshiro Ono

Abstract

A series of animal experiments has been conducted using monkeys in order to investigate a threshold for the occurrence of brain damage in head injuries.

Brain concussion is evaluated as a reasonable criterion for brain damage. On the other hand, brain contusion takes place in different incidence and distribution influenced by the participation of rotational acceleration and the direction of the impact delivered on the head.

So far, a brain seems more vulnerable to sagittal impact than lateral, as far as the degree of brain concussion is utilized as the criterion of brain damage in head injury.

The experiment is still in progress, and the conclusion will be achieved only after further experimentation.

Introduction

From both a medical and engineering point of view, one of the most important and yet unsettled problems in advanced industrial development is head protection from an accident. A variety of clinical and pathophysiological manifestations take place in head injury, in many ways primarily of the many types and forms of impact delivered to the head.

As a dynamic mechanism of head injury, translational acceleration impact in combination with rotational at the moment of impact take part in production of brain damage.

From a pathological point of view, the intracerebral pressure gradient theory on the one hand (1), and the intracerebral shear strain theory on the other (2), have been believed to explain concussion and contusion resulting in brain damage. Taking these dynamic studies and clinicopathological theories of head injury into consideration, many researchers, utilizing theoretical analyses, animal experiments and even human volunteers, have diligently sought to establish a threshold beyond which brain damage and death are likely to occur.

A majority of these investigations have been conducted effectively and successfully by engineers and medical doctors working in close cooperation. Accumulated achievements now provide a clue to what safety standard in head protection is to be used, not only in traffic, but also in an industrial environment.

We have been carefully studying the pathomechanism and dynamics of craniocerebral injury using primates, human skulls, human dummies and mathematical models for more than 15 years (3) (4) (6) (8) (9). The experiments have been conducted in effective collaboration with engineers working in the University of Tokyo and the Japan Automobile Research Institute (JARI) near Tokyo over a period of 6 years, and, for the purpose of our research at JARI, new impactor apparatus was introduced to produce head injury in animals: A series of experiments is still in progress.

A number of different medical and engineering research goals are in view, but the burden of this report is limited to the question of the relative seriousness of sagittal and lateral impact.

Our experimental research, now in progress, is composed of two steps using monkeys (Macaca fuscata, Macaca mulatta, Macaca fasicularis and Papio cynocephalus).

In the first step, the significance of translational impact, rotational impact and the combination of these two has been investigated separately in regard to production of brain injury in three groups, A, B and C. All impacts were delivered on a frontal or occipital area of the head.

In the second step, lateral impact was delivered to the head by way of contrast with the group C experiment in the first step.

Arrangement and Method

First step experiment

Group A: A new impactor apparatus consisting of a slider mounted on a 12-in. HYGE sled was introduced to produce head injury in animals. When the sled is pushed by a thrust column powered by HYGE air compressor, the slider on the sled travels along a slider guide, a pin impinges against a lead block and the whole sled system, with the monkey, runs straight on a railway (Figure 1).

Masking of the face and forehead of the animal is accomplished by means of a plaster-of-Paris mask to prevent a contact phenomenon.

Group B: An impactor apparatus used in the group B experiment consists of a monkey chair device, and an impactor ejection arrangement, driven by compressed air. A monkey is seated in the chair with its head immobilized by a head impact mask (Figure 2).

Upon impact, the head mask rotates around the neck C_{6-7} and the body pivots around the hip. Finally the body comes to rest at an angle of 60 degrees.

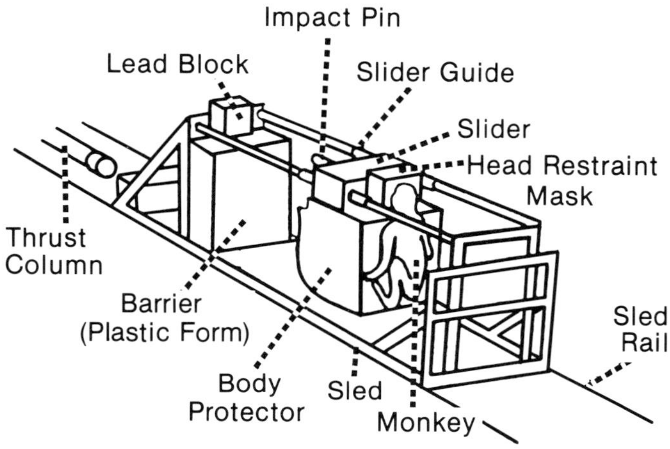

a. Overall View of Experimental Set-Up of Newly Developed Impact System on HYGE Sled

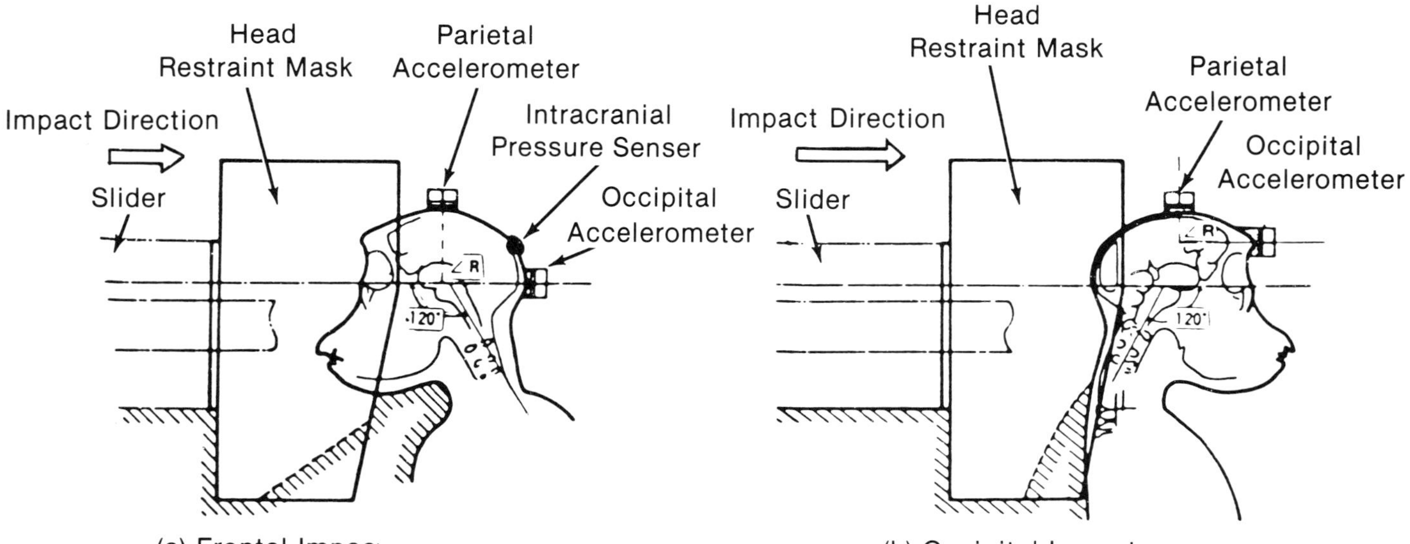

(a) Frontal Impact (b) Occipital Impact

b. Translational Head Impact Test Configuration and Set-Up for Masking of Subject's Head

Figure 1. Group A Experiment

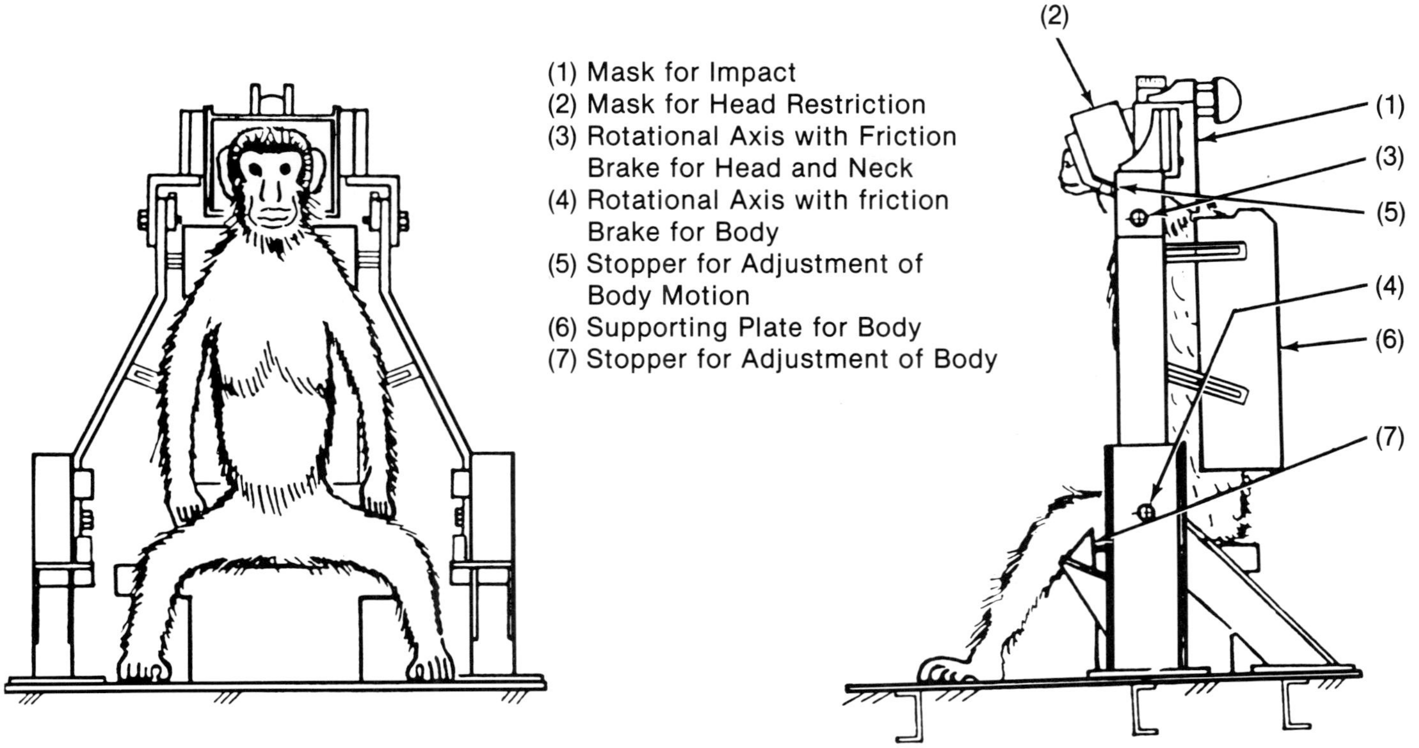

a. Rotational Head Impact Test Configuration and Set-Up for Masking of Subject's Head

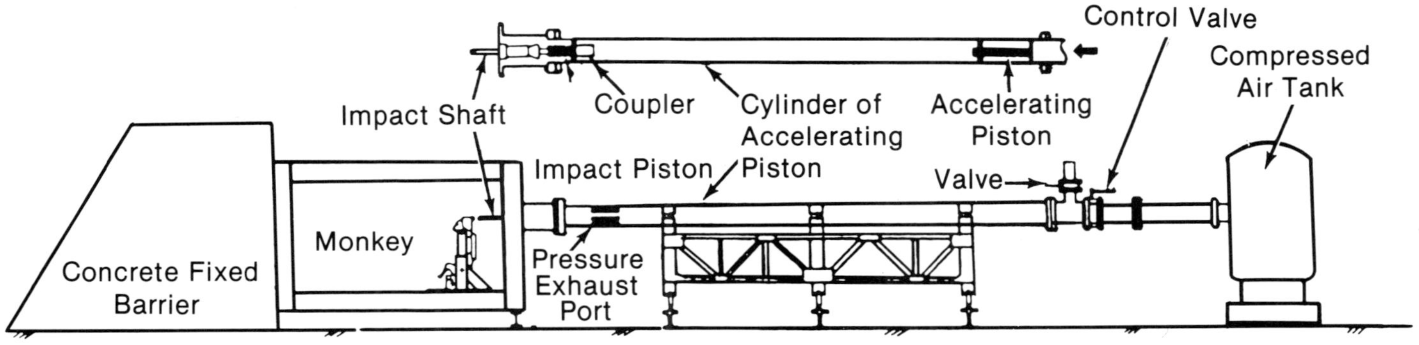

b. Illustration of the Impactor System for Rotational and Direct Head Impact

Figure 2. Group B Experiment

The mechanism provides an almost purely rotational acceleration impact on the occipital region of the head.

Group C: An impactor ejection arrangement is the same as in the group B experiment except that the impactor head is covered with a rubber block which is designed to accommodate adequately the whole of the monkey's head (Figure 3).

A restraint device for the monkey holds the free head of the subject in position for the impact and then gradually absorbs kinetic energy impacted to the subject.

This system provides a condition of mainly rotational, less translational acceleration impact on the head, similar to actual accidents.

Second step experiment

The same restraint device and impactor ejection apparatus as in the group C experiment is used for our second step experiment of lateral impact. A monkey is seated in a lateral sitting position on the chair device, and an impact is delivered on the head at the lateral zygomatic area (Figure 4).

Results

The discussion in this report is limited to the corelation of a dynamic condition imparted to the head, and the injury induced to the brain, of the subject, leaving aside other data obtained in the experiments (Figures 5, 6).

Head acceleration and brain concussion: Severity of concussion was judged according to the following signs immediately after the impact.

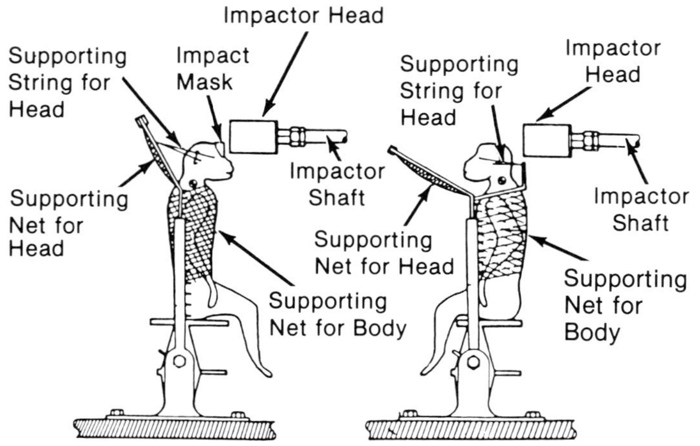

Set-Up Restraint System

Figure 3.Group C Experiment

a. loss of the corneal reflex persisting for at least 20 seconds;
b. apnea persisting for at least 20 seconds;
c. moderate or severe abnormality of the blood pressure.

Blood pressure abnormality was shown in three types: mild, moderate and severe in combination with some range of bradycardia as illustrated in Figure 7. Taking these three signs into consideration, the grade of concussion was estimated by means of four criteria.

0: none of the three signs applies.
1: one of the three signs applies.
11: two of the three signs apply.
111: all three signs apply.

Sixty-three frontal and 59 occipital impacts were delivered to 63 subjects in total in the three groups of the first-step experiment. Thirty lateral impacts were delivered to 10 subjects in the second-step experiment.

Figure 8 illustrates comparison between averaged acceleration-duration of the monkey's head and grades of concussion in occipital as well as frontal impact in the group A, B and C experiment. Incidence of concussion can be distributed along a curved line representing the threshold of concussion, which is more clear in occipital impact than in frontal. Because the group C experiment comes closest to the situation corresponding to actual head injury, the next illustration (Figure 9) is composed of results obtained only in group C. The threshold of concussion is estimated to be almost the same in both occipital and frontal impact. The incidence of severe concussion, however, is much higher in the case of occipital impact.

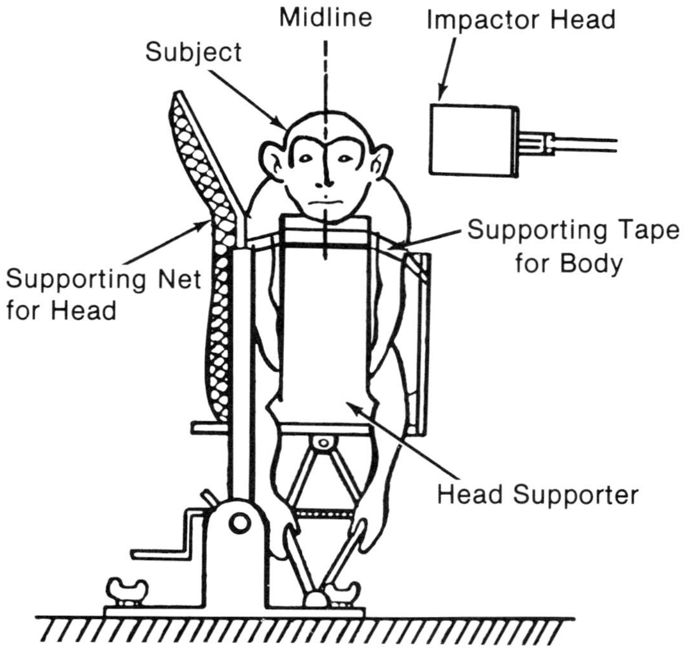

Figure 4.Second Step Experiment Set-Up Restraint System

Physical Measurements

	Velocity	Acceleration	Intracranial Pressure	Motion	Dimensions Recorded by X-Ray
Group A	Sled	Head (X, Z Axes) Slider (X Axis) Sled (X Axis)	Epidural Space	Head (4000 f/s) Head and Body (2000 f/s)	Location and Direction of the Attached Accelerometers Skull Diameter Thickness of Skull Bone
Group B	Impactor Head Mask	Head (X, Y, Z Axes; 9 ch) Head Mask	—	Head (4000 f/s) Head and Body (2000 f/s)	Location and Direction of the Attached Accelerometers Skull Diameter Thickness of Skull Bone
Group C	Impactor	Head (X, Y, Z Axes; 9 ch)	—	Head (4000 f/s) Head and Body (2000 f/s)	Location and Direction of the Attached Accelerometers Skull Diameter Thickness of Skull Bone

Figure 5.

Biological Observations

1) Physiological Survey
   Vital Signs (Respiration, Pulse Rate, Blood Pressure, ECG)
   EEG
2) Biochemical Survey
   Blood Gas Analysis (PO_2, PCO_2, PH)
3) Neurological Survey
   Eye Movement, Blinking, Pupillary Response
   Light Reflex, Corneal Reflex, Behavioral Response to Pain
   Occulocephalic Response
4) Pathological Survey
   Autopsy Examination
   Optical Microscopic or Electron Microscopic Examination

Figure 6. Biological Observations

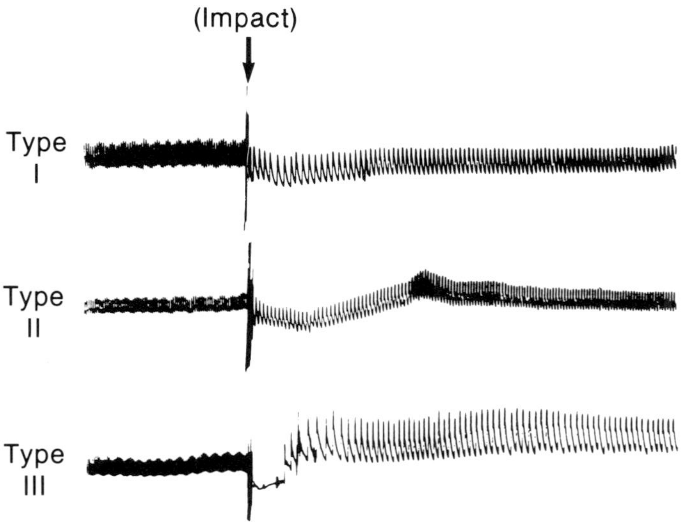

Figure 7. Pattern of Blood Pressure After Concussion

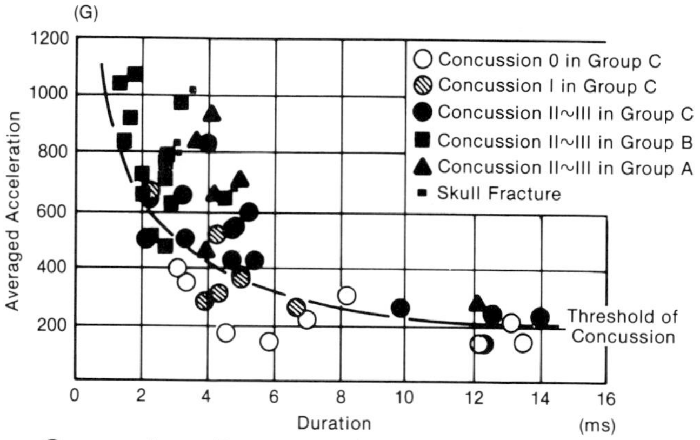

a. Comparison Between Averaged Acceleration-Duration of the Monkey Head and Grades of Concussion in Occipital Impact Among Three Groups (A, B, C)

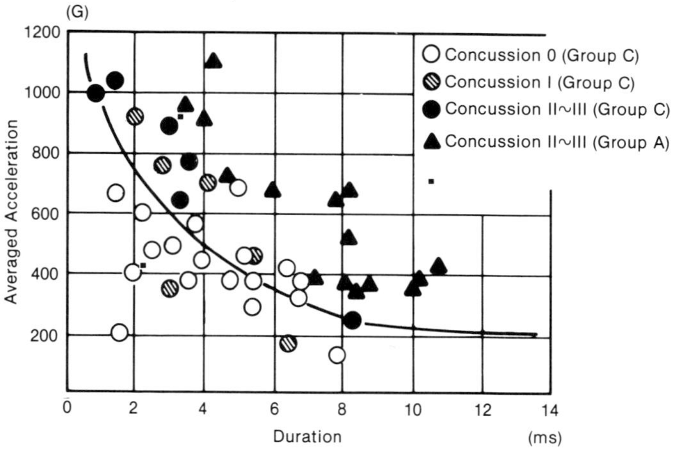

b. Comparison Between Averaged Head Acceleration-Duration and Grades of Concussion in Frontal Impact (Groups A and C)

Figure 8. Results in the Group A, B and C Experiments

Figure 10 demonstrates the similar correlation obtained in our second-step experiment, lateral impact; and the line of the threshold of concussion estimated in the first experiment is put in. Because the second-step experiment is preliminary at present, the illustration is somewhat confusing. Nevertheless, the threshold of concussion in lateral impact seems higher than the one obtained in sagittal impact.

Head acceleration and brain contusion: As for brain contusion, translational acceleration impact alone did not produce any contusion at all, even though all the 24 subjects fell into severe concussion.

In the group B experiment, cortical contusion predominantly in the parasagittal region and by contrecoup was produced in 7 out of 12 nonfractured subjects (Figures 11, 12).

In the group C experiment, contrecoup contusion was visualized in 3 out of 14 nonfractured subjects (Figure 13).

It is very interesting and surprising to note that in cases of lateral impact, the distribution of hemorrhage is quite different from that observed in the first-step experiment.

Intramedullary petechial hemorrhage was brought on frequently, irrespective of either severity of concussion following lateral impact or presence of skull fracture (Figures 14, 15).

Discussion

A great variety of brain injuries and accompanying clinical manifestations brought about in head injury are basically classified into two groups: primary and secondary. Brain injuries produced in close and immediate correlation with an impact on the head are considered to be primary, whereas brain injuries augmented by intracranial secondary pathology, e.g., edema, ischemia, hematoma, infection, etc., or by extracranial complications such as circulatory failure due to chest injury, are classified as secondary. The severity of head injury depends upon various combinations of all these types of brain damage, but the problem of head protection is mainly that of the prevention of primary brain damage.

As for primary brain damage, the presence of skull fracture, especially of a comminuted type, complicates brain damage in many ways by the penetration of bone fragments. Therefore, it seems possible to evaluate the severity of head injury on the basis of the presence or absence of skull fracture alone, but this report is principally concerned with the evaluation of primary brain damage precluding skull fracture.

In order to evaluate the severity of head injury, initial loss of consciousness from a clinical point of view, and brain contusion from a pathological point of view, seems very common and clear characteristics for every researcher. However, the pathophysiology and

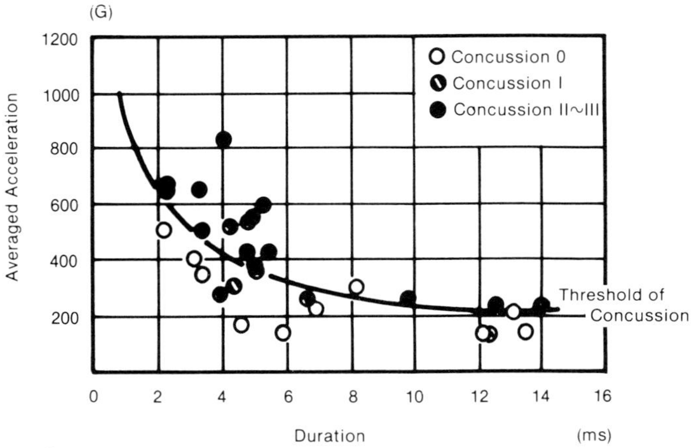

a. Correlation Between Averaged Head Acceleration-Duration and Grades of Concussion in Occipital Impact (Group C)

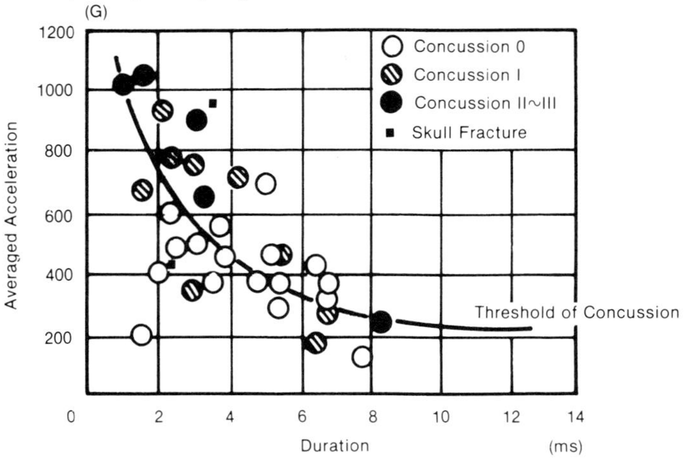

b. Correlation Between Averaged Head Acceleration-Duration and Grades of Concussion in Frontal Impact (Group C)

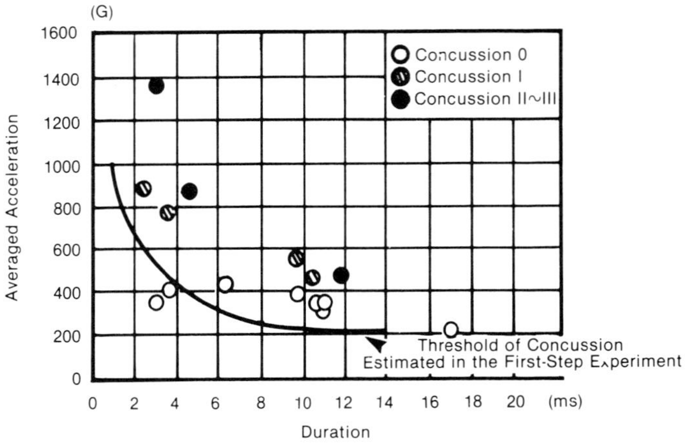

Figure 10. Results in the Second Step Experiment

mechanism of brain concussion is not yet fully understood. Moreover, the mechanism by which brain contusion is produced is also disputed as, for example, by the cavitation theory (1), and the shear strain theory (2)(7)(11). It is difficult, therefore, to agree that the same physical rule, operating through the same mechanism, contributes to both manifestation of brain concussion and production of brain contusion.

Keeping these considerations in view, we conducted the group A and B experiments in the first step using monkeys. Although severe brain concussion was observed equally both in A and in B experiments, no brain contusion was brought on in A. This consequence means that the physical rule which results in brain concussion is not the same as the one which produces brain contusion: it is the rotational acceleration impact on the head which plays a main role in producing brain contusion.

Then, what is the correlation of rotational acceleration impact with brain concussion or contusion?

In the group B and group C experiments, brain concussion without skull fracture was equally observed, even though its incidence seems to be influenced by the rotational component of the impact.

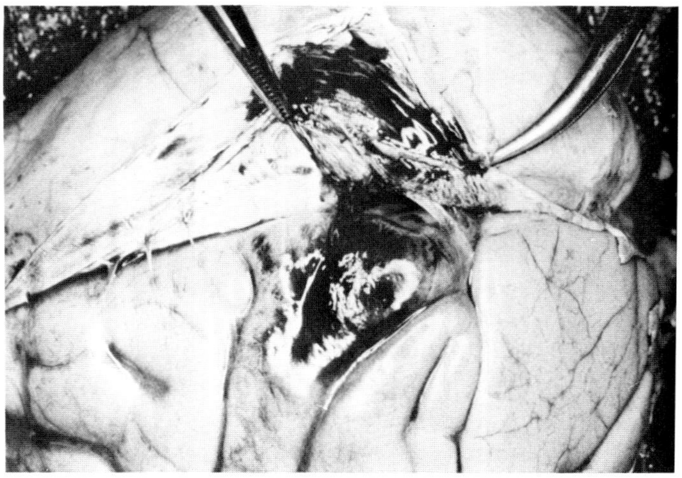

Figure 11. Parasagittal Contusion in Group B

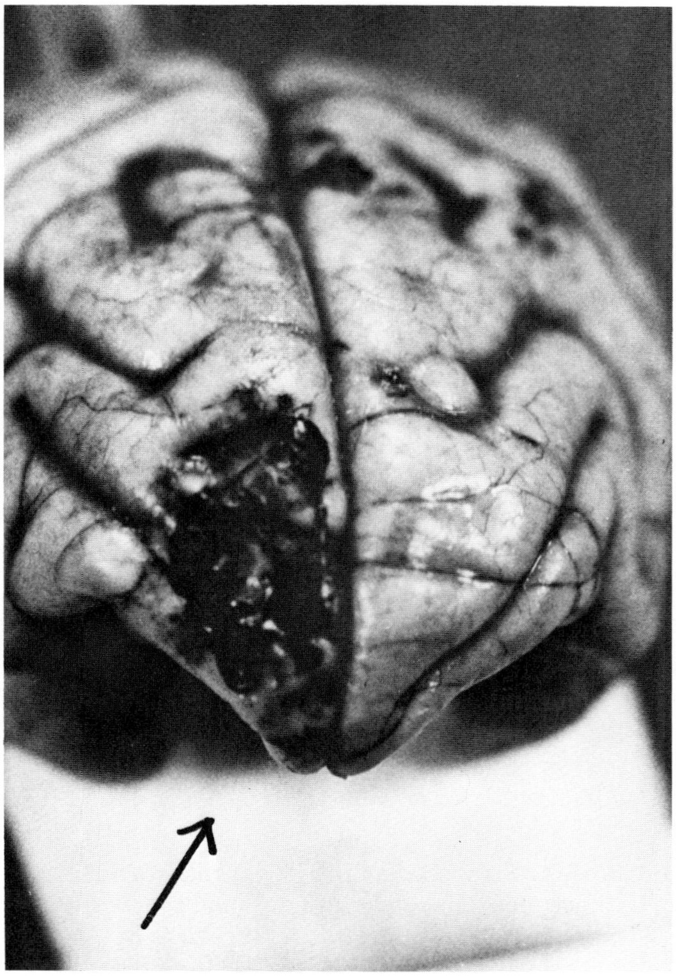

Figure 12. Contrecoup Contusion in Group B

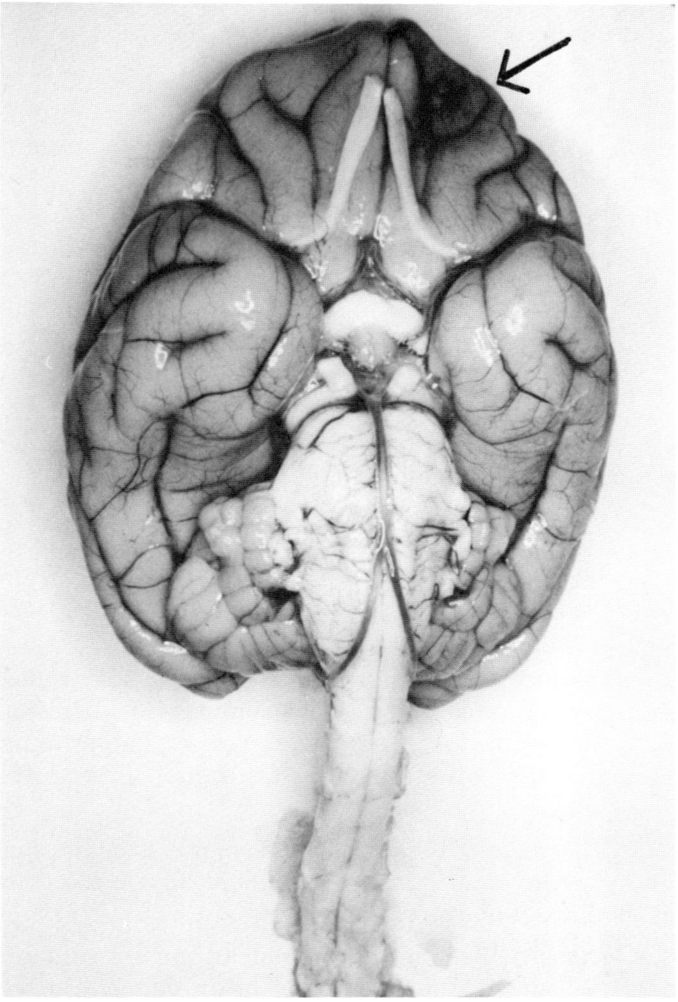

Figure 13. Contrecoup Contusion in Group C

As for brain contusion, contrecoup lesion was equally produced in both groups.

In addition, parasagittal brain contusion was remarkable in 5 out of 12 nonfractured subjects in group B, almost pure rotational acceleration impact being delivered on the head. The latter is defined as gliding contusion after Lindenberg, and brought about by effect of shear strain, as Ommaya has pointed out already in his literature (7).

These consequences suggest that incidence and distribution of brain contusion is influenced clearly by the rotational component of the impact. It is not appropriate, therefore, to appreciate brain contusion as severity of brain damage in correlation with impact delivered on the head, unless either of the translational and rotational components of the impact is assessed exactly in every experiment.

On the other hand, because brain concussion was brought on in a similar way in the group A, B and C experiment, it is conceivable to accept degree of concussion as a severity index of brain damage produced by impact.

After ardent discussions in regard to the evaluation of brain concussion and contusion as a severity index of brain damage resulting from impact to the head of monkeys, we proceeded to the next step of the experiment.

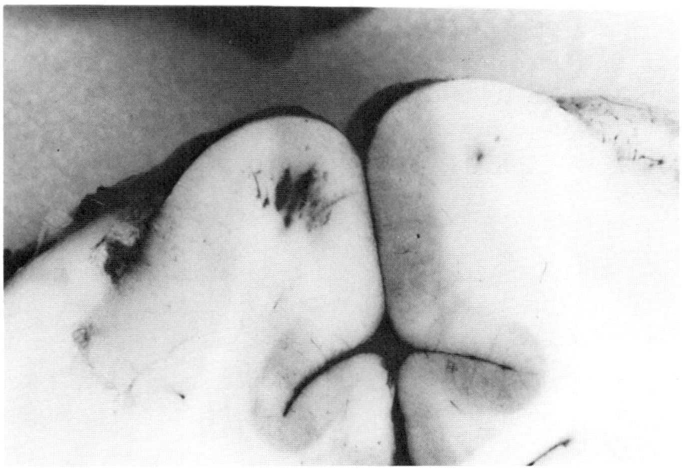

Figure 14. Intramedullary Hemorrhage (Lateral Impact)

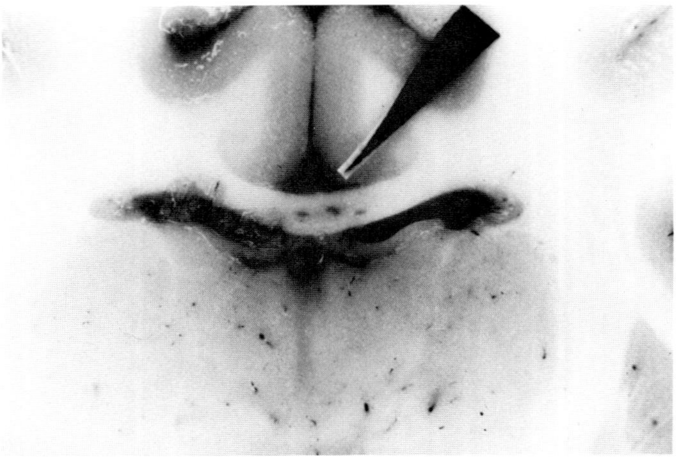

Figure 15. Hemorrhage in the Corpus Callosum (Lateral Impact)

The results obtained in the second-step experiment were very provocative for us, even though not conclusive at present.

Intramedullary petechial hemorrhage and contusion predominated pathology in comparison with what was observed in the group C experiment. The dynamic measurements were almost in the same range in the two groups.

It is suggested again that incidence and distribution of brain contusion are dependent on the direction of the impact delivered to the head.

When the degree of brain concussion is evaluated as a measure of the severity of brain damage in our animal experiments, the head seems more vulnerable to sagittal impact than lateral.

The Wayne State Tolerance Curve (WTC) has been one of the most commonly known criteria to qualify a human head tolerance to impact force. Gadd Severity Index and Head Injury Criterion are also introduced from WTC. All these criteria deal with the significance of the frontal impact alone.

As far as we know, the only criterion which deals with frontal as well as lateral impact is the Mean Strain Criterion (MSC) presented by Stalnaker and McElhaney (10). According to MSC, a brain is more vulnerable to lateral impact. This is just the opposite to our experimental results. Recently Nahum reported experimental studies of side impact to the human skull (5), too.

The animal experiments undertaken by Stalnaker and McElhaney were different from ours in the following criteria.

i) Severity of head injury was scaled partly on the basis of pathology of the damaged brain. Our criteria were based on concussion alone.

ii) They included brain damage combined with skull fracture.

iii) The Maximum Strain Criteria for frontal impact was estimated theoretically with the aid of Maximum Strain Curve, and no animal experimentation was undertaken as for frontal impact.

A brain is a complex composite of the cerebrum, cerebellum and brain stem. Therefore, even though brain parenchyma is equally vulnerable to strain in all directions, it is not certain that the whole brain responds to impact in a same way in all directions.

All these differences in combination may contribute to the controversial situation between their investigation and ours.

References

1. Gross AG: A new theory on dynamics of brain concussion and brain damage. *J Neurosurg 15*:548–561. 1958
2. Holbourn AHS: Mechanism of head injuries. *Lancet ii*: 438–441. 1943
3. Kohno H, Nakamura N, Hirakawa K, et al.: Experimental head injury and concussion: morphologic changes and pathophysiologic responses following translational acceleration in primates (in Japanese). *Neurol Med Chir (Tokyo) 19*:781–791. 1979
4. Masuzawa H, Nakamura N, Hirakawa K, et al.: Experimental head injury and concussion in monkey using pure linear acceleration impact. *Neurol Med Chir (Tokyo) 16*:77–90. 1976
5. Nahum AM, Ward C and Raasch FD: Experimental studies of side impact to the human head. *24th STAPP Car Crash Conference (Detroit)*. 1980
6. Nakamura N, Hirakawa K, Masuzawa H, et al.: Experimental head injuries and concussion using translational acceleration impact. *The International Conference on Neurotraumatology (Cairo)*. 1978
7. Ommaya AK and Gennarelli TA: Cerebral concussion and traumatic unconsciousness. *Brain 97*: 633–654. 1974
8. Ono K, Kikuchi A, Nakamura M, et al.: Human head tolerance to sagittal impact reliable estimation deduced from experimental head injury using subhuman primates and human cadaver skull. *24th STAPP Car Crash Conference (Detroit)*. 1980
9. Sekino H, Nakamura N, Kanda R, et al: Experimental head injury in monkeys using rotational acceleration impact. *Neurol Med Chir (Tokyo) 20*: 1980 (in Japanese)
10. Stalnaker RL, McElhaney JH and Robert VL: MSC tolerance curve for human head impact. *ASME Winter Annual Meeting (Washington)*. 1972

11. Unterharnscheidt F and Higgins LS: Traumatic lesions of brain and spinal cord due to nondeforming angular acceleration of the head. *Texas Reports on Biology and Medicine 27*:127–166. 1969

Discussion

Dr. Tarriere: Speaking about head injury, the first thing I wish to discuss is the risk of injury to the head and neck if there is no direct head impact. I have found a 1979 paper by Wilkie, Mendelson, Stapp and Melvin and they report some cases of injuries without impact. In our studies we categorize injuries in frontal, in lateral and in rear collision, and only in the case of frontal collision have I ever seen a case of head or neck injury when there is no head impact. In lateral is quite different, i.e., no head injury. Some of this data was presented at the last Stapp conference.

Dr. Ommaya: I think we have about five minutes. I know I would like perhaps to ask Al to comment on what he has heard from Dr. Tarriere just now. Do you have any points to make right now?

Dr. Burstein: Although I'll touch on it in a little more detail when I talk about injury criteria, I do want to call your attention to the fact that we have been looking at some very diverse injury mechanisms for the neck as compared to a more homogeneous type of loading situations that are involved in head injury. I want to call your attention to the fact that we are looking at the head, which was obviously an inertial loading system in some of those latter films, and we were looking at the trunk, which was depicted as the inertial loading system in some of the earlier work, especially the football work. Due to this fact that you have a very different system, you don't have the uniform homogeneous isotropic sphere that everyone likes to start out with when we talk about head injuries. Rather, you've got perhaps two uniform homogeneous isotropic spheres and in between those two spheres are all the information that you are seeking to find.

I want to bring out the fact that you are looking at much more complex systems in the very simplest form. In this very simple form, you can break them down to a first order analysis. I would also point out the fact that the same is true when we look at injury mechanisms where the statement was made that in some cases you don't see bone fractures and in some cases you do see bone fractures. I hope you realize that you're not looking at contradictions but you are looking at the difference between hanging and compressing the neck, and I think that those differences should be obvious, and when we talk about criteria for injury I hope you are not going to be too disappointed if I don't write down a single expression that equals zero and when it's met, that is the criterion for injury.

Dr. Goldsmith: I would like to make a comment regarding Mr. Tsongos' remarks on helmets. When you use a helmet, you have primarily the intent of protecting the head. This is the normal use of the helmet. Now he says that you do not injure the neck or don't increase the potential of injury to the neck if you wear a helmet, but the very fact that you add mass and inertia in what is essentially a very complicated spring would seem to me to increase the loading on that spring. I have asked some of my more mathematically inclined colleagues, that if given two arbitrary criteria for, let us say, head and neck injury could they come up with some kind of optimum design for a helmet so as to give you maximum protection for the head and minimum added potential for injury to the neck.

I was wondering if you would care to comment on that?

Mr. Tsongos: My statement was based on statistical evidence rather than medical evidence, and we found that the helmet really did not increase the number of neck injuries. Helmeted and nonhelmeted riders did not have significant difference statistically in the neck injuries. There was, however, a great difference in the number of head injuries.

So my statement was based on statistics rather than clinical facts.

Professor Hugh Hurt probably can comment on this also.

Professor Hurt: I would like to add to Dr. Tsongos' comments that the typical motorcycle accident does not involve large inertial loadings of the neck from head motions as in the case Dr. Ewing discussed where the person being restrained, has large inertial loadings placed upon the body, putting large loads on the neck and so forth. In the typical motorcycle accident the motorcycle victim's head makes contact with the automobile involved in a collision, with the pavement or the curb, or a tree, post, a rock, and in that way there is subsequent neck motion as a result of that impact directly applied to the head.

In the cases which we examined under those particular types of loadings, those mechanisms which protect the head from injury also reduce or attenuate the subsequent motion of the neck. So that in those cases with the motorcycle accident the inertial loadings of the neck from the helmet mass is essentially trivial.

The helmets do perform a function of protecting the head and, in addition, produce a reduction of neck injuries, but it's strictly because of the particular motions involved in the motorcycle accident.

SESSION 2, PART 2:

Physiopathology and Biomechanics of Neck Injury

Session 2, Part 2

Physiopathology and Biomechanics of Neck Injury

Introduction
Dr. A. K. Ommaya

Physiopathology and Biomechanics of Neck Injury

This session was chaired by Dr. A. K. Ommaya who reviewed some of the historical and conceptual aspects of research in this area. A paper embodying these comments and reviewing cervical injury mechanisms in detail plus a comprehensive bibliography of neck injury mechanisms and management will be included in a separate report. In the interim a brief bibliography of some of the important papers available is appended here.

Bibliography

Kazarian L. & Graves G.A., "Compressive Strength Characteristics of Human Vertebral Column," *Spine* 2, 1-14, March 1977.

Banze, R.J., and Ardran G., "Experimental Production of Forward Dislocation in the Human Cervical Spine," *J. Bone and Joint Surgery* 60-B, 239-245, May 1978.

Huelke, D.F., O'Day, J., Lawson, T.E., Barhydt, W.H., and Mendelson, R.E., "Cervical Injuries in Automobile Crashes," Report No. UM-HSRI-80-40, Highway Safety Research Institute, University of Michigan, Ann Arbor.

Van Eck, P.J., Chaffin, D.B., Foust, D.R., Baum, J.K. and Snyder, R.G., "A Bibliography of Whiplash and Cervical Kinematic Measurement," Report prepared for the Insurance Institute for Highway Safety, Washington, D.C.

The Human Neck—Anatomy, Injury Mechanisms and Biomechanics *Publication No. SP-438.* Society of Automotive Engineers, 400 Commonwealth Drive, Warrendale, PA 15096. March 1979. Includes articles by:

- Huelke, D.F., "Anatomy of the Human Cervical Spine and Associated Structure (HS-026 180)
- Huelke, D.F., Moffat, E.A., Mendelson, R.A., and Melvin, J.W., "Cervical Fractures and Fracture Dislocations—An Overview" (HS-026-181)
- Huelke, D.F., Mendelson, R.A., States, J.D., and Melvin J.W., "Cervical Fractures and Fracture Dislocations Sustained without Head Impact" (HS-026-182)
- Mendelson, R.A., "Anatomy and Trauma of the Cervical Spinal Cord," (HS-026-183)
- Moffat, E.A., and Schulz, A.M., "X-Ray Study of the Human Neck During Voluntary Motion," (HS-026-184)
- States, J.D., "Soft Tissue Injuries of the Neck," (HS-026-185)
- Melvin, J.W., "Human Neck Injury Tolerance," (HS-026-186)
- McElhaney, J., Snyder, R.G., States, J.D., and Gabrielsen, M.A., "Biomechanical Analysis of Swimming Pool Injuries," (HS-026-187)

Portnoy, H.D., McElhaney, J.D., Melvin, J.W., and Croissant, P.D., "Mechanism of Cervical Spine Injury in Auto Accident," Proceedings American Association for Automotive Medicine, 1971.

Roaf, R.A., "A Study of the Mechanics of Spinal Injuries," *J. Bone and Joint Surgery,* 42B, 810-823, 1960.

Culver, R., Bender, M. and Melvin, J.W., "Mechanisms, Tolerances and Responses Obtained in Neck Injury by Superior-Inferior Head Impact," HSRI Report No. UM-HSRI-78-21, May 1978.

Mertz, H.J., and Patrick, L.M., "Strength and Response of the Human Neck," Proceedings of the 15th Stapp Car Crash Conference, SAE, November 1971.

Ommaya, A.K., Langwieder, K., Backaitis, S., Partyka, S., and Fan, W., "Comparative Studies in the U.S. and Federal Republic of Germany," Proceedings of the 9th International E.S.V. Conference, Kyoto, Japan, 1982.

Levy, L., "An Unusual Case of Flexion Injury of the Cervical Spine," *Surgical Neurology,* Vol. 17, No. 4, p. 255-259, 1982.

Physiopathology and Mechanisms—Neck Injury

Claude Tarriere

Our epidemiological study indicates that severe neck injuries are very exceptional in the absence of direct head impact. The most common neck injury observed is the subjective syndrome of neck pain, AIS=1 which occurs in about 7 to 8% of the victims in frontal collisions, 20% in lateral collisions and 18% in rear collisions. An experimental study of lateral collisions has permitted a measure of the behavior of the neck with or without head impact (with and without neck bending limitation). Table No. 39 gives the amplitude of the sideway bending of the head for different cadaver and dummy tests. All these tests are reconstruction of actual lateral collisions.* Details are given in Appendix I. Figure 25 is of particular interest in that it describes the relative movement head-thorax and head-lateral wall. It appears that sideway bending of the neck could reach 80 without neck injury. In one case, such a bending angle produces brain injuries (504/Citroen LN case): the angular rotation speed reached 40 rd/s in this case.

An experimental study of frontal collisions with rear passengers wearing only a lap-belt produced some severe neck injuries when there was direct impact of the head against the padded top of the front seats. Among 8 subjects, 6 sustained very severe neck injuries (AIS 5 or 6); 6 sustained spinal fracture and 3 had complete medulla section. The neurological results are not available for the two last subjects. Two subjects were indemn. A frontal collision reconstruction (Renault 12/Chrysler 180) in which the driver of the Chrysler 180—who was wearing his belt with too much slack—sustained a direct neck impact against the steering wheel. It resulted in a fracture of the odontoid vertebra with displacement and a section of the medulla. The maximum head acceleration was 280 g and the HIC was 5800.

Another frontal collision reconstruction (Renault 12/Renault Florida) shows neck injuries for both frontal occupants. The unbelted driver sustained a direct neck impact against the steering wheel, inducing an odontoid fracture with an important displacement, a C_1–C_2 luxation and very severe neurological lesions (AIS=6). The maximum acceleration reached 220 g and an HIC of 2000. The unbelted right front occupant sustained a direct head impact, inducing a fracture of the body of C_1 and C_3 and a C_3–C_4 luxation with neurological injuries (AIS=6); the HIC was 4000.

*These reconstructions are a part of the KOB program. The complete report can be requested from BAST, in Koln, Germany.

Appendix I

Reconstructions—3rd cadaver reconstruction of the 504/LN accident—

The partial ejection which occurred during this accident, resulted in different behavior to that observed for the other reconstructions, and different injuries. The extensive rotation of the head, without a violent impact, is no doubt responsible for the peripheric hemorrhage observed, as well as for the two small injuries to the cerebral trunk (AIS=4). The thorax, which was not held by the belt, swung around the door, which resulted in extensive, yet localized, thoracic deflection. These particular kinematics, combined with the good bone condition of the subject, led to very slight injuries (1 rib fracture) despite the high thoracic deflection.

The case of this test is to be isolated from the others. It did, however, enable us to observe an original type of behavior in a side collision. It would be interesting to compare this observation with other accidentological data which are available for unbelted occupants of side collisions, in order to ascertain whether this behavior is frequent or it is simply the result of a particular set of circumstances.

If this observation is repeated, it will provide complementary information about the role played by safety belts in side collisions.

Analysis of neck's behavior—Comparison between human subjects and dummies—

(a) In these series of reconstructions, we have not observed neck injuries on the victims of the real accident, like on the subjects of the cadaver tests. We have been able to estimate the amplitude of the lateral bending by measuring the maximum angle between the axis of thorax and head for the reconstructions Peugeot 304/Renault 15 and Peugeot 504/Peugeot 504. These values are collected in Table 1.

(b) If we consider the whole reconstructions Peugeot 304/Renault 15, we can observe that there are important differences between the head kinematics of dummies and cadavers. The head impact velocity against the side of the vehicle is slightly higher in the case of the cadaver (2.3 m/s for the cadaver and 1.8 m/s for the dummy). In addition, the angle of the head in relation to the

Table 1. Amplitude of the Sideways Bending of the Head.

		Angle Head/Thorax	Belted Subject	Bending Limited by Impact With the Wall
304/R15	Dummy Test No. 2	30°	Yes	Yes
	Dummy Test No. 3	39°	Yes	Yes
	Aprod Test No. 3	60°	Yes	Yes
	Cadaver Test No. 1	81°	Yes	Yes
504/LN	Dummy Test No. 1	10°	Yes	No
	Dummy Test No. 2	10°	Yes	No
	Dummy Test No. 3	40°	No	No
	Cadaver Test No. 1	10°	Yes	Yes
	Cadaver Test No. 2	10°	Yes	Yes
	Cadaver Test No. 3	>75°	No	No
504/504	Dummy Test No. 1	50°	No	Yes
	Dummy Test No. 2	49°	No	Yes
	Dummy Test No. 3	48°	No	Yes
	Cadaver Test No. 1	27°	No	Yes
	Cadaver Test No. 2	48°	No	Yes
	Cadaver Test No. 3	33°	No	Yes

chest at time of impact is 80 in the case of cadavers, whereas it is only 35 in the case of the dummy. The dummy's neck is much stiffer than that of the cadaver, and this stiffness minimizes the sideways bending of the head and the severity of head impact as one can see by considering the angle values at impact.

(c) In whole reconstructions Peugeot 504/Citroen LN, we have observed under the test conditions of cadaver tests 1 and 2, a slight impact of the head against the lateral window. This impact did not cause craniocerebral injuries. The lateral window was not broken. The window frame is deflected outside. The window also limits the lateral bending of the head and helps prevent cervical injuries likely to result from excessive sideways bending of the head such as that observed for the cadaver test No. 3 (head/thorax angle greater than 75 in test No. 3 as compared with 10 in the two other cadaver tests).

These observations tend to show that a head impact in lateral collisions can prevent excessive sideways bending of the neck and thus reduce the possibility of neck injury.

It has to be noted that 10 of sideways bending of the neck for cadavers where the head motion is limited by impact, is not equivalent to the same 10 observed for the dummy without head impact. In that case, it is the stiffness of the neck which limits bending while, in the first case with cadavers, it was the impact against the wall.

Concerning the Peugeot 504/Peugeot 504 reconstructions, there has been initiated a detailed analysis of head and thorax kinematics for cadaver test No. 1 (the film on this test comprises a comprehensive view illustrating the various positions of the "thorax-neck-head" system). Figure 1 illustrates the deformations of the B-pillar and of the thorax-neck-head system between the time of shoulder-wall contact and the time when the head sustains a maximum lateral bending. The events represented in relation to a mark related to the ground are explained below:

time 0: shoulder-wall contact and beginning of thoracic deflection.

+7 ms: speeding of sternum higher portion (close to the neck), materialized by B-target.

+10 ms: speeding of the median portion of thorax (illustrated by A-target) and beginning of thorax side motion.

+14 ms: the head being still motionless, thoracic deflection comes near to its maximum level whereas the thorax continues its side motion. The neck (illustrated by C-target) is submitted to a deflection which generates shearing stresses likely to create cervical injuries.

+18 ms: thoracic deflection comes to an end, which results in an increased side motion of thorax and speeds up the head (materialized by D- and E-targets), which sustains a sideways bending towards B-pillar.

+22 ms: the intrusion of B-pillar at head level provides a head impact with the B-pillar whereas the thorax pursues its side motion which reaches 46 mm. Since the intrusion speed of B-pillar is lower than thorax motion speed, the side bending of the head is continued despite the impact with B-pillar.

+38 ms: the sideways bending of the head has reached its maximum level.

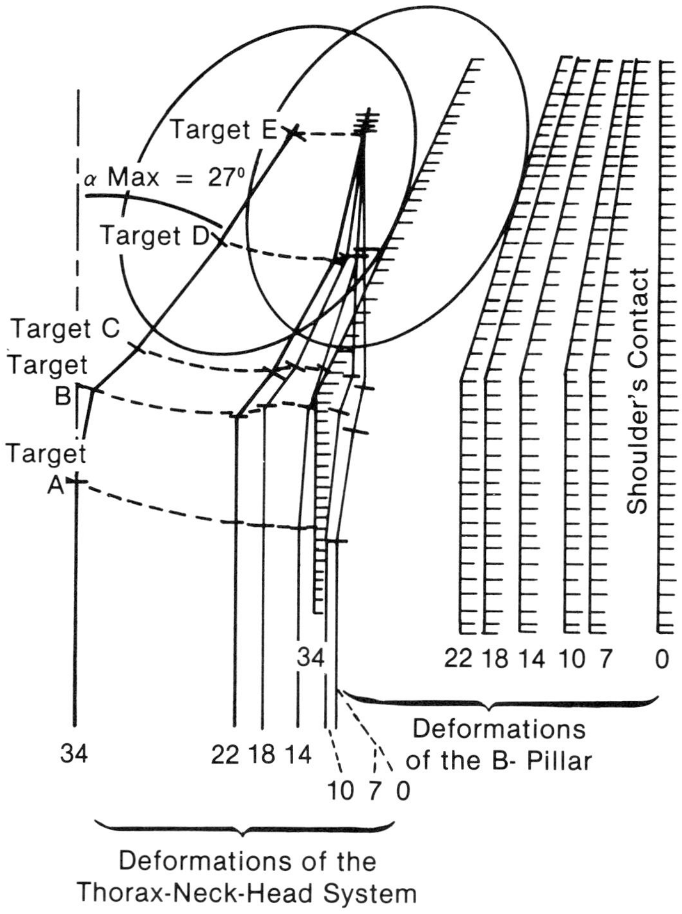

Figure 1.

The previous description illustrates again that it is the head impact which limits bending. Such an impact was observed in all cadaver tests, excepted cadaver test No. 3 of Peugeot 504/Citroen LN reconstruction. This explains why no cervical lesions were observed, either in actual victims or in cadavers.

In terms of human tolerances, observed head sideways bendings up to 80 have been observed (Peugeot 304/Renault 15) without any cervical or brain lesions. (In this case, this 80 amplitude was obtained despite the head contact.)

However, when the sideways bending is not limited by the impact of the head, brain or cervical lesions may result. This was more particularly observed in cadaver test No. 3 of Peugeot 504/Citroen LN reconstruction in which the bending angle was greater than 75.

Vehicle deformations

Every reconstruction was judged satisfactory as concerns the deformation of the side-wall of the struck car, particularly at the level of the occupant seated nearside to impact. The damage to both struck and striking car were correctly reproduced with reference to true-life accidents. A good repeatability has been obtained for every accident in both dummy and cadaver tests, which gives a satisfactory accuracy for research tools available by means of actual collisions reconstructions.

However, we have to emphasize that even if the deformations are correctly reproduced at the level of the occupant seated to the right of the impact and that it is sufficient to estimate that the reconstruction is satisfactory, some differences were observed; for instance, at the level of the rear of the struck vehicle in Peugeot 304/Renault 15 reconstructions, since the right front side frame of the Peugeot struck the Renault 15 on the very rigid spot where the rear suspension axis is attached. These very precise impact conditions are difficult to reproduce: such a type of impact affects the damage to the side-wall for it concerns rigid points.

If a selection of real side collisions to be reconstructed had to be made, we would choose those where the rigid parts of the striking vehicle do not cause an interaction with the rigid parts of the struck vehicle such as B-pillar or the rigid spot where the rear suspension axis is attached, in order to avoid impacts particularly difficult to reproduce.

Particular kinematics of occupant or vehicle

Some reconstructions carried out within the frame of this program demonstrated particular kinematics of occupants or vehicles which are described below:

—The comparative analysis to the subject's behavior in the Peugeot 504/Citroen LN reconstruction illustrated the role played by safety belts in side collisions with respect to an occupant located at right angle to the impact.

—From the partial ejection of body segments observed in some reconstructions Austin Mini/Ford Capri, it appears mandatory to equip the side collision dummy with articulated arms, proper to simulate such ejections. These reconstructions showed, too, the need to equip the vehicles with special windows in order to prevent such ejections and the injuries susceptible to result from such a collision.

—Such a risk was particularly illustrated by the reconstruction in which the struck vehicle underwent a half-turn. It has been possible to reproduce this vehicle kinematic, which is not unusual in real-world accidents.

Five actual side collisions were reconstructed with Part 572 dummy, cadavers and, in the case of the Peugeot 304/Renault 15 collision, with an APROD dummy.

The reconstructions supply a basis for reflection upon human tolerances, as upon protection criteria for side collisions, by enabling a comparison of the behavior of all the surrogates (dummies and cadavers) among themselves and, in reference with the actual victims, in very realistic conditions.

The five actual accidents have been duplicated with a good general faithfulness, which gives a satisfactory accuracy for research tools available by means of actual collision reconstructions.

In terms of human tolerance, these reconstructions improve knowledge of admissible levels in side collisions:

—High HIC levels (one was about 1980) were associated with an absence of cerebral injuries on cadavers. It shows that the HIC tolerance level is probably above 1500.

—For the thorax, the value of 30% of thoracic deflection proposed as the limit corresponding to 7–8 rib fractures constitutes probably an underestimation with respect to the real resistance of living people.

—For the pelvis, the 3-ms acceleration which was measured, leads one to believe that the impact tolerance may be above 100 g.

Concerning the behavior of the Part 572 dummy, these reconstructions have given a clear demonstration that the Part 572 dummy is unsuitable for use in side collisions. The almost complete absence of thoracic deflection, added to the stiffness of the neck, gives an unrealistic behavior which did not provide information about protection criteria for the head and thorax. On the other hand, this dummy and the cadavers act similarly as concerns the pelvis, and the 3-ms acceleration which was measured enables us to think that the protection criterion for the pelvis may be at 100 g.

The small number of tests using APROD (3 for the Peugeot 304/Renault 15 reconstruction) prevents us from drawing definitive conclusions. The satisfactory behavior of the APROD in side collisions indicates that it would be possible to define more precisely protection criteria, based on more numerous tests.

We found a clavicle fracture which had been already observed in some true-life side collision cases, in four cadaver tests, for the impacted-side passenger, and in two cadaver tests, for the opposite-side passenger, (it would be the result of an interaction between the two front passengers).

(In a more extended reconstruction program involving tests external to the KOB program, 36% of cadavers (25 reconstructions) had a clavicle fracture (9).)

Hence, it appears mandatory to equip the side collision dummy with arms and shoulders realistic enough to be able to reproduce the large loads transmitted by the arm and shoulder at the moment of impact.

In the real victims, like in the subjects of cadaver tests, rib cage lesions are not associated with intrathoracic lesions. It is an explanation and a justification that the thoracic tolerance is defined in terms of bony injuries (rib fractures, sternum fractures, clavicle fractures).

No cervical injury was observed for the victims of the actual accident and the cadavers of the reconstructions. The main reason seems to be that the lateral head impact, by limiting the sideways motion of the head, protects the cervical spine.

The limitation of the sideways bending of the head and neck can also protect the brain if the head impact is sufficiently absorbed by deformability of the wall.

In fact, the only brain injuries found on cadavers are due to a large magnitude of the sideways rotation of the head without impact.

The observation of the partial ejection of the arm and/or head in two tests shows again the need to equip the dummy with an articulated arm and points up the need to design the lateral window to prevent risk of lesions associated with such ejections.

The risk of total ejection of an occupant or of partial ejection of a body segment is probably higher if the lateral collision is continued with a half or complete turn of the vehicle. This last phenomenon, which we have observed in several tests of the Austin Mini/Ford Capri reconstruction, is not unusual in the real-world accident. It appears with a frequency of 8% (52/645 side collisions) in the side collisions sample analyzed by Peugeot/Renault.

The comparative analysis of the cadavers' behavior in a series of reconstructions (Peugeot 504/Citroen LN) displays the prominent part taken by the seat belt in the protection of an occupant seated nearside to impact. This concerns only an above-mentioned observation, but is very interesting and quite original.

The reconstruction test series validates the better accuracy of actual collision characteristics estimated by well-trained accident investigation teams (violence of the collision or angle between two vehicles, for instance).

References

1. B. Friedel, "Research Association for Biomechanics at the Federal Highway Research Institute," in Proceedings of IRCOBI Meeting, September 1977, edited by the IRCOBI Secretariate, ONSER, 109, ave. Salvador Allende, 69500 Bron, France.
2. D. Cesari, Dr. E. Friedel, A. Heger, G.M. Mackay, C. Tarriere, R. Weissner, "Preliminary Report about the Work of the Joint Biomechanical Research Project (KOB)," Proceedings of the 7th E.S.V. Conference, Paris, June 1979, edited by the U.S. Department of Transportation, DOT-NHTSA, Washington, D.C. 20590, USA.
3. G. Walfisch, A. Fayon, C. Tarriere, C. Got, A. Patel, "Travaux effectués pour disposer d'un mannequin et de critères convenables pour améliorer la protection en choc latéral," in Ingenieurs de l'Automobile, S.I.A., no. 3, March 1979, p. 230.
4. A. Fayon, Y.C. Leung, R.L. Stalnaker, G. Walfisch, M. Balthazard, C. Tarriere, "Presentation of Frontal and Side Impact Dummy Defined from Human Data and Realized from a Part 572 Basis," Proceedings of the 7th ESV Conference, Paris, June 1979, edited by the U.S. Department of Transportation, DOT-NHTSA, Washington, D.C. 20590, USA.
5. J. Sacreste, A. Fayon, C. Tarriere, "Analysis of Data Connected with Fractures Observed in Simulations of Impacts Performed with Instrumented Cadavers," Proceedings of the 4th International IRCOBI Conference on the Biomechanics of Trauma, Goteborg, Sweden, edited by IRCOBI Secretariate, ONSER, 109 ave. Salvador Allende, 69500 Bron, France, Sept. 1979.
6. C. Thomas, J.Y. Foret-Bruno, F. Hartemann, C. Tarriere, "Influence of age and restraint force value on the seriousness of thoracic injuries sustained by belted occupants in real accidents," Proceedings of 4th International IRCOBI Conference on the Biomechanics of Trauma, Goteborg, Sweden, Sept. 1979, edited by IRCOBI Secretariate, ONSER, 109 ave. Salvador Allende, 69500 Bron, France.
7. G.G. Schmidt, "The age as a factor influencing soft tissue injuries," in Proceedings of the 4th International Conference on the Biomechanics of Trauma, Goteborg, Sweden, Sept. 1979, edited by IRCOBI Secretariate, ONSER, 109 ave. Salvador Allende, 69500 Bron, France.
8. C. Got, A. Patel, A. Fayon, C. Tarriere, G. Walfisch, "Results of experimental head impacts on cadavers, the various data obtained and their relations to some measured physical parameters," Proceedings of the 23rd Stapp Car Crash Conference, SAE paper 780 887, SAE.
9. C. Tarriere, G. Walfisch, A. Fayon, J.P. Rosey, "Synthesis of human tolerance obtained from lateral impact simulations," Proceedings of the 7th ESV Conference, Paris, June 1979, edited by U.S. Department of Transportation, NHTSA, Washington, D.C. 20590, USA.
10. T.A. Gennarelli, A.K. Ommaya, L.E. Thibault, "Comparison of translational and rotational head motions in experimental cerebral concussions," Proceedings of the 15th Stapp Car Crash Conference, Nov. 1971, edited by SAE.

Preliminary data of 100 autopsies. Procedure for a detailed layer by layer autopsy for head and neck trauma.

Irving Rehman, Ph.D., F.I.C.S.
Thomas T. Noguchi, M.D.

With the cooperation of: Los Angeles County Medical Examiner-Coroner Facility; The Life Foundation of Medicine and Law, Inc.; Dr. Carley Ward; and Professor Harry H. Hurt, Jr., Traffic Safety Center, University of Southern California

A program of study of Motorcycle Trauma is being carried on jointly by the Traffic Safety Center of the University of Southern California under the direction of Professor Harry H. Hurt, Jr. and at the Los Angeles County Medical Examiner-Coroner Facility under the direction of Thomas T. Noguchi, M.D., Chief Medical

Examiner-Coroner. The development of the specialized autopsy "Procedure for a detailed layer by layer head and neck autopsy for trauma" and the head and neck autopsies were done by Irving Rehman, Ph.D., Deputy Coroner-Medical Examiner. Financial support has been provided by the U.S. Department of Transportation.

The preliminary data reported in this paper consist of a consecutive series of 100 autopsies taken from 292 motorcycle fatalities occurring in Los Angeles County in the period between July 1, 1979 and March 22, 1981. The motorcycle victims in this study range in age from 15 to 75 years in age, consisting of 87 males and 13 females. Since this program is still in progress, no extensive analysis of the considerable data obtained is available at this time.

A team approach is employed. The University of Southern California Investigative Team of the Traffic Safety Center is notified of the accident, and they will immediately visit the scene of the fatal accident to determine the cause, photograph and record the factors concerned as well as interview witnesses, etc. This information will be correlated with the autopsy data to provide comprehensive information concerning cause and effect.

The victim's body is brought to the Coroner's Facility where further documentation and examination, including x-rays and photography, is done. A complete autopsy of the trunk and of the head and neck is done. The head and neck portion of the autopsy is done in a layer by layer manner as described in the "Procedure for a detailed layer by layer autopsy for head and neck trauma."

Although several studies concerned with motorcycle trauma and fatalities have been reported, no detailed studies of soft tissue trauma to the head and neck have been so specifically oriented. Most of the studies and the data and analyses have been directed toward skeletal or intracranial trauma.

Generally, motorcycle accidents result in more serious injuries because of the higher speeds, poorer driver visibility and exposure and less protection as has been pointed out by Zettas, Zettas and Thanasophon (1).

King (2) has stressed the greater frequency of trauma to the chest, abdomen and limbs with less emphasis on the head and neck. He reports only a single neck injury in a series of 102 trauma cases.

The difficulty and often inability to accurately ascertain soft tissue injury or presence of trauma result in an inaccuracy in diagnosis and data accumulation. Since many of the soft tissue injuries involving tearing, laceration, hemorrhage, hematoma, etc., are missed, emphasis was placed upon identifying skeletal and cranial trauma through x-ray, CAT scans and some angiography. Many deeper lying structures that have been traumatized leading to lacerations, contusions, etc., producing hemorrhage and hematoma may be completely missed because there is no clearly evident or superficial or surface indication. Considerable morbidity may result from head and neck injuries according to Doolittle, Brown and Boshell (3). Such deeper lying injuries may not be readily evident to the emergency room physician in his preliminary examination and may lead to serious posttraumatic sequelae.

Smith, Dehner (4) and Haddad (5) in their studies have attributed the most frequent site of injuries to the head and neck. In another study on motorcycle injury patterns in Victoria reported by Trinca and Dooley (6) consisting of a series of 100 consecutive fatalities, 58 cerebral injuries included 47 skull fractures and subluxations of cervical vertebrae. They stressed the fact that most of the victims died of serious head injuries. Only one case of severe brachial plexus damage and no cervical spine injuries were noted in the non-fatal accidents. Andrew (7) found that in four fatalities there was significant head injury. Two brachial plexus injuries resulted from a head-on collision between two motorcycles.

In reviewing the literature on motorcycle trauma it was noted that very few references were made to soft tissue trauma. It soon became evident in this study of this autopsy material that considerable soft tissue trauma occurs that may be completely missed because of the inability to adequately visualize this trauma by the usual radiographic techniques. The more specialized techniques of subtractive angiography and computerized axial tomography (CAT scan) are expensive and may not be readily available. Hemorrhages and hematomas occurring within the carotid sheath, although having possible serious consequences, are not easily identified in the living state.

The following specialized autopsy procedure was developed at the Los Angeles County Medical Examiner-Coroner Facility to perform a "Detailed Layer by Layer Autopsy Procedure for Head and Neck Trauma" Rehman (8). The usual autopsy does not include a detailed dissection of the head and neck. The area above the sternum and clavicles is more or less a "no man's land" in that the requirement to do a detailed autopsy of the head and neck is not necessary to determine the cause of death in a forensic autopsy. The tongue, pharynx, larynx, trachea and esophagus are removed at the Los Angeles Medical Examiner-Coroner Facility as part of the routine autopsy. However, this does not expose soft tissue trauma in the musculature, vessels, glands and posterior part of the neck. The deeper lying structures, nerves and their roots, i.e., the brachial plexus, phrenic nerves and sympathetic trunks and sympathetic ganglia, are not seen at all and their physiologic effects in relation to trauma cannot be projected or actually anticipated.

In autopsies concerned with motorcycle fatalities one must be aware of the modus operandi of the motorcycle driver and rider and in general the difference in attitude of the motorcyclist in relation to his or her vehicle and the environment in which they find themselves. High speeds are the rule rather than the exception and therefore more severe accidents occur. The driver or rider will usually continue the direction of the motorcycle and impact an object with his head and neck in the greatest percentage of cases so that much more severe injuries and trauma will occur in this region of the body. Since the head essentially consists of a ball approximately eight to twelve pounds in weight at the end of a flexible shaft, the neck, then both head and neck, must be treated as a single unit in doing an autopsy. The structures within the neck affect trauma to the skull and its contents, i.e., the brain. These autopsies were performed with unit concept in mind and therefore resulted in a more detailed autopsy, done in a layer by layer manner both anteriorly and posteriorly, as well as the interior of the cranium and its contents.

Procedure for a Detailed Layer by Layer Autopsy for Head and Neck Trauma

The layer by layer autopsy of the neck should be done in a detailed manner from the superficial to the deeper structures of the anterior, lateral and posterior aspects of the neck to determine the soft tissue damage, hemorrhage and hematoma, lacerations and presence of fractures of skeletal structures.

The superficial examination should include charting and recording of all bruises, contusions, lacerations, fractures, etc., preceding the autopsy of the trunk as outlined in the "Army Method."

Should the autopsy of the trunk be done prior to the neck layer by layer autopsy, the following modification is recommended. The manubrium sterni should be transected at its middle and the lower half of the manubrium sterni and the body of the sternum removed with the rib cage so that the clavicles, first ribs and upper half of the manubrium sterni remain intact to preserve the integrity of the shoulder girdle and cervical structures for the "layer by layer" neck autopsy.

Anterior Layer By Layer Cervical Autopsy

Determine the mobility of the head and neck in flexion, extension and lateral bending and rotation.

Place the body in the supine position with a block beneath the shoulders to elevate the head and extend the neck.

Examine the sternum, clavicles, anterior and lateral neck for lacerations, contusions, abrasions, etc.

Make an oblique incision through the skin and platysma, paralleling and slightly below the clavicles across the sternum, extending from one shoulder tip to the other. This incision lies immediately below the clavicles and passes across the manubrium sterni. This forms the upper part of the normal autopsy incision, that however is extended further laterally to the acromiom processes to facilitate the reflection of the skin and platysma up over the chin. The sternomastoid muscles can now be examined at their sternal and clavicular origins for evidence of tearing, rupture or hemorrhage indicative of hyperextension (Plate 1).

Detach the sternomastoid muscle from their sternal and clavicular origins and reflect them upward toward their insertion at the mastoid process (Plate 2).

The lower part of the carotid sheaths are now exposed beneath the strap or ribbon muscles of the neck, i.e., sternohyoid, omohyoid, sternothyroid and thyrohyoid muscles. These muscles may be reflected cranially or caudally (Plate 3).

The carotid sheaths should be examined for hemorrhage and trauma to the contents, i.e., carotid artery, internal jugular vein and vagus n. for evidence of laceration, compression, hemorrhage or hematoma.

The sympathetic trunk, deep to the carotid sheath, can now be examined with emphasis on the area of the superior cervical ganglion deep to the angle of the mandible.

Retract the carotid sheaths and contents laterally to more fully expose the hyoid bone, thyroid and cricoid cartilages, pharynx and larynx, trachea and esophagus for fractures, contusions, abrasions, hemorrhage and hematoma. Palpate the hyoid bone, thyroid and cricoid cartilages for fractures (Plate 4).

Examine the thyroid gland and tracheo-esophageal grooves for the recurrent laryngeal n.

Retract the trachea and esophagus to the opposite side. Examine the root of the neck, i.e., the supraclavicular triangle for brachial plexus and stellate ganglion trauma (Plate 5).

Examine the parotid and submandibular areas. Examine the anterior, lateral and posterior walls of the pharynx, larynx, trachea and esophagus (Plate 6).

Section the trachea and esophagus at the level of the suprasternal notch of the sternum or at the level of the seventh cervical vertebra. Examine their interiors as they are turned upward (Plate 7).

Identify the carotid tubercle (C_6) and examine the vertebral vessels as they pass from the subclavian artery and vein into the costotransverse formen of C_6 (Plate 8).

Examine the longus colli muscles, the anterior longitudinal ligament and the bodies and discs of the cervical vertebrae. The prevertebral fascia can now be examined for subfascial hemorrhage possibly involving the underlying phrenic nerve and sympathetic trunk on the scalenus anterior muscle. The roots and trunks of the upper portion of the brachial plexus should be examined at this time.

The posterior triangle, bounded by the sternomastoid and trapezius muscles and the clavicles can now be examined. Observe the condition of the cervical vertebral column at the base of the skull after removal of the cervical viscera (Plate 9).

The tongue, pharynx, larynx, trachea and esophagus can now be removed by detaching these structures from the mandible and base of the skull for more thorough examination of their interior and exterior. The jugular veins and carotid arteries should be left intact if possible to facilitate subsequent enbalming of the head and neck.

Examine the remainder of the anterior surface of the cervical vertebral column to the base of the skull. The sympathetic trunk and superior cervical sympathetic ganglion can be seen at this stage.

Posterior Cervical Layer by Layer Autopsy

Place the body in the prone position.

Examine the skin and superficial aspect of the neck from the external occipital protuberance to the spine of the seventh cervical vertebra. Soft tissue trauma should be looked for in the following steps.

A longitudinal midline incision is made through the skin and superficial fascia to the underlying spines of the cervical vertebra extending from the external occipital protuberance to the spine of the seventh cervical vertebra (Plate 10).

The skin and superficial fascia are reflected laterally to expose the trapezius muscles (Plate 11).

Reflect the trapezius muscles laterally to expose the splenius capitis and cervicis muscles (Plate 12).

Reflect these muscles to expose the semispinalis capitis and cervicis muscles. (Plate 13).

Turn the semispinalis muscles laterally and examine the short rotators, cervical spinous processes and suboccipital muscles in the suboccipital triangle (Plate 14).

Remove the short lateral rotators and the ligaments and soft tissues for lacerations, tears, hemorrhage, etc. The laminae and spines should be examined for fractures, etc. Extend the removal of the short rotators laterally beyond the articular processes to examine the facets and nerve roots (Plate 15).

Reflect the suboccipital muscles and examine the atlanto-occipital and atlanto-axial articulations. The ligaments should be carefully examined for tears and hemmorrhage indicative of hyperflexion.

Clean the lateral processes of the atlas and examine the vertebral vessels as they pass along the upper margin of the lateral processes of the atlas (Plate 16).

The laminectomy cut should be done bilaterally, approximately one and one-half cm. lateral to the base of the cervical spinous processes and extend from the base of the skull through the lamina of the seventh cervical vertebra. Free the posterior part of the atlanto-occipital capsul or ligament from its attachment to the foramen magnum and turn the laminae and spines caudally to uncover the cervical spinal canal.

Examine the dura for tears and the epidural and subdural spaces for hemorrhage and hematoma, spinal cord injury or compression, etc.

Transect the cervical spinal cord at the level of C_7 and the cervical nerve roots bilaterally at their intervertebral exits from the cervical spinal canal.

Carefully cut the dura from its attachment at the foramen magnum to completely free the cervical spinal cord for later removal with the brain as a single unit (Plate 17).

Expose and cut the cervical nerve roots in order to reflect the cervical spinal cord and dura cranially to expose the posterior longitudinal ligamentum flavum, tectorial membrane, and the bodies and intervertebral discs of the cervical vertebral column (Plate 18).

Upon completion of this posterior portion of the neck layer by layer autopsy, replace the cervical spinal cord in the canal, the cervical laminae and spines and posterior cervical musculature covering the vertical column and canal, and approximate and suture the posterior skin.

The body can now be replaced in the supine position for completion of the removal of the brain and cervical spinal cord.

This completes the anterior and posterior cervical layer by layer neck autopsy.

Scalp, Skull and Interior of Cranium

Reflect the scalp, remove the calvarium and observe the interior of the cranial cavity, brain, etc. Examine the surface of the brain for lacerations, contusions and evidence of subarachnoid hemorrhage. Cut any remaining attachments of the dura mater to the margin of the foramen magnum, the petrous and tympanic portions of the temporal bones and carefully evaluate the brain removing it posteriorly. Removal of the brain and cervical spinal cord as a unit and reflection of the dura from the anterior, middle and posterior cranial fossae will complete the layer by layer head and neck autopsy.

Head and Neck Trauma—Preliminary Data of 100 Autopsies

Hyperflexion	61
Hyperextension	61
Neck—laceration	18
Face—laceration	21
Ext. Auditory Canal:	
Hemorrhage—right	26
Hemorrhage—left	31
Mandible—fracture	29

Testing for hyperflexion and hyperextension in the motorcycle fatality resulted in a greater frequency than had been expected. This may have been the result of the more relaxed condition and loss of tonicity occurring in the cervical musculature postmortem.

External auditory canal hemorrhage usually was indicative of a basilar fracture being present within the middle cranial fossa. Mandibular fracture or laceration over the mandibular area usually pointed toward a skull fracture.

Anterior Neck

Sternomastoid m.—laceration	30
Sternomastoid m.—hemorrhage	48
Ribbon (strap) mm.—hemorrhage	44
Ant. neck—massive hemorrhage	7
Supraclavicular triangle:	
Hemorrhage—right	37
Left	36

Anterior neck trauma, although not often visible superficially, produced considerable sternomastoid and ribbon muscle lacerations and hemorrhages at the sternal and clavicular origins of these muscles due to hyperextension and rotation of the head and neck. Trauma in the supraclavicular and posterior triangles, unless extensive, was also difficult to identify. This hemorrhage was also associated with vertebral vessel lacerations causing hemorrhage in the supraclavicular and posterior triangles. The vertebral vessels pass directly from the firmly attached arching portion of the subclavian vessels to the costrotransverse foramen of C_6 and are therefore readily susceptible to stretching in hyperextension. The resultant stretching and hemorrhage may invade the carotid sheath, surround the roots of the brachial plexis and extend both superficial and deep to the prevertebral fascia to involve the phrenic nerve, sympathetic trunk, stellate and superior cervical sympathetic ganglia.

Hemorrhage and hematoma in the submandibular region as a result of mandibular fracture and extension of prevertebral trauma may pass into the floor of the mouth, pharynx and larynx or thyroid capsule and gland and paratracheal and esophageal areas. Identification and localization of such traumatic sequelae may be extremely difficult to identify.

An interesting and unexpected finding was the number of cases having oedema in the ary-epiglottic folds of the larynx and the correlation with the length of hospitalization had the victim initially survived the accident.

The anterior exposure of the vertebral column revealed few vertebral column skeletal fractures or intervertebral disc separations.

Posterior Neck

Trapezius m.—hemorrhage	4
Splenius Cap. and Cerv. mm. hemorrhage	3
Semispinalis Cap. and Cerv. mm. hemorrhage	20
Suboccipital Triangle:	
Hemorrhage—superficial	4
Hemorrhage—deep	39
Post. Vertebral Vessels laceration and hemorrhage	28
Atlanto-occipital Articulation:	
Hemorrhage	39
Separation	20
Atlanto-axial Articulation:	
Hemorrhage	33
Separation	22
Cervical Vertebral Canal—hemorrhage:	
Epidural	24
Subdural	16
Subarachnoid	2
Cervical Spinal Cord:	
Soft	8
Transected	9
Cervical Vertebrae—fracture: C_1–8, C_2–6, C_3–1, C_5–1, C_6–4, C_7–1	
Cervical Disc—fracture C_6	3
Cervical Spinal Canal—hemorrhage	3
Post. Longitudinal Lig.:	
Laceration	26
Hemorrhage—deep	45
Tectorial Membrane:	
Laceration	42
Hemorrhage	37
Ligamentum Flavum:	
Laceration	30
Hemorrhage	46

Hemorrhage and hematoma were found only infrequently in the posterior neck muscles in this series of autopsies. This however did not apply to the deeper part of the suboccipital triangle in which the vertebral vessels are to be found. These vessels are vulnerable to trauma as they leave the costotransverse foramen of C_2 (axis) and pass medially over the lateral process of the atlas into the foramen magnum. Laceration of these vessels can readily occur in hyperflexion with hemorrhage infiltrating and surrounding the first and second cervical nerves at the intervertebral foramina and also extend on to and into the atlanto-occipital and atlanto-axial capsules, ligaments and articulations. Stretching and laceration of these articular ligaments and capsules is clearly seen in the increased separation between the occiput and atlas and the atlas and axis that may occur in hyperflexion.

Examination of the upper cervical vertebrae, i.e., C_1 and C_2, is more easily accomplished in this posterior approach which may account for the greater number of fractures noted. Motorcycle fatalities usually may be associated with higher velocities in a forward direction and therefore greater head impacts may result with trauma to the vertebral column. Table 1 and associated Plates 19 through 25 illustrate some typical injuries which have been observed.

Scalp

Frontal area—laceration	20
Temporal area:	
Laceration	9
Hemorrhage	21
Parietal area:	
Laceration	11
Hemorrhage	11
Occipital area:	
Laceration	9
Hemorrhage	10
Subaponeurotic area: hemorrhage	38

Reflection of the scalp anteriorly and posteriorly revealed frequent subaponeurotic hemorrhage that extended laterally into the temporal area and infiltrated the temporal muscles. Scalp lacerations were frequently present extending to the underlying skull and associated with subaponeurotic hemorrhage. Frontal impacts produced many lacerations of the supraorbital areas with hemorrhage extending into the orbits.

Skull

Supraorbital area—fracture	12
Frontal area—fracture	9
Parietal area—fracture	16
Temporal area—fracture	17
Occipital area—fracture	11
Cranial Cavity—hemorrhage:	
Epidural	8
Subdural	45
Subarachnoid	34
Basilar Artery—laceration	12
Vertebral Artery—laceration	8
Supraorbital—fracture	19
Anterior Cranial Fossa—fracture:	
Transverse	4
Longitudinal	5
Middle Cranial Fossa—fracture:	
Radiating	13
Transverse (hinge)	43
Longitudinal	20
Posterior Cranial Fossa—fracture:	
Radiating	8
Transverse	2
Longitudinal	6
Odontoid process—fracture	13
Subluxation—occiput on atlas	12
Transverse and alar ligs. of atlas lacerations and stretching	18

The various skull fractures found in this series occurred in a relatively small number of fatalities. These data differ somewhat from the descriptions and reports of the Police and Sheriff's investigators. The data accumulated by the Investigative Team of the Traffic Safety Center of the University of Southern California are considerably more detailed and accurate and when correlated with the autopsy findings should be extremely important in determining the role played by the neck structures in influencing and producing skull and brain trauma.

The high incidence of odontoid fracture, subluxation and tearing of the alar and transverse ligaments of the atlas and axis may be due to the greater velocities and lesser protection afforded the motorcyclist than is the case with the vehicular driver or occupant. It was noted that in a number of basilar transverse or hinge fractures in the middle cranial fossa that the basilar and vertebral arteries were lacerated or transected.

The fractures occurring in the anterior, middle and posterior cranial fossae produced concommittent trauma to the cerebral hemispheres, cerebellum, pons, medulla, brain stem, etc. The brain was removed with the cervical spinal cord as a single unit and subsequently examined by the neuropathologist.

The preliminary data reported in this paper of the layer by layer detailed head and neck autopsy indicate the need for more thorough autopsies of the head and neck in vehicular and motorcycle accidents and resultant trauma.

The data obtained in this program of study of 292 motorcycle fatalities is in the process of being compiled, computerized and analyzed and will be reported in detail when the program is completed.

References

1. Zettas JP, Zettas P and Thanasophon B: *J Trauma 19*:11. 1979
2. King P: *Aus NZ J Surg 49*:2. Apr 1979
3. Doolittle RP, Brown RT and Boshell A: *Pedriatrics 64*:6. Dec 1979
4. Smith BH, Dehner LP: *Military Med 134*:1477. 1969

Table 1. Common Injuries Found in Motorcycle Trauma

Plate No. 19	Massive Anterior Neck Hemorrhage
Plate No. 20	Sternomastoid Muscle—Laceration of Sternal Head and Hemorrhage Infiltration
Plate No. 21	Hemorrhage and Hematoma Infiltration of Carotid Sheath
Plate No. 22	Fracture of Body of 6th Cervical Vertebra Hemorrhage Infiltration of Walls of Vertebral and Subclavian Arteries
Plate No. 23	Hemorrhage in the Submandibular Region and the Floor of the Mouth Hematoma Surrounding the Trunks of the Brachial Plexus
Plate No. 24	Supraclavicular Triangle and Carotid Sheath Hemorrhage Cervical Vertebral Column Hemorrhage
Plate No. 25	Suboccipital Triangle Hemmorrhage Vertebral Vessel Laceration—Posterior Cervical Spine Fracture and Hemorrhage Muscle Laceration and Hemorrhage

5. Haddad JP, et al.: *J Trauma 16*:550. 1976
6. Trinca GW and Dooley BJ: *Aus NZ J Surg 49*. 1979
7. Andrew TA: *Injury 10*:317. 1979
8. Rehman I: Detailed layer by layer head and neck autopsy. *Report to Head and Neck Injury Criteria Workshop and Dept. of the Navy*. 1978

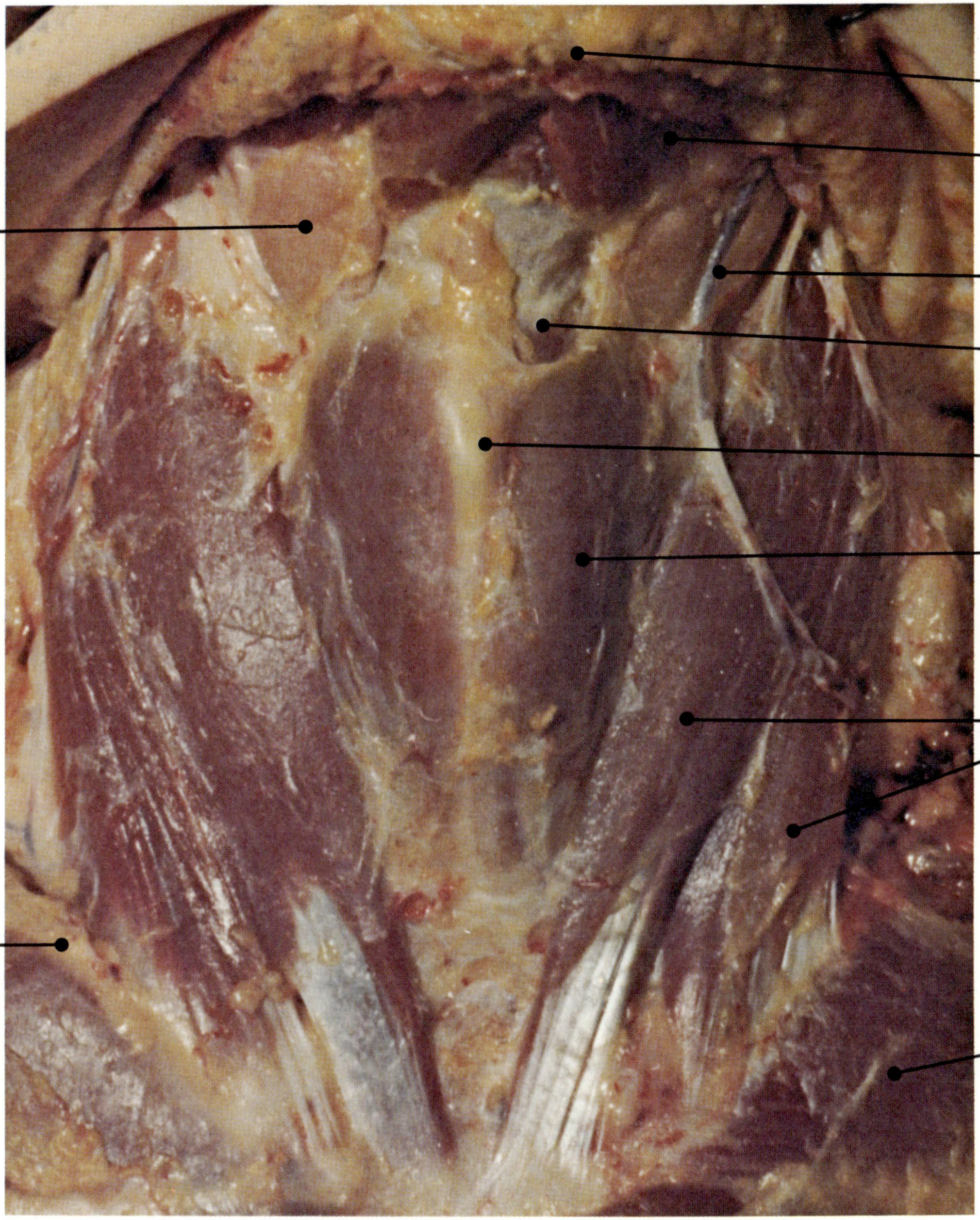
Mandible
Digastric m.—Ant. Belly
Submandibular Gland
Ext. Jugular v.
Hyoid Bone
Thyroid Cartilage
Sternohyoid m.
Sternomastoid m.
Clavicle
Pectoralis Major m.

Plate No.1

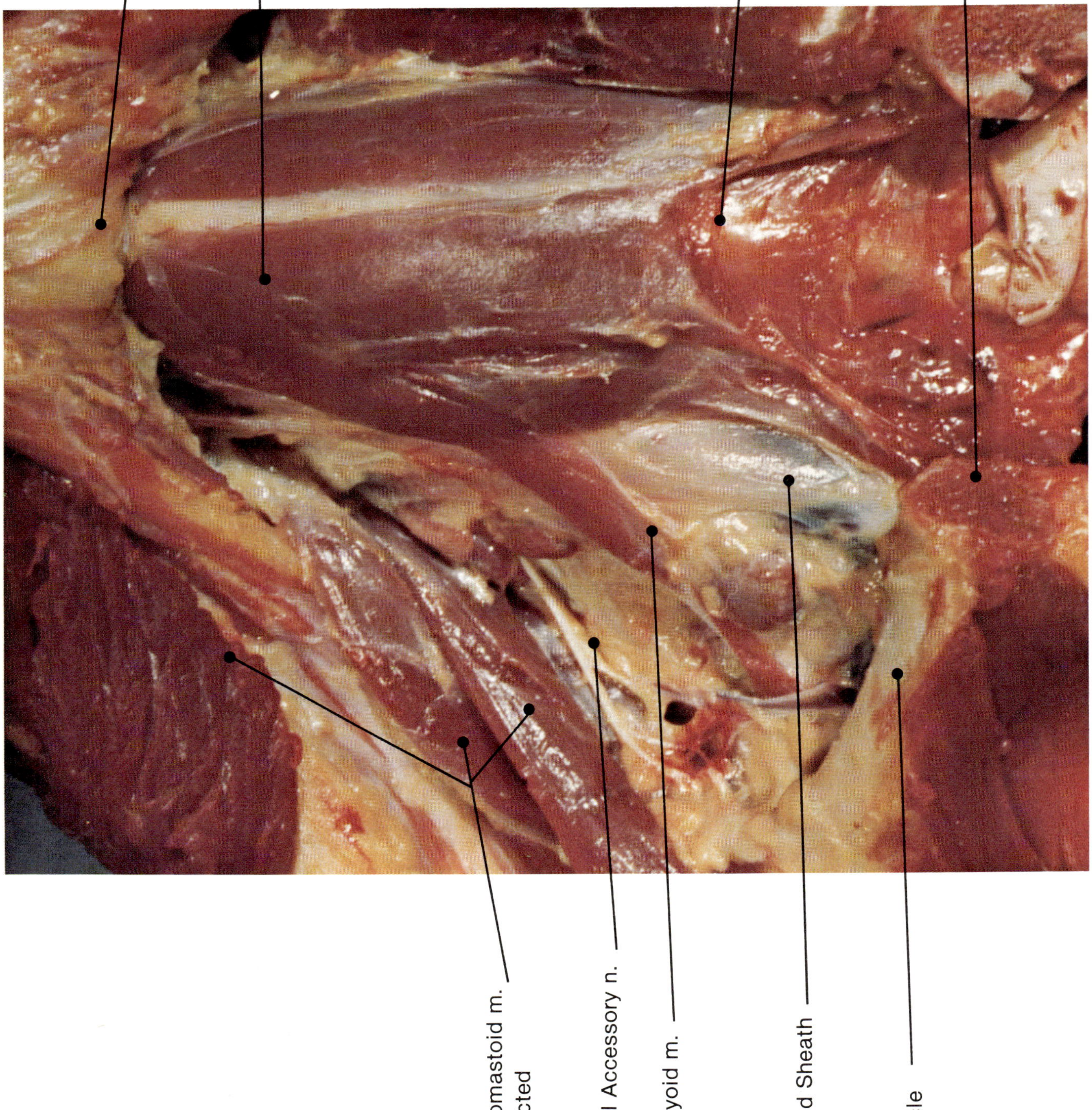
Mandible
Sternohyoid m.
Cut End of Sternohyoid m.
Cut End of Clavicle
Sternomastoid m. Retracted
Spinal Accessory n.
Omohyoid m.
Carotid Sheath
Clavicle

Plate No. 2

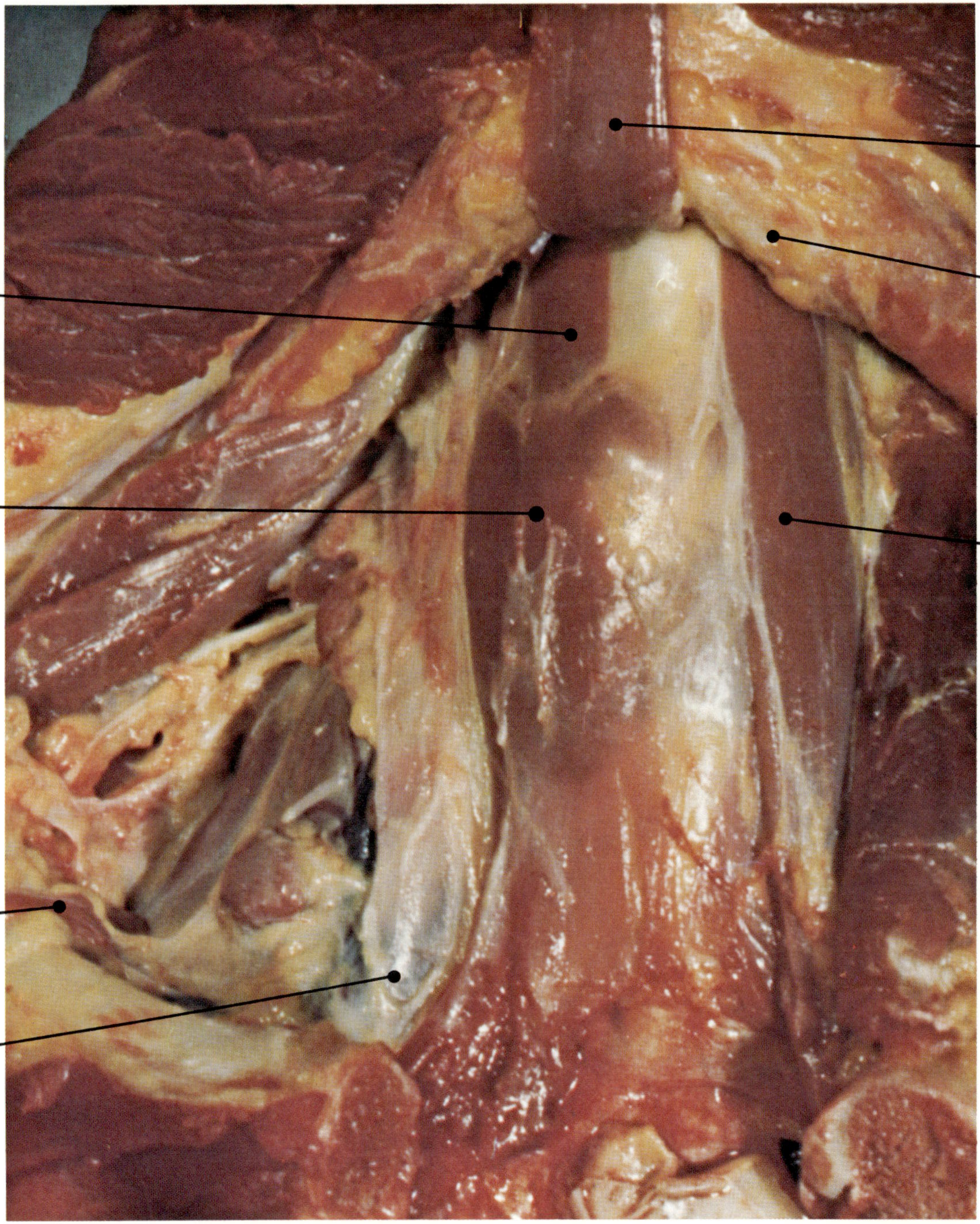
Sternohyoid m.—
Reflected Upward
Thyrohyoid m.
Mandible
Sternothyroid m.
Sternohyoid m.
Omohyoid m.—
Cut and Retracted
Int. Jugular v.

Plate No. 3

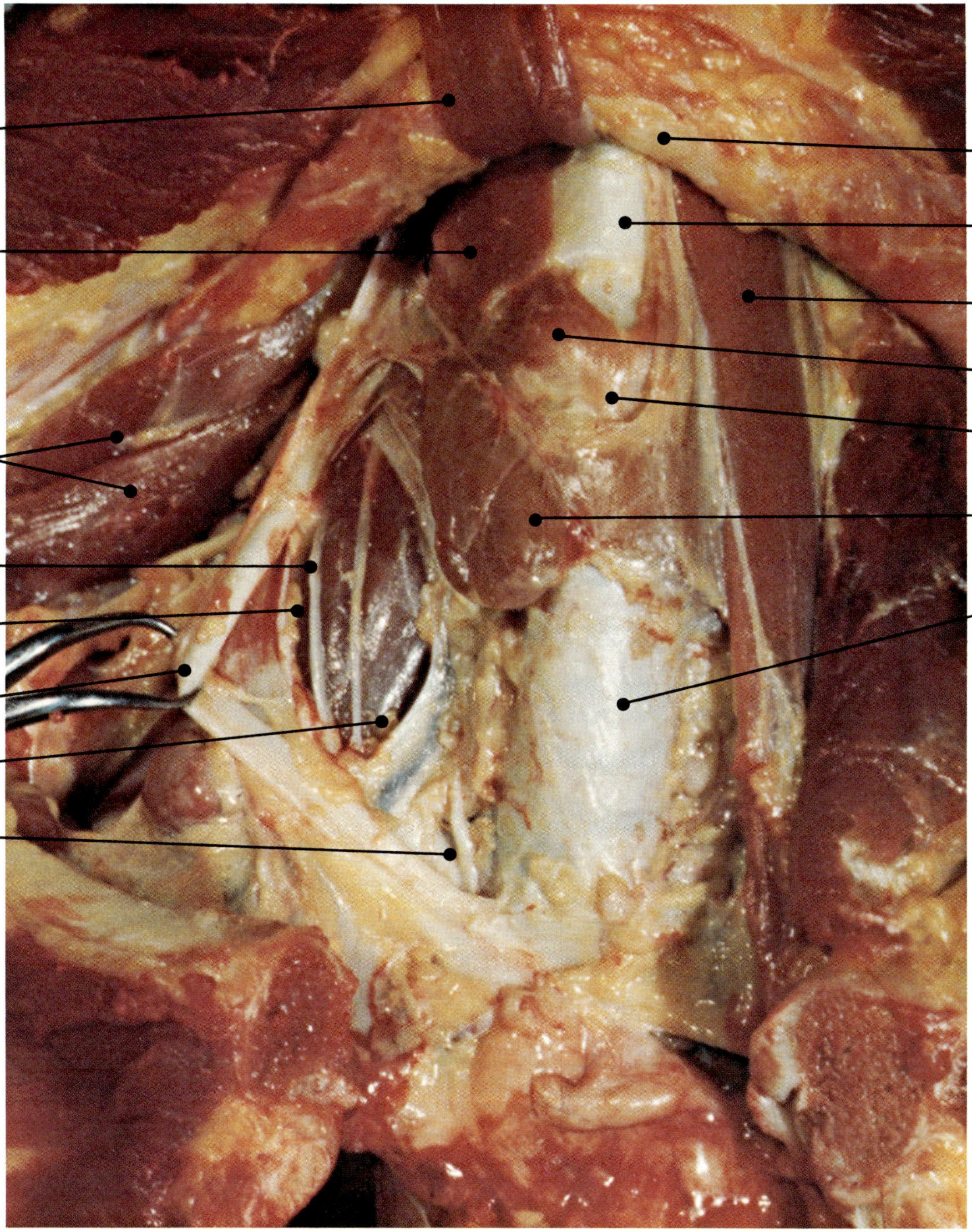
Sternohyoid m.—
Retracted Upward
Thyrohyoid m.
Sternomastoid m. Reflected
Scalenus Ant. m.
Phrenic n.
Carotid a.—Retracted
Sympathetic Trunk
Recurrent Laryngeal n.
Mandible
Thyroid Cartilage
Sternohyoid m.
Cricothyroid m.
Cricoid
Thyroid Gland
Tracea

Plate No. 4

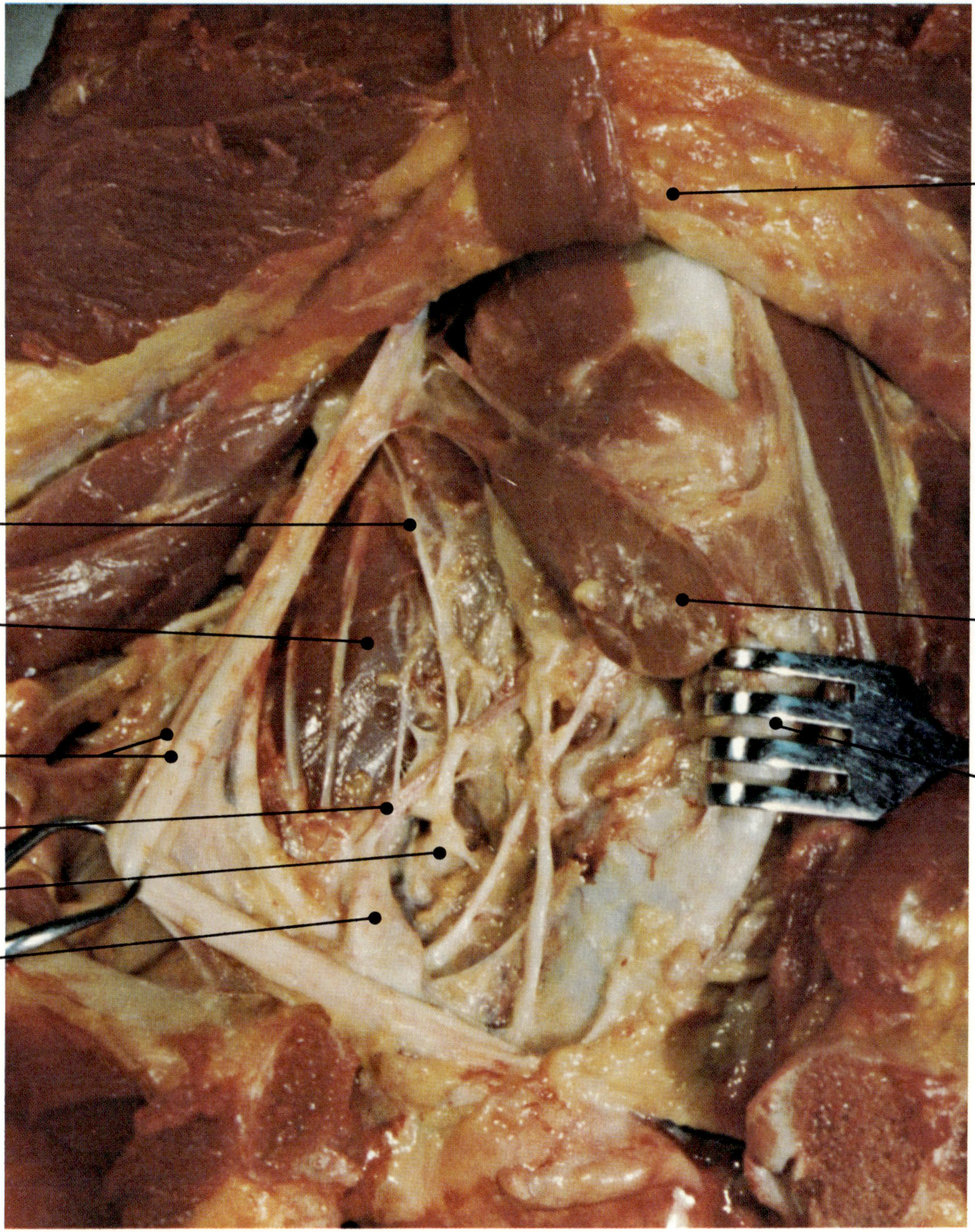

Mandible
Sympathetic Trunk
Thyroid Gland—Retracted
Scalenus Ant. M.
Carotid a. & Vagus n.
Retracted Laterally
Trachea—Retracted
Vertebral a.
Stellate Ganglion
Subclavian a.—Retracted

Plate No. 5

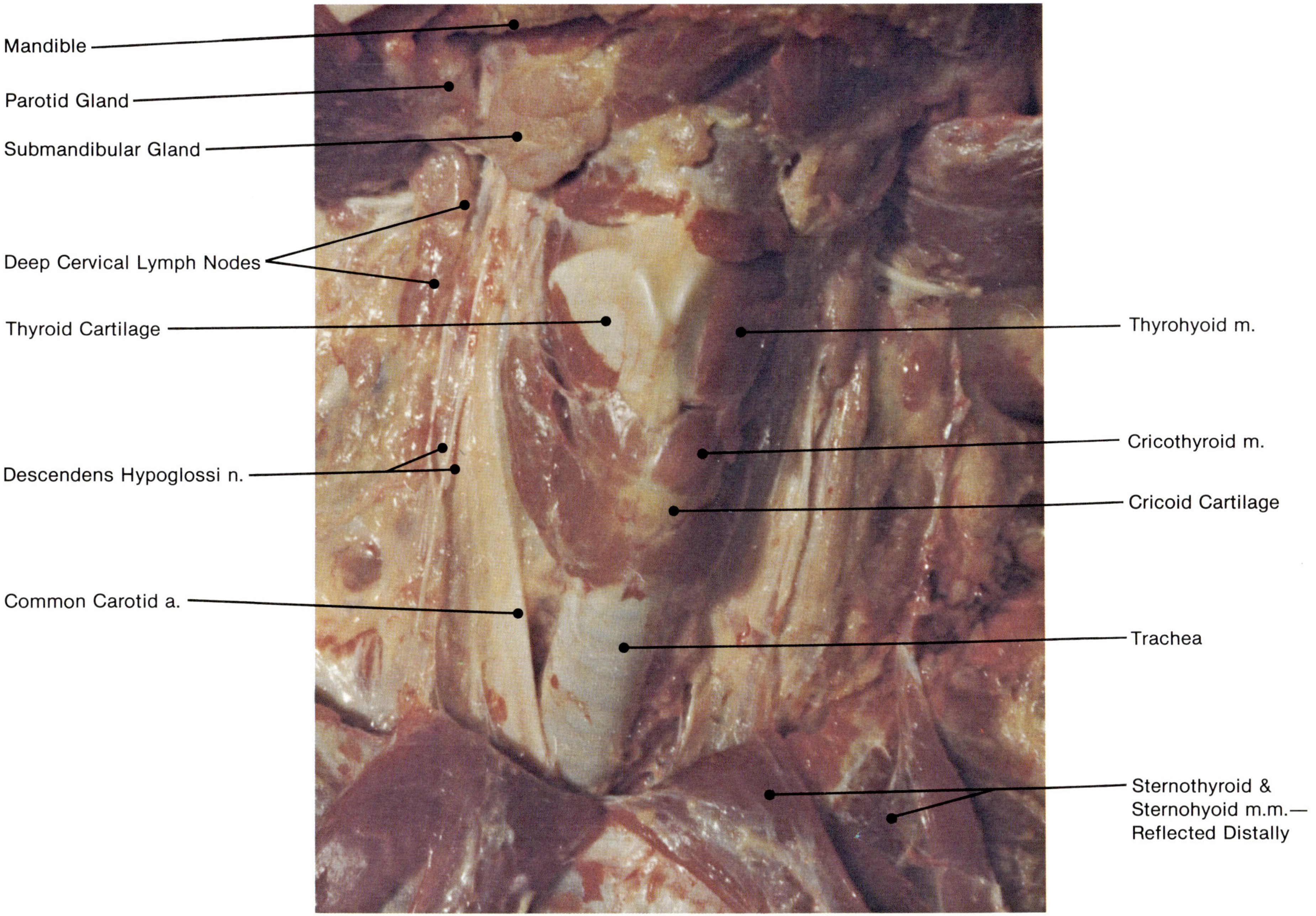
Mandible
Parotid Gland
Submandibular Gland
Deep Cervical Lymph Nodes
Thyroid Cartilage
Descendens Hypoglossi n.
Common Carotid a.
Thyrohyoid m.
Cricothyroid m.
Cricoid Cartilage
Trachea
Sternothyroid &
Sternohyoid m.m.—
Reflected Distally

Plate No. 6.

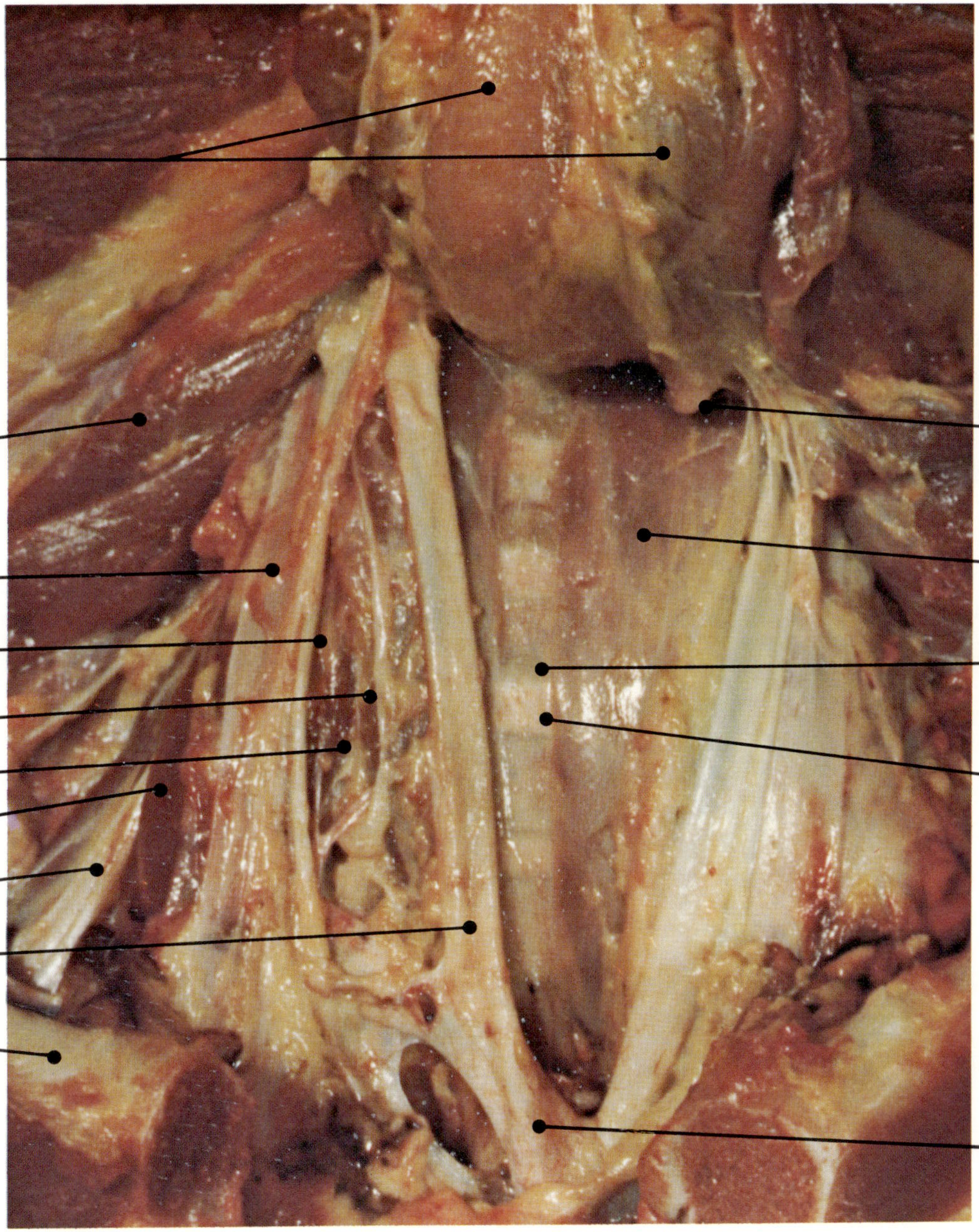
Trachea and Esophagus—Cut and Reflected Upward
Sternomastoid m.—Reflected
Int. Jugular v.
Vagus n.
Sympathetic Trunk
Longus Colli m.
Scalenus Ant. m.
Brachial Plexus
Common Carotid a.
Clavicle
Cornua of Hyoid Bone
Longus Colli m.
Body of Cervical Vertebra
Cervical Disc
Innominate a.

Plate No. 7

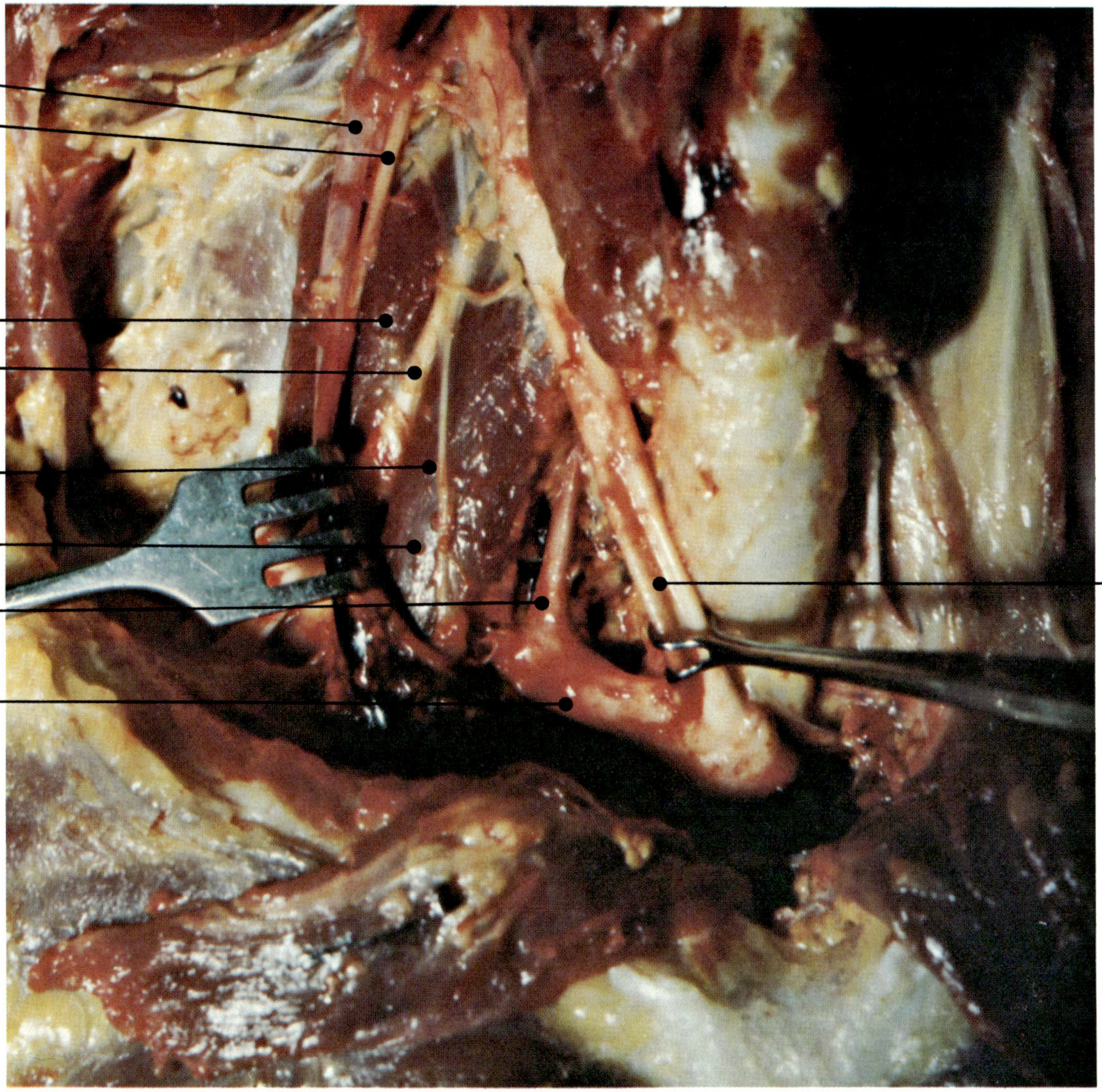

Int. Jugular v.
and Vagus m.
Retracted
Scalenus Medius m.
Brachial Plexus—
Upper Roots
Phrenic n.
Scalenus Ant. m.
Vertebral a.
Subclavian a.
Common Carotid a.
—Retracted

Plate No. 8.

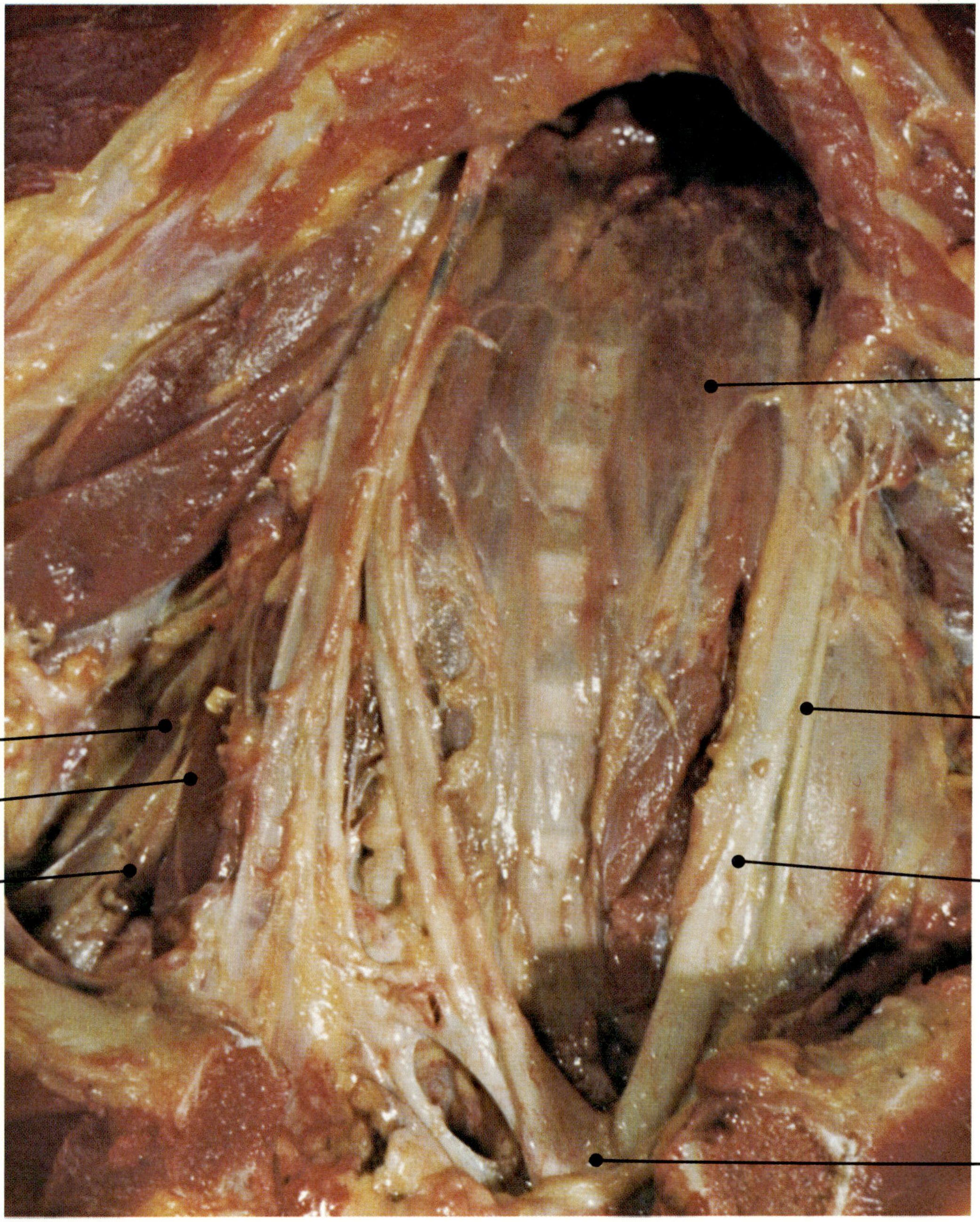
Longus Colli m.
Vagus n.
Lt. Common Carotid a.
Aortic Arch
Scalenus Medius m.
Scalenus Ant. m.
Brachial Plexus—Trunks

Plate No. 9

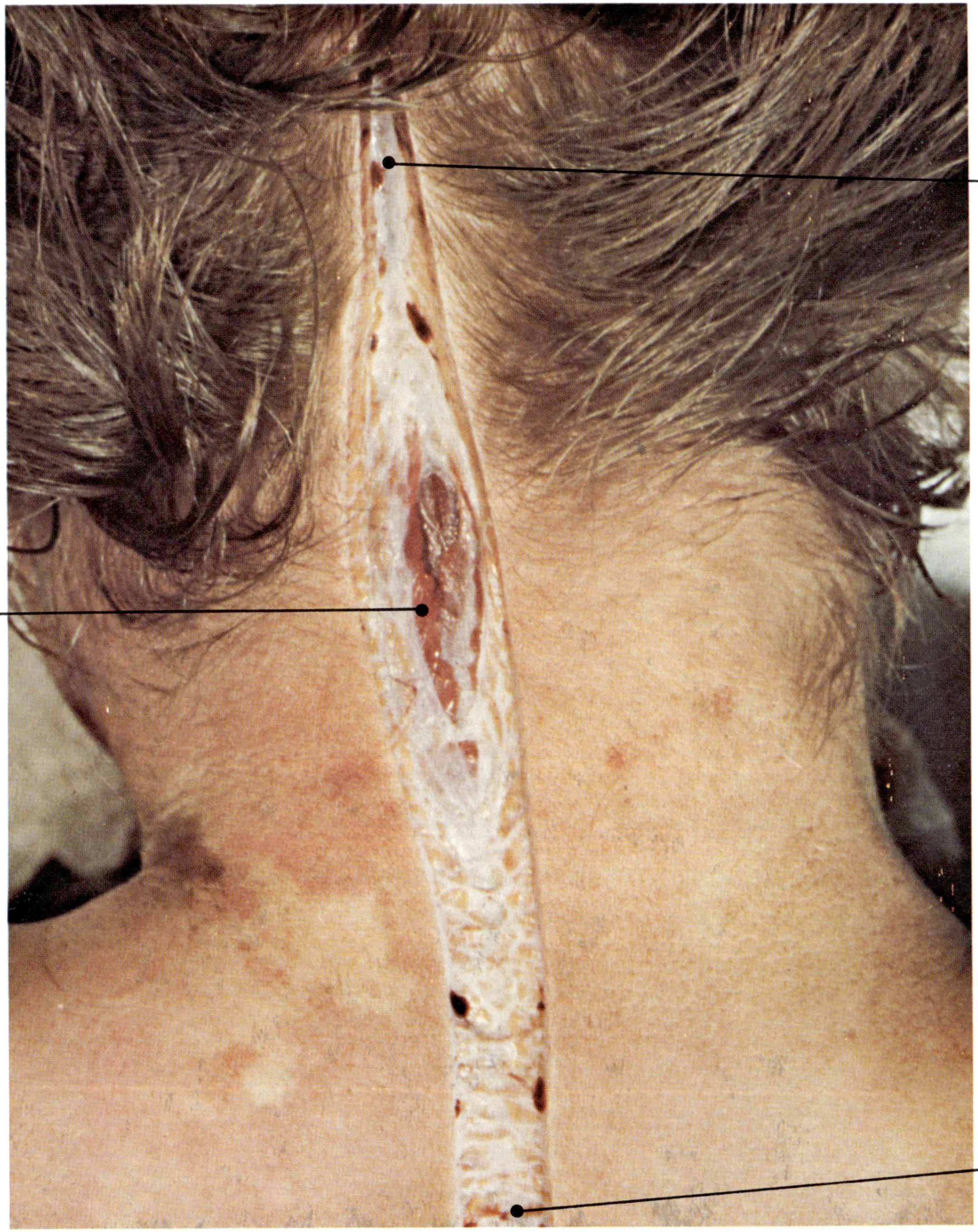

Posterior

Plate No. 10

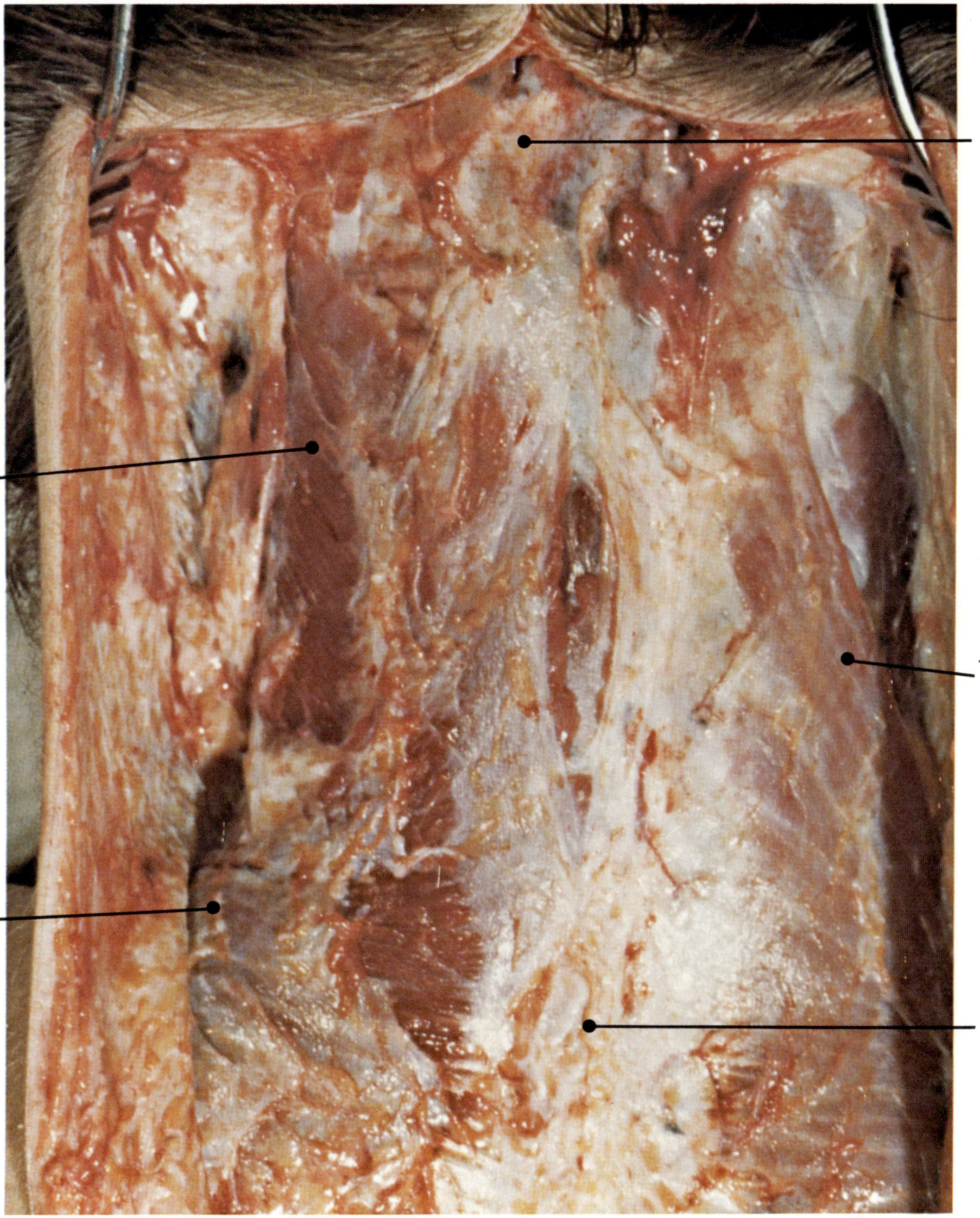
Ext. Occipital Protuberance
Splenius Capitis m.
Trapezius m.
Trapezius m.—Cut
Spine—7th Cervical Vertebra

Plate No. 11

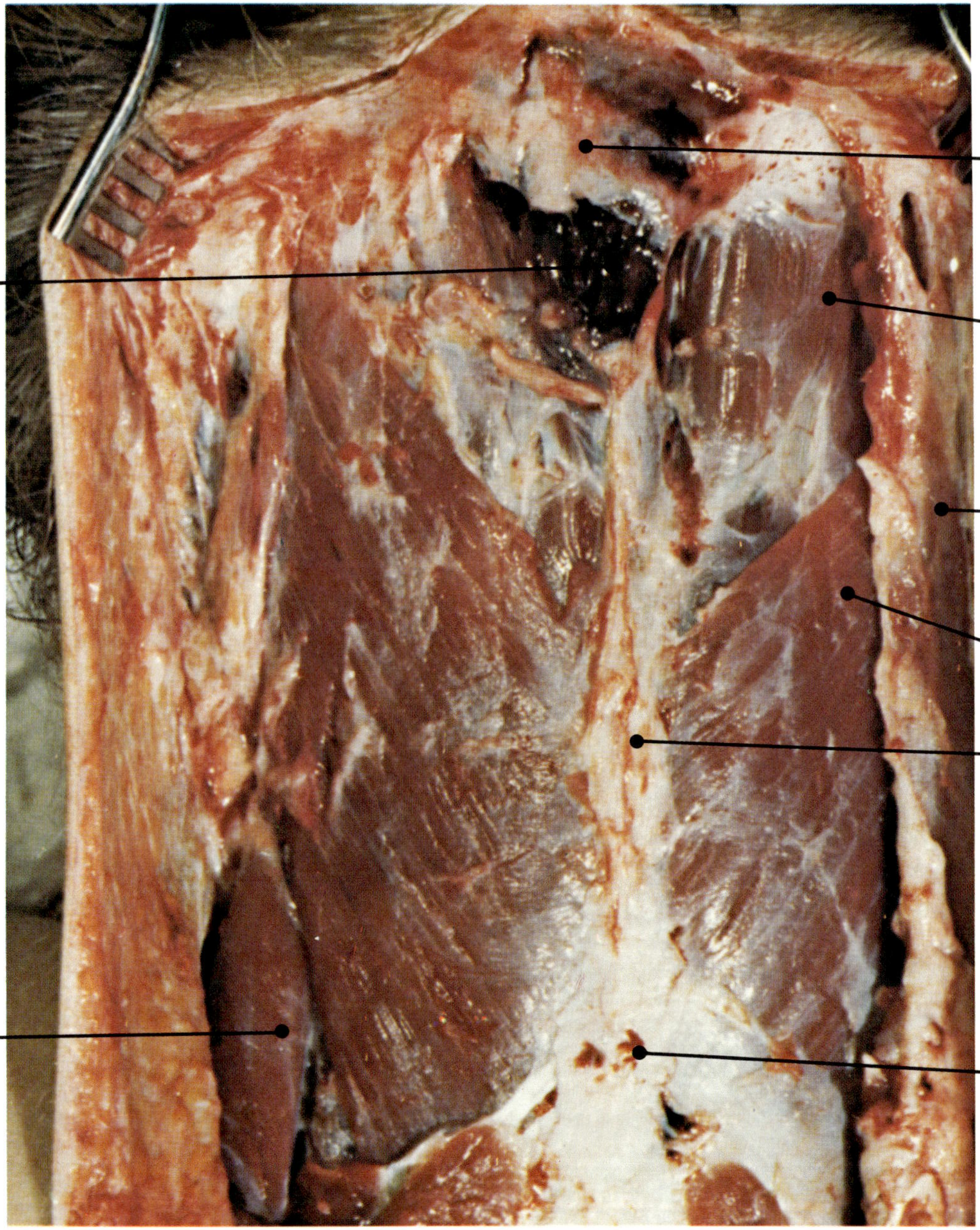
Ext. Occipital Protuberance
Suboccipital Hemorrhage
Semispinalis Capitis m.
Trapezius m.—Reflected
Splenius Capitis m.
Ligamentum Nuchae
Trapezius m.—Turned Laterally
7th Cervical Vertebral Spine

Plate No. 12

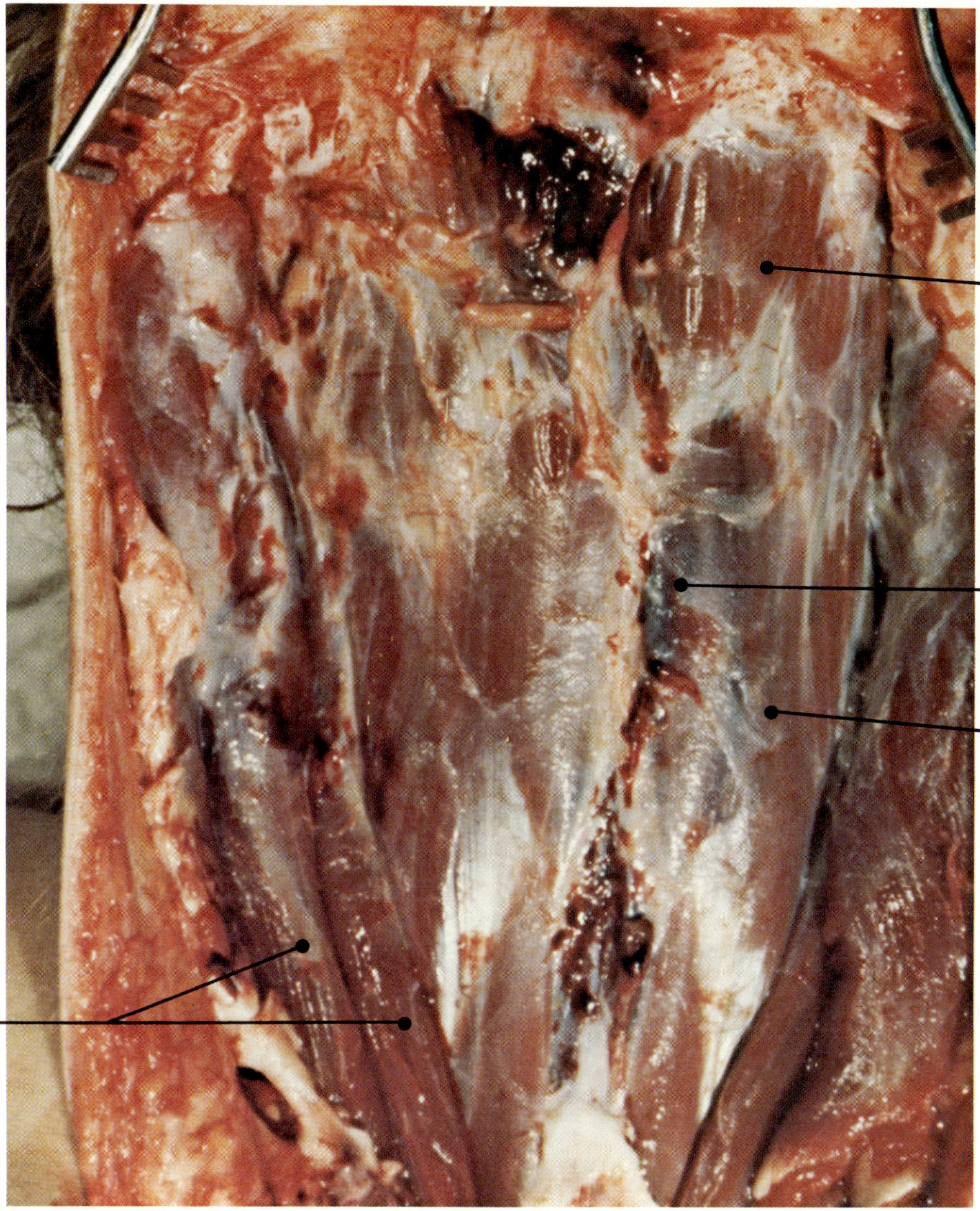
Semispinalis Capitis m.
Intramuscular Hemorrhage
Semispinalis Cervicis m.
Splenius Cervicis and Capitis m.m.—Reflected

Plate No. 13

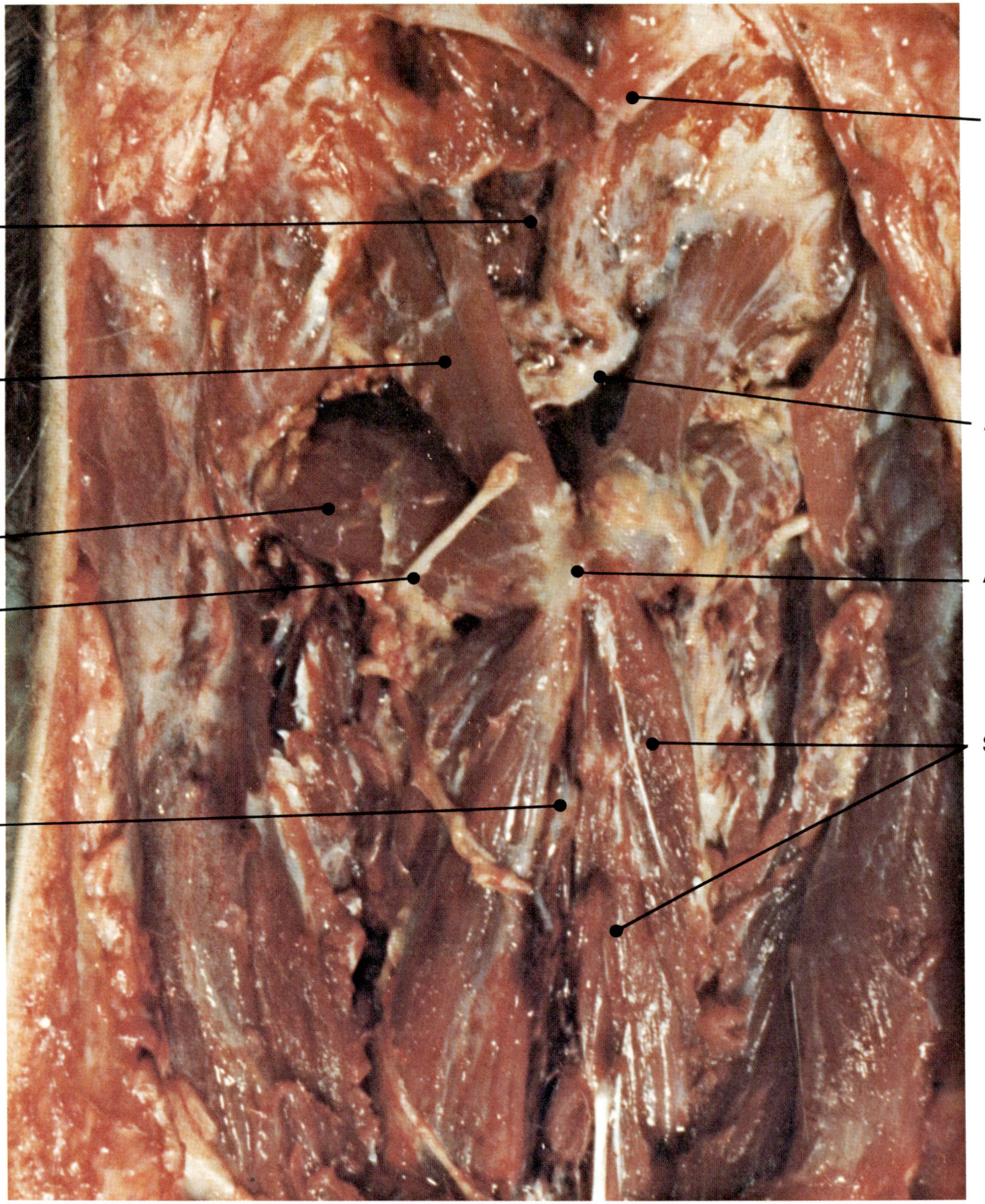
Ext. Occipital Protuberance
Rectus Capitis Posterior Minor m.
Rectus Capitis Posterior Major m.
Atlas
Inf. Oblique m.
Axis
2nd Occipital n.
Short Rotators
Cervical Spines

Plate No. 14

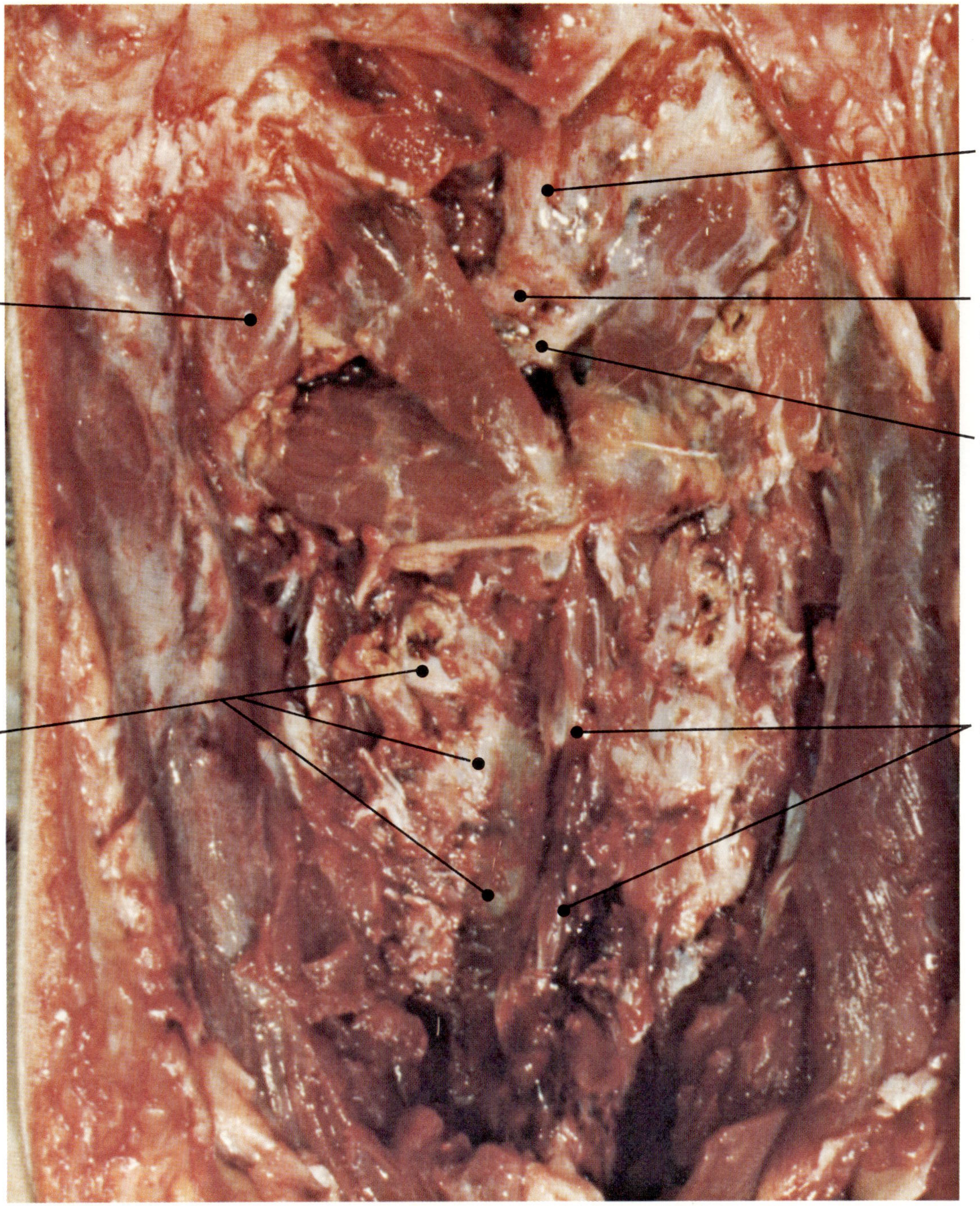
Ext. Occipital Protuberance
Superior Oblique m.
Atlanto-Occipital Articulation
Atlas
Laminae-Cervical Vertebra
Cervical Spines

Plate No. 15

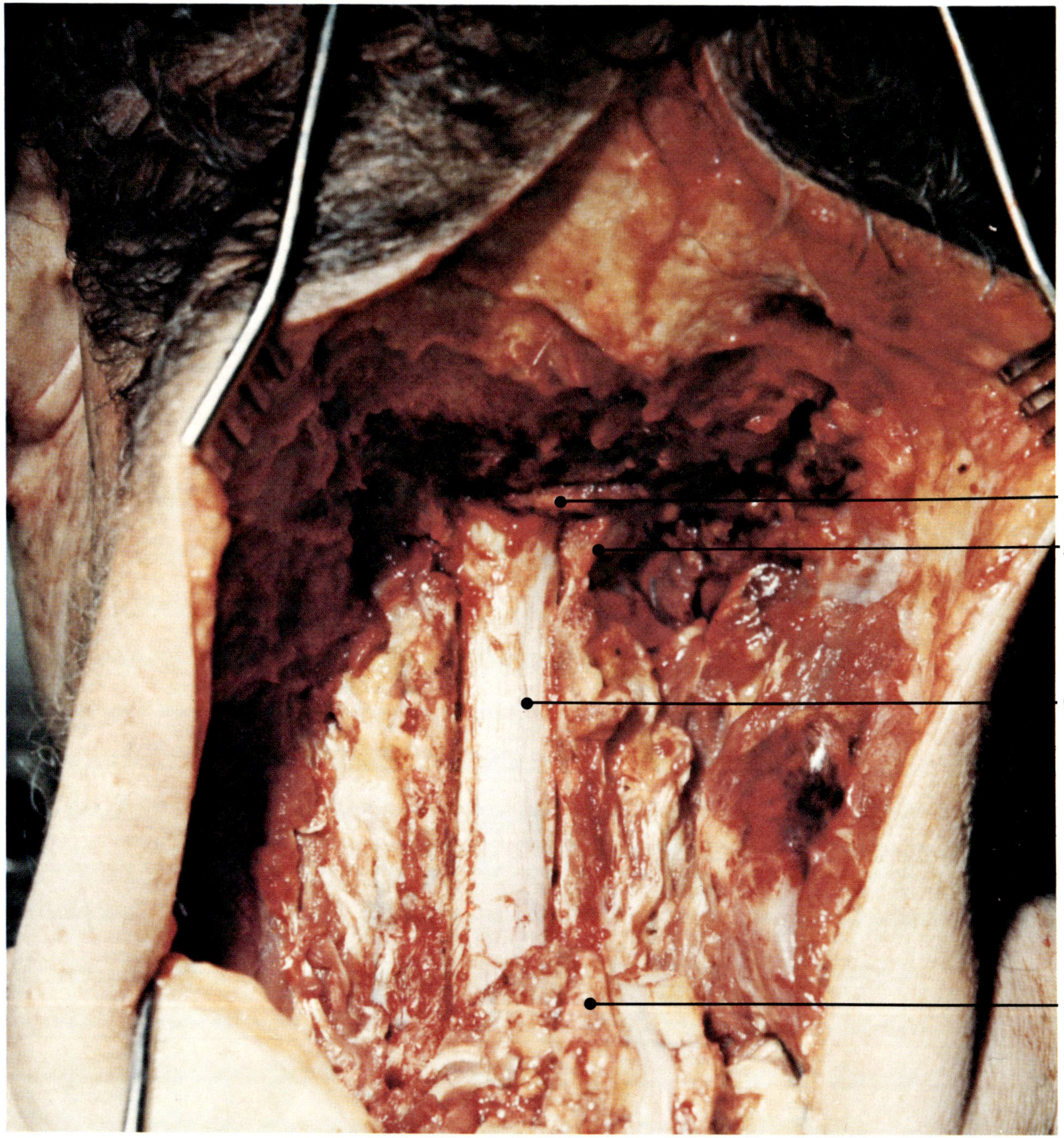
Vertebral a.
Axis
Cervical Dura
Cervical Spines and Laminae—Reflected Caudally

Plate No. 16.

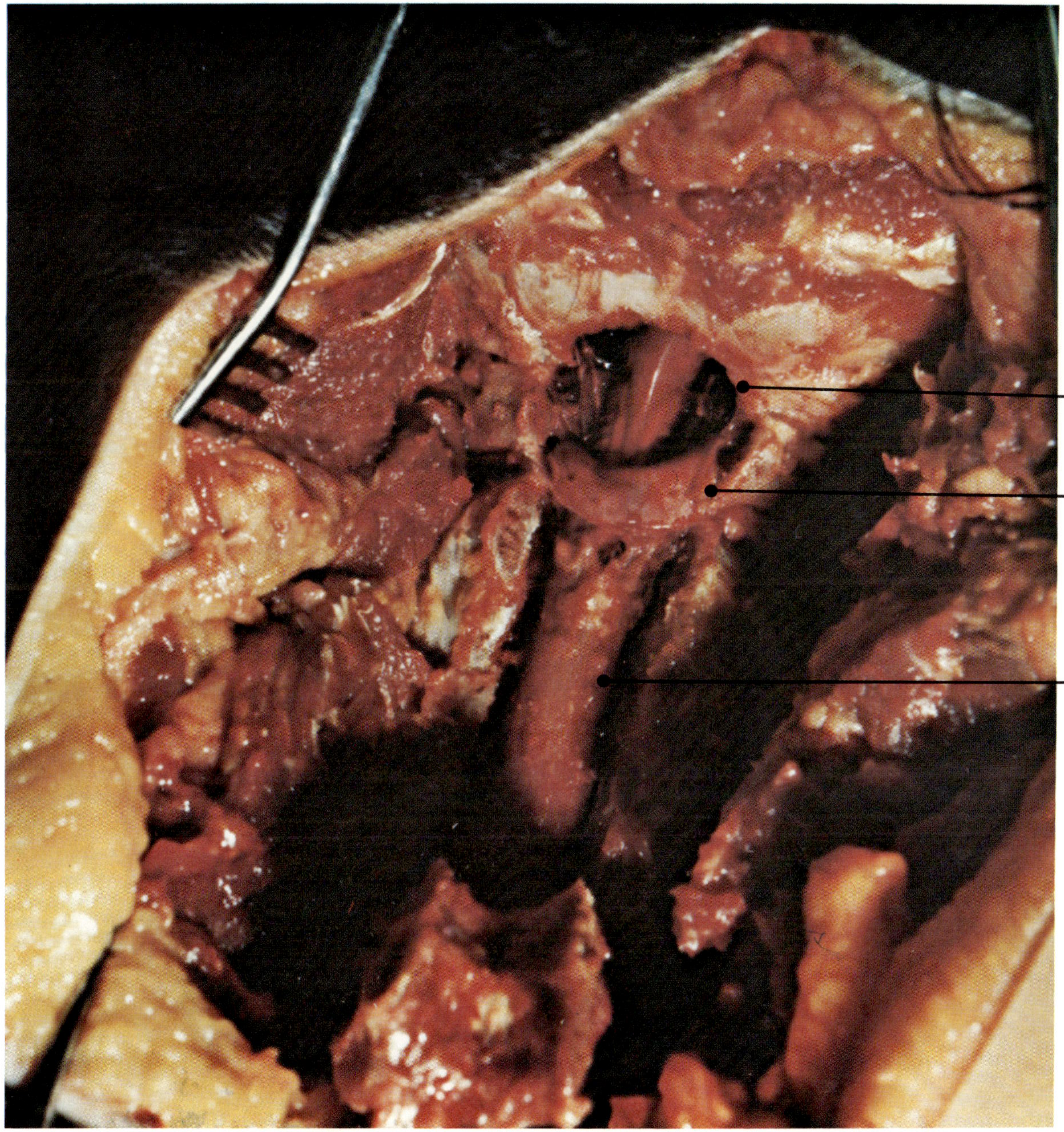

Plate No. 17

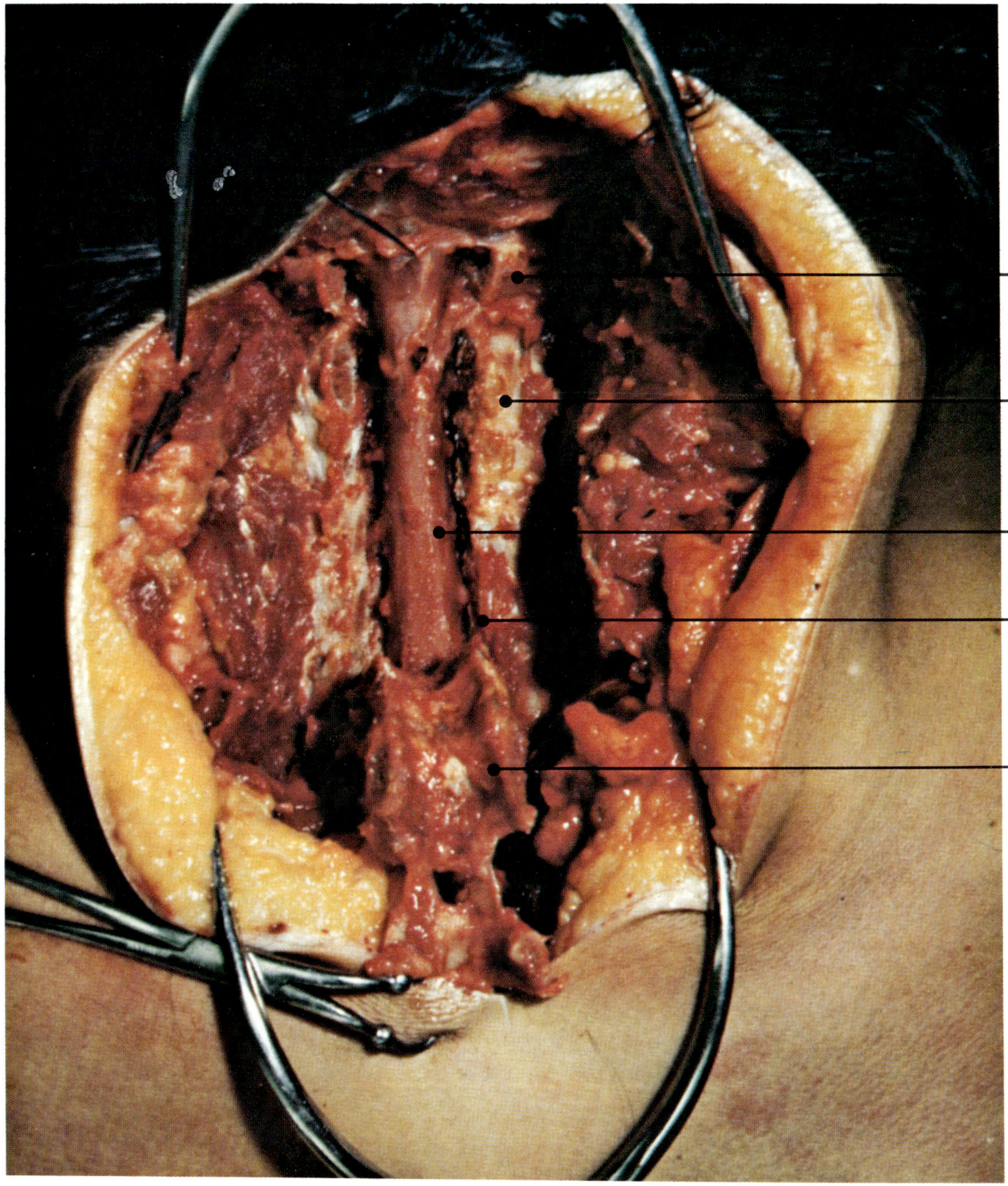
Lateral Process of Atlas
Axis
Spinal Dura
Cervical Nerve Roots
Laminectomy—Spines and Lamina

Plate No. 18

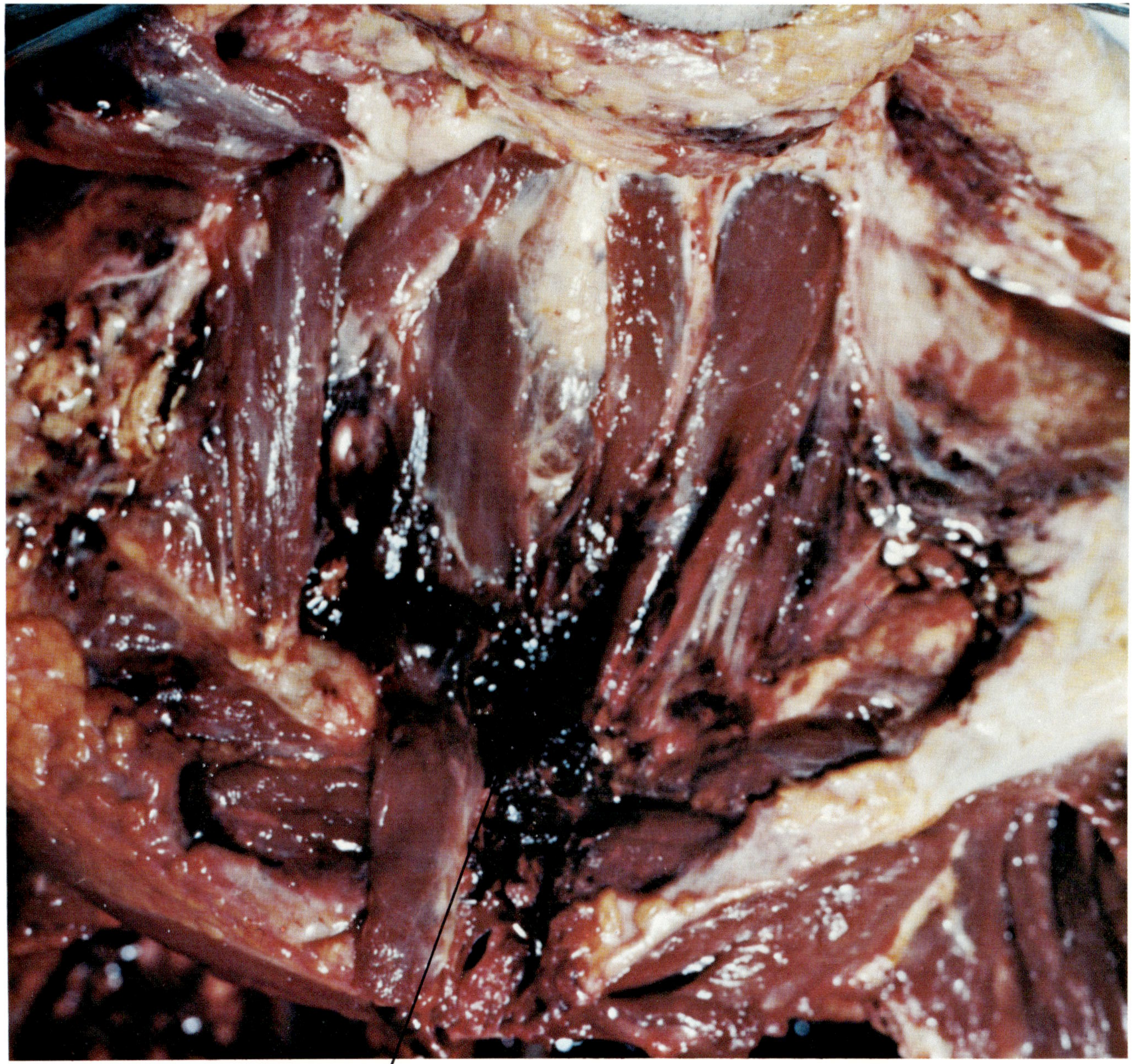

Massive Hemorrhage—Anterior Neck

Plate No. 19

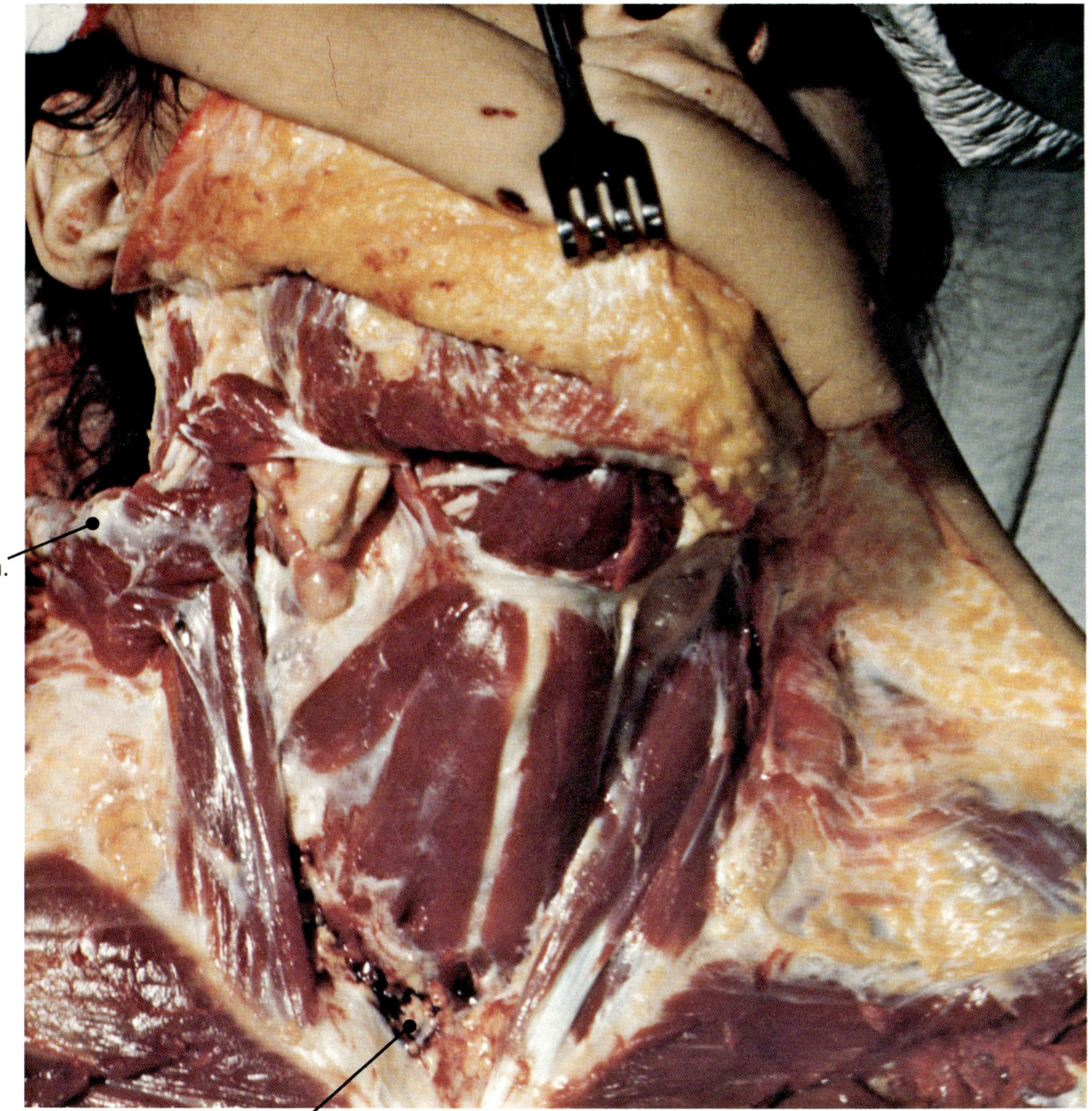
Sternal Head—
Sternomastoid m.
Sternomastoid m. Hemorrhage
Sternal Head Laceration
(Sternal Head Retracted)

Plate No. 20.

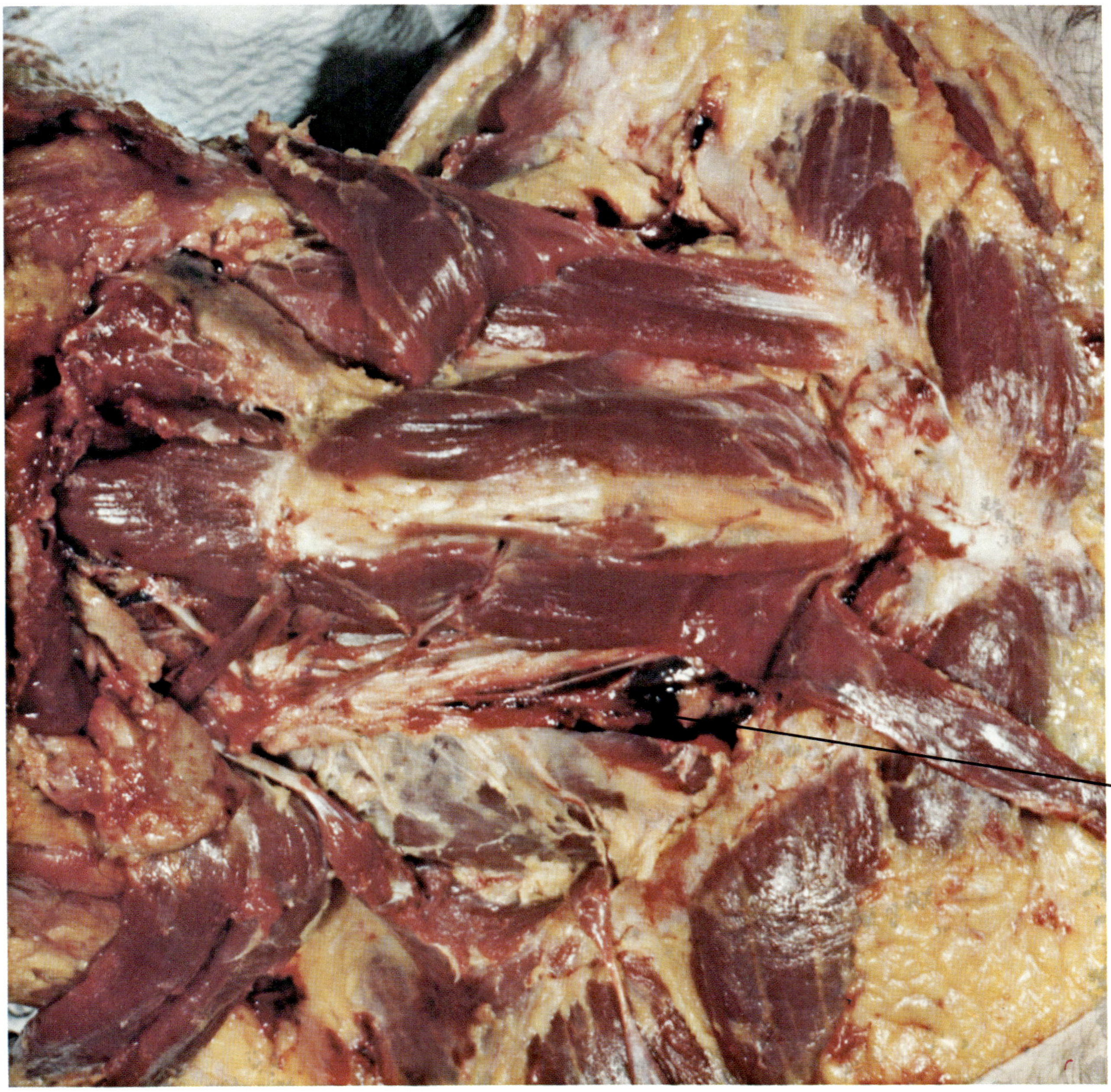

Plate No. 21

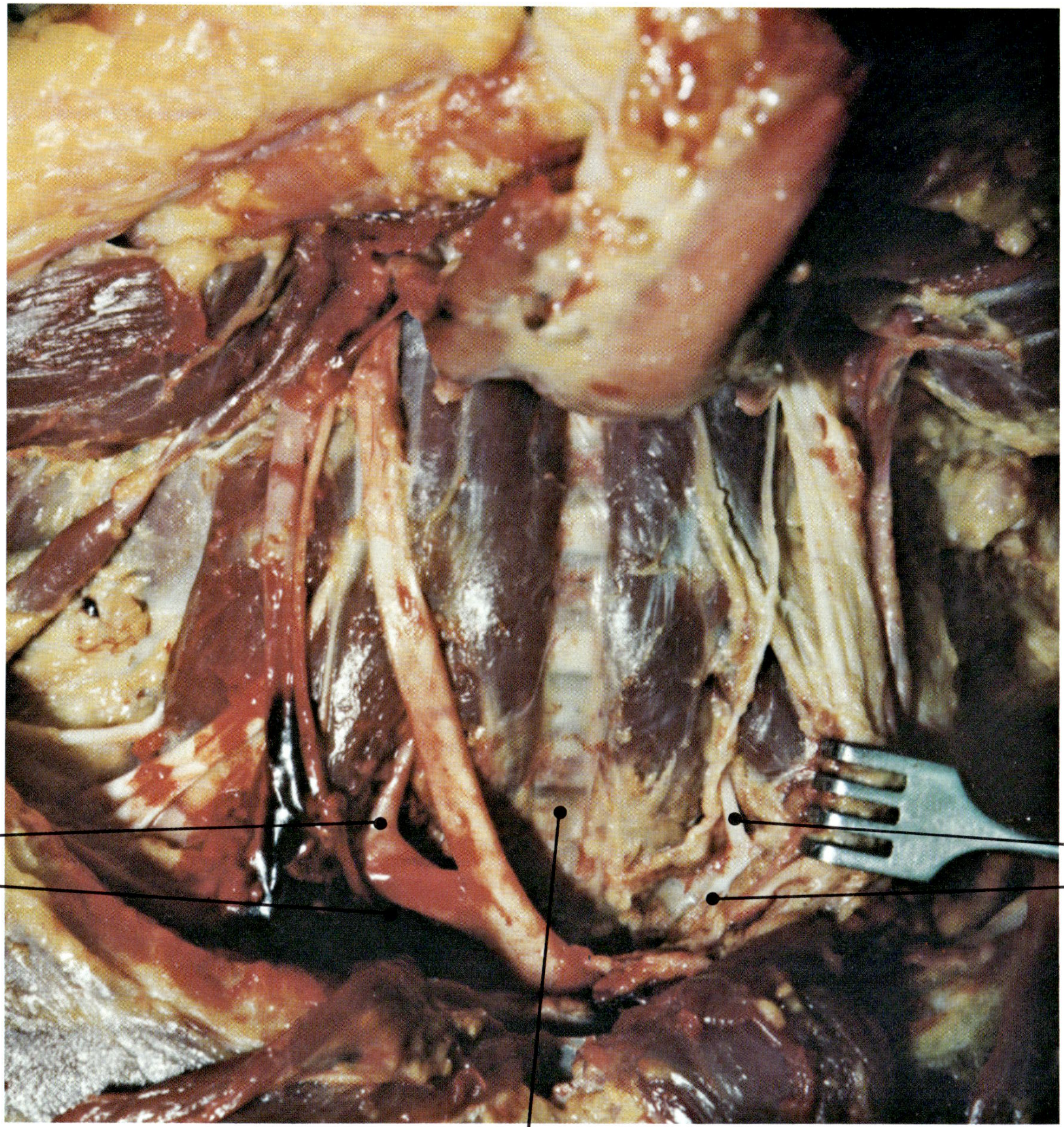
Vertebral a.—
Subclavian a.—Walls Infiltrated with Hemorrhage
Vertebral a.—
Subclavian a.—Normal
Fracture C_6 Vertebra Vertebral Vessel Hemorrhage

Plate No. 22

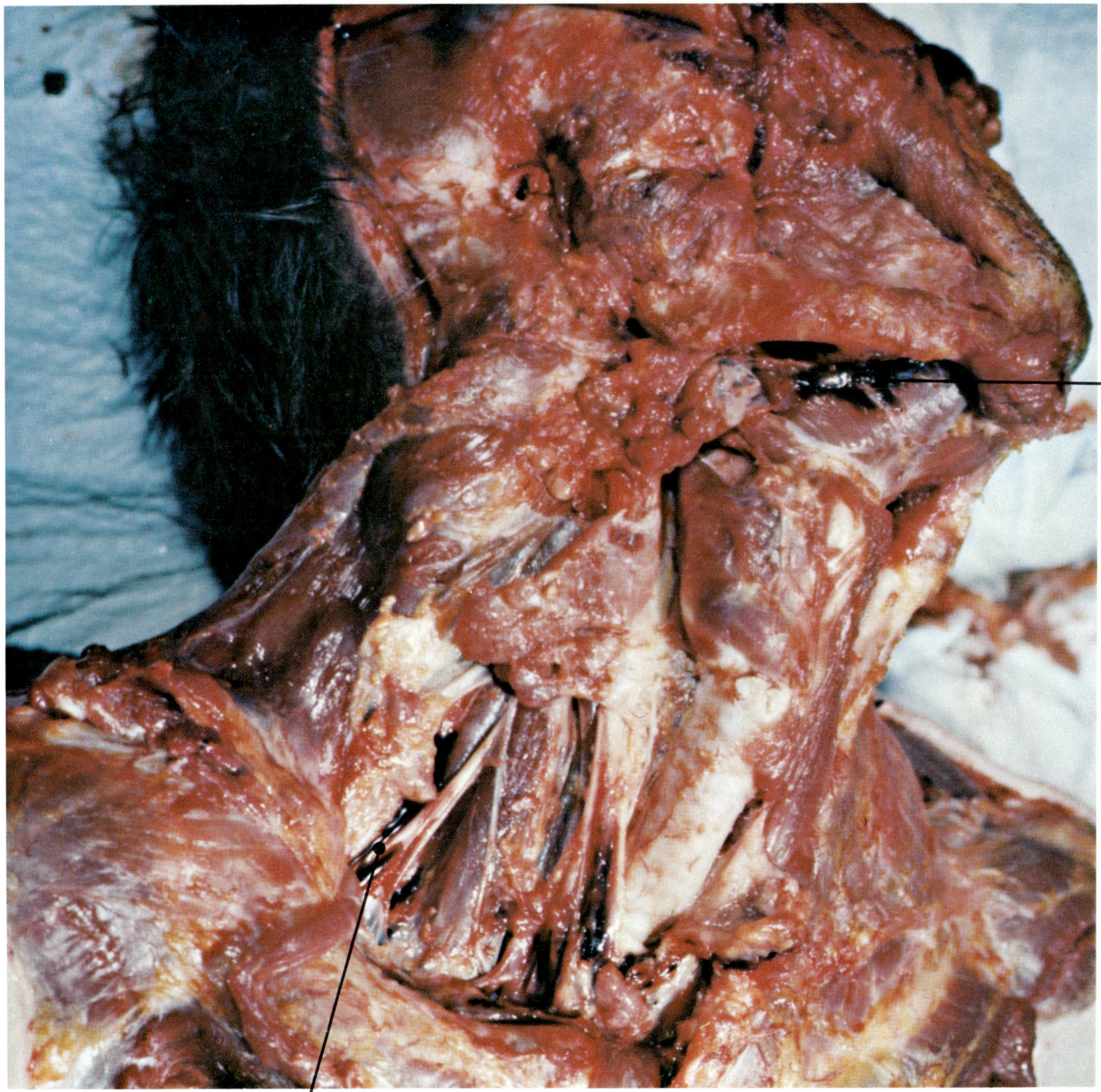

Plate No. 23

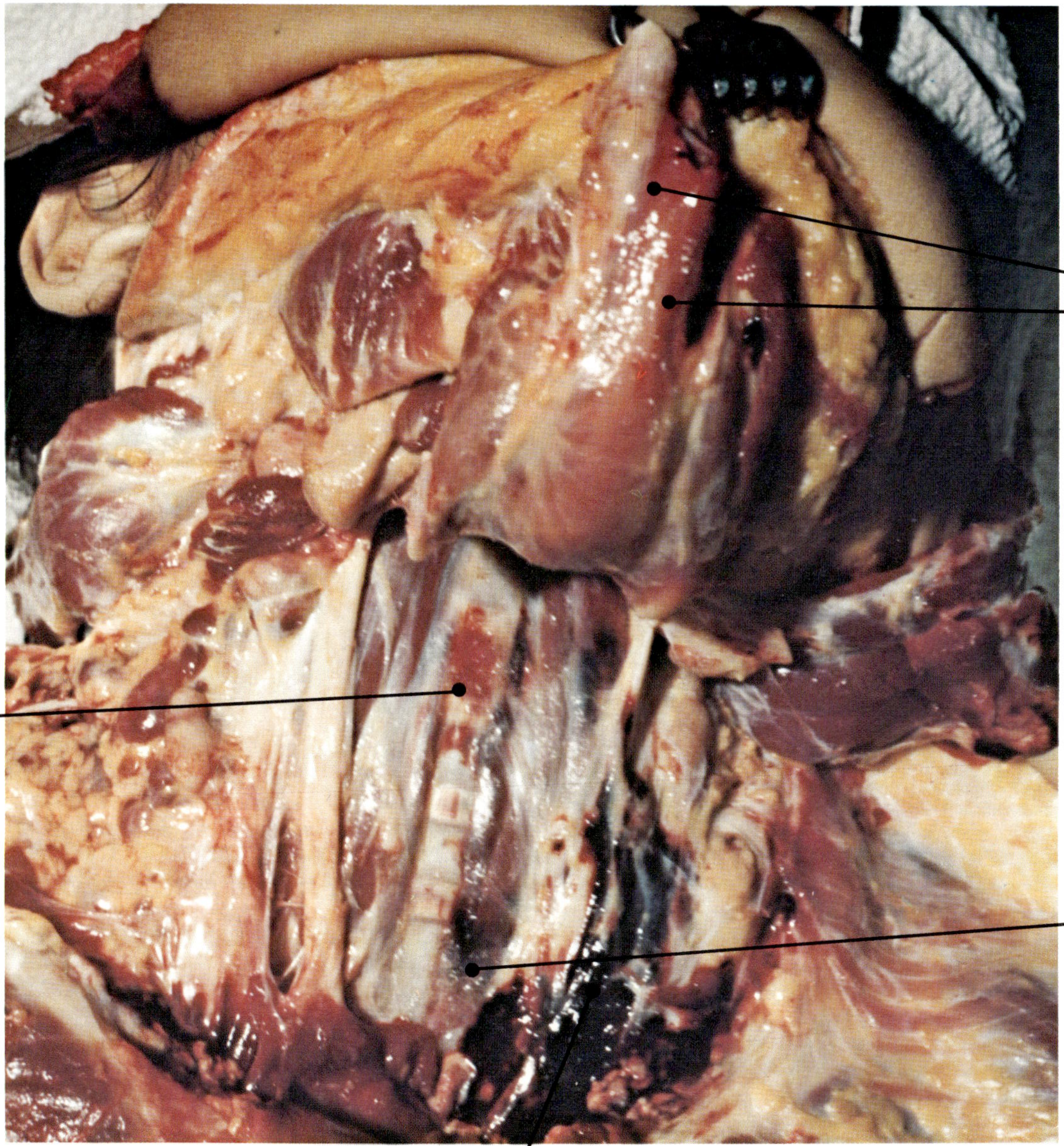
Trachea and
Esophagus—Retracted
Upward
Cervical Vertebral Column
Hemorrhage
Longus Colli m.—
Laceration and
Hemorrhage
Supraclavicular and Carotid Sheath Hemorrhage

Plate No. 24

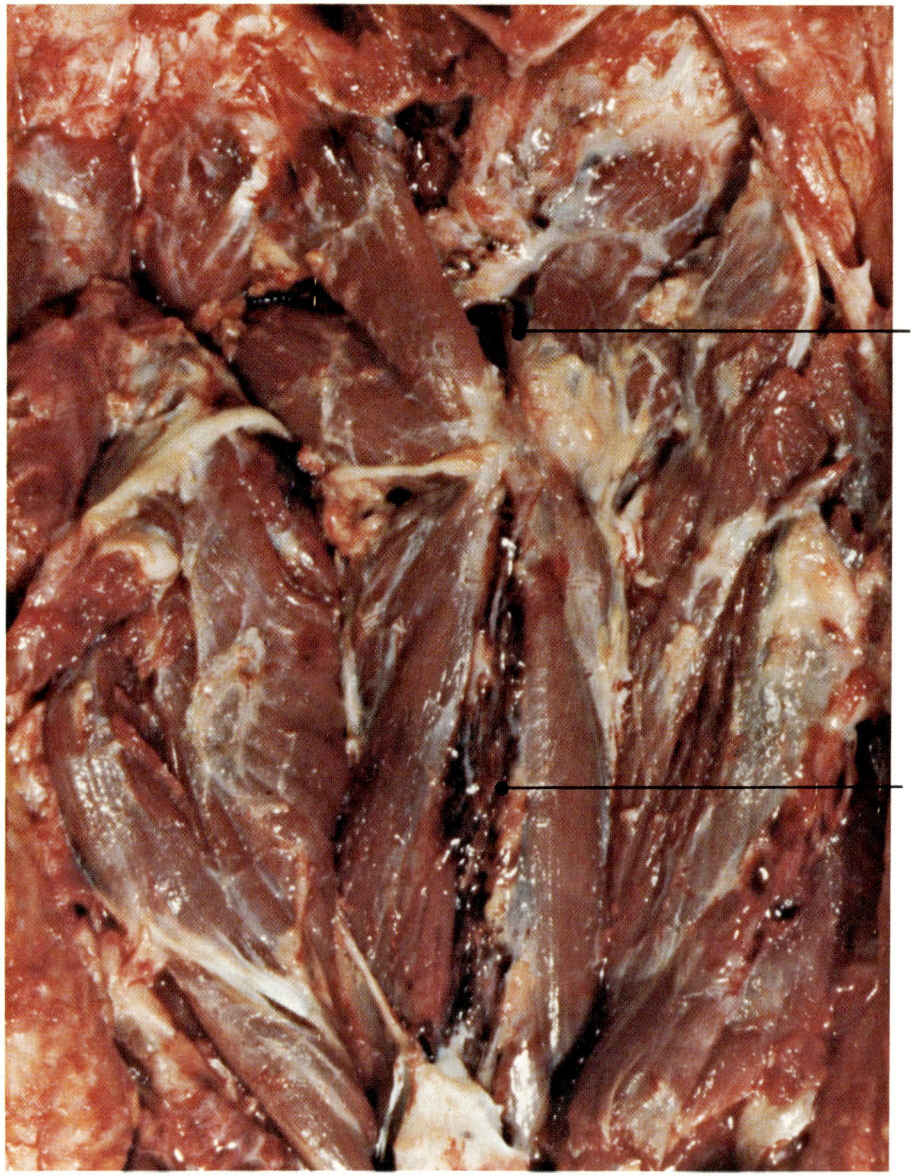

Vertebral Vessel Hemorrhage (Suboccipital Triangle)
Cervical Spines—Fractures and Hemorrhage

Plate No. 25

The Biomechanics of Neck Injury from Direct Impact to the Head, Experimental Findings

V. R. Hodgson, Ph. D.
L. M. Thomas, M.D.

1. Introduction

There has been considerable work done regarding mechanics of injury to the neck, particularly the cervical spine, but most of the findings have been deduced from static experiments on portions of the spine. The mechanics of dynamic experiments have been held back primarily because of the difficulties in visualizing or measuring the injury process. The intent of this paper is to show some of the techniques we have recently used to observe and quantify injury parameters which have been found to affect outcome of an impact to the head relative to neck injury (1). These include:

1. Impact location
2. Line of action
3. Energy level
4. Concentrated versus distributed loading
5. Initial neck curvature
6. Protective gear

This list is by no means exhaustive and other factors such as readiness, age, conditioning, neuro-muscular reactions and anatomical and physical strength variations, etc., each of which is a study in itself, can combine to make understanding of neck injury mechanisms, determining tolerable limits, and devising protection, a very formidable problem.

2. Loading Conditions

2.1 Axial Loading

We became interested in the study of neck injury primarily because of injuries which occurred in football and the apparent lack of understanding of neck injury to a person wearing protective headgear. Based on the studies of Blyth and Mueller (2) and Torg, et al. (3), the majority of neck injuries in football are due to axial-compression loading. It is also assumed to be a major mode of injury in motor vehicle collisions. To investigate this type of loading, our two approaches have been through use of the Hybrid III dummy which has a load indicating neck including axial compression, a-p shear and bending moment about an axis perpendicular to the sagittal plane and embalmed human cadavers using various techniques to study and measure spine movement under load, both static and dynamic. These techniques have included cutting down one side of the neck soft tissue to expose parts of the bony spine from C1 and C7 and monitoring the movement by means of high speed cameras operated at 500–1000 fps during impact; static x-rays and cineradiography of intact cadaver necks during static or quasi-static loading; and strain gages mounted on the anterior surfaces of the vertebral bodies and near the articulating facets during static and dynamic loading.

2.1.1 **Static Loading** (Figure 1) is the setup used to load intact cadavers through a head fixture in the static plane both axially and anterior to the cervical axis, and loading through a fixed or free clevis attached to the head fixture. It has been discovered in some preliminary dynamic tests that when the impact surface gripped the head the effect was to restrict the amount of rotation (nodding) of the head at the atlanto-occipital axis. Distributed impacts appeared to prevent flexion of the upper cervical and cause further curvature in a usually existing lower cervical flexure. On the other hand, concentrated impacts, especially if they are anterior to the cervical spine axis, which is very often the case for forward facing motion, produced high cervical flexion (in general the line of action is not in the sagittal plane or axially aligned, and torsion will occur along the cervical spine with minimum resistance in the upper part). As illustrated in Figure 1, these loading conditions were simulated statically by means of a clevis fixture which was allowed to be free or locked to simulate concentrated and distributed loading, respectively. In Figure 2 are shown plots of deflection versus loading, displaying the basic difference between axial loading (assumed to be aligned with the centroidal axis of the cervical spine) and loading parallel but anterior to the cervical spine, with a free clevis in either case. The axial loading (Curve 1) produced an essentially linear relationship between displacement and force, indicating that the bone was transmitting the internal force (stress) through the bodies and the articulating facets (0–18 percent) (4). Anterior loading produced compression-flexion of the spine and the resultant nonlinear curve indicative of bone and ligament (posterior longitudinal, interspinous and supraspinous ligaments) loading. The basic differences between these two modes of loading are that with the true axial loading failure will be bone stress related and can probably be predicated by the intensity of external loads. When the load is applied off axis the injury is most likely to be related to

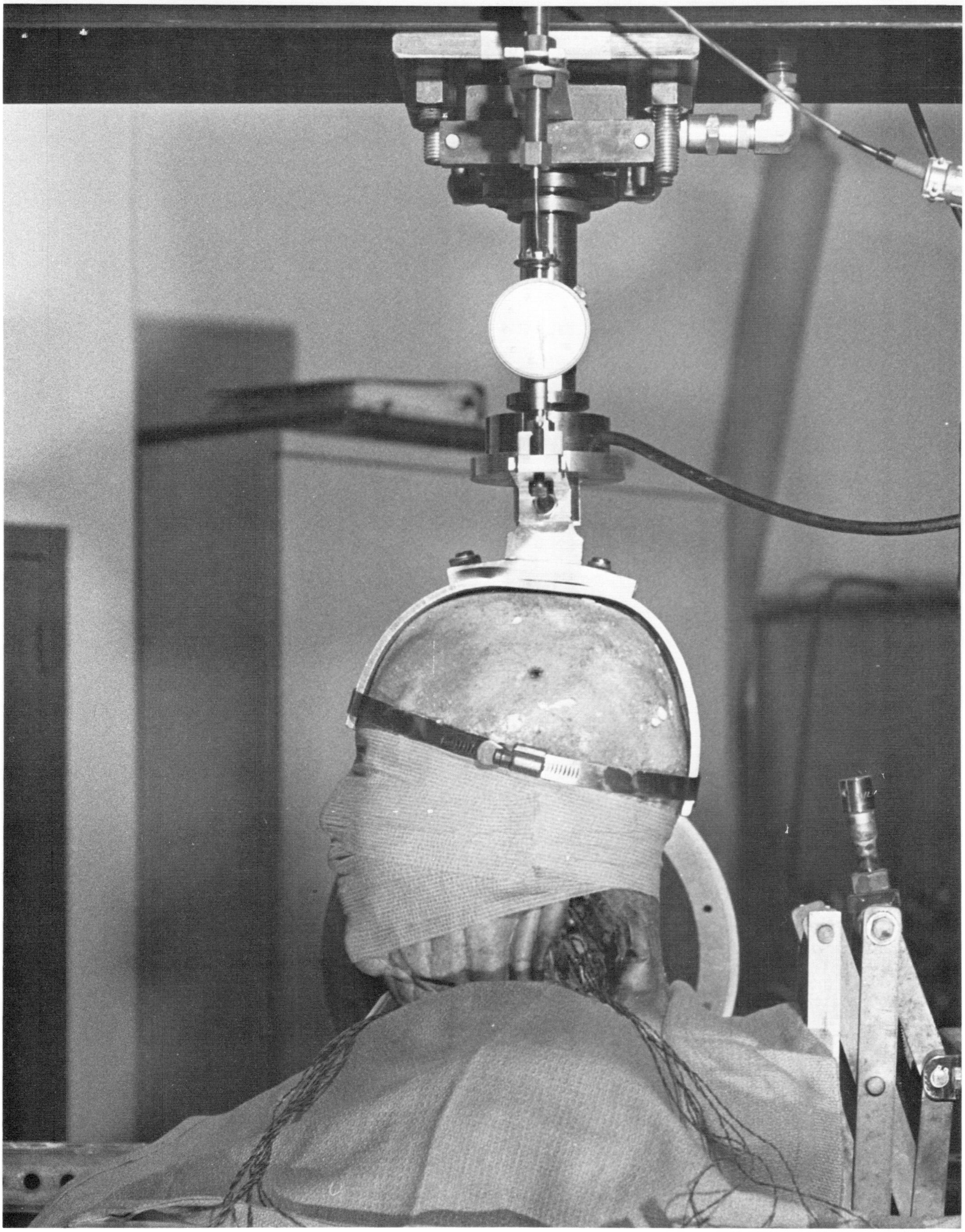

Figure 1.

stress in the ligaments supporting the integrity of the spines, either due to tension in the above mentioned ligaments, or due to posterior-anterior shear which becomes a larger component of the internal resistance to loading as the neck is bent in flexion.

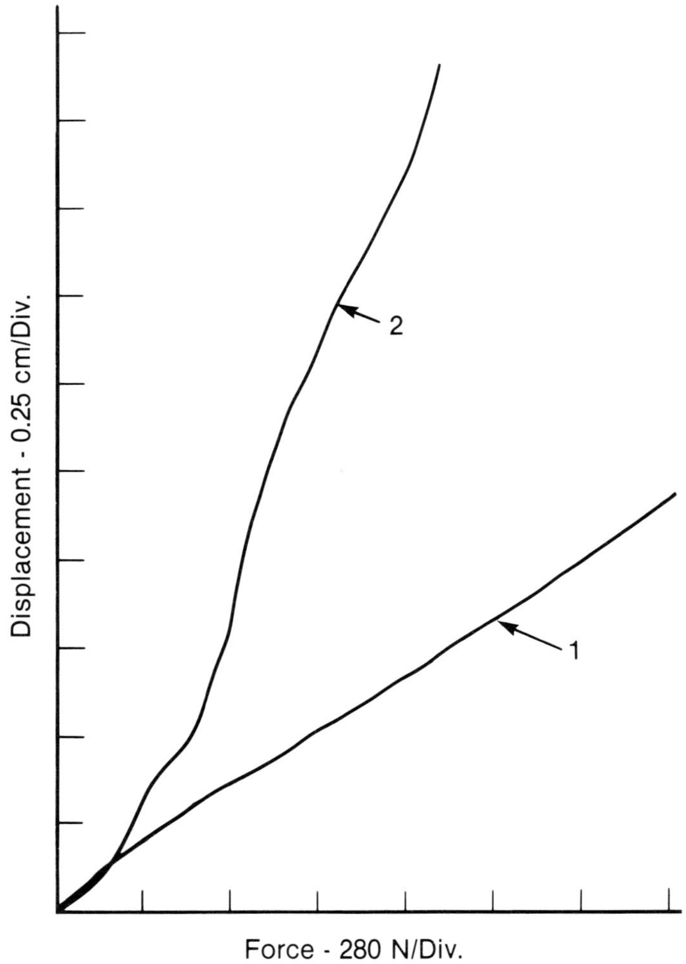

Figure 2.

Figures 3a-d show the effects of the four static loading conditions on three strain gage measuring locations on the anterior surfaces of the vertebral bodies. Three strain gage locations are ordinarily not adequate to define the flexure of the neck and expected failure location, but in conjunction with a hemisectioned neck and photographic coverage they are helpful in describing the failure tendencies under these loading conditions and as predictors for neck distortion and failure sites under similar dynamic loading conditions.

2.2.2 Dynamic Distributed Loading—A blocking-tackling device was introduced to teach the techniques of these maneuvers in football under dynamic conditions. It was alleged to have caused several neck injuries (5) to players who struck the moving tackling dummy with their lowered heads. This appeared to present one method of indirectly obtaining human tolerance to axial loading and to determine if protective helmets could have an attenuating effect on internal forces in the neck due to crown loading. A Hybrid III dummy was strapped in a supine position to a light pallet on a roller bearing conveyor in the path of the tackling bag which was propelled into the crown of the dummy at various load intensities up to and beyond that used in the field (Figure 4). Neck loads and head accelerations were measured and recorded for various orientations of the body.

The major findings in this study (6) were that the football helmets which were resilient were all similar in their effect and attenuated neck axial force compared to wearing no helmet at all. The only helmet which produced significantly higher axial force was a polystyrene-covered crash helmet which was considerably firmer and provided less take-up distance between the shell and the dummy head crown than its resilient football helmet counterparts. Tolerance curves were published from this work in terms of time above load versus axial load, in the Hybrid III dummy

Clevis Free, Axial Loading, Initially Upper Cervical Extension

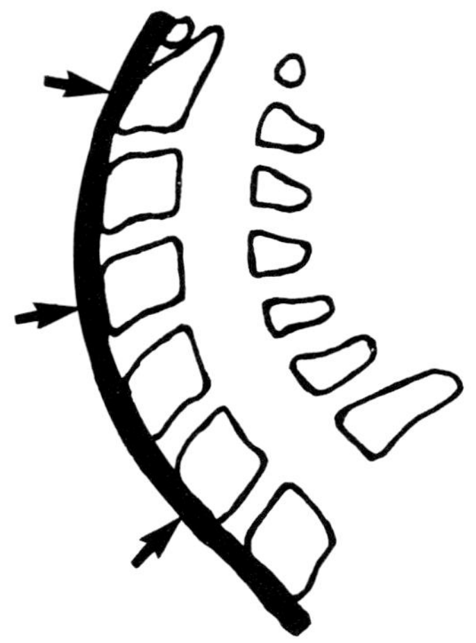

250* Tension (T)
700 T
480 Compression (C)

Predicts Mid-Cervical Anterior Longitudinal Ligament Failure/ Dislocation

Figure 3a.

Clevis Free, Axial Loading, Initially Straight Spine.

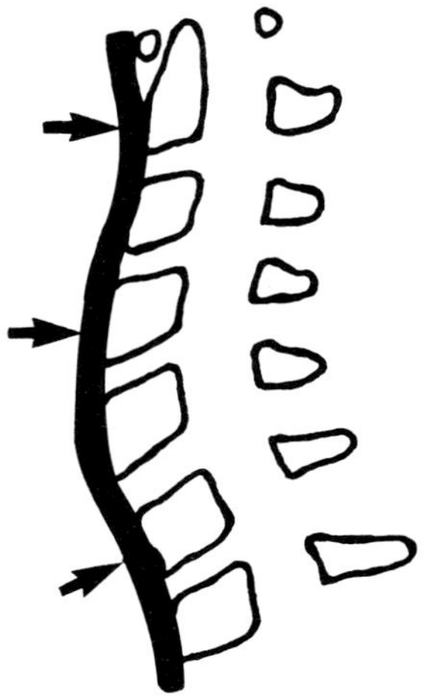

960 C
250 T
680 C

Predicts Upper Cervical Fracture/Dislocation

Figure 3b.

*Units of Strain.

Clevis Free, Anterior Loading, Initially Straight Spine (Simulates Concentrated Impact Which Allows Head to Nod).

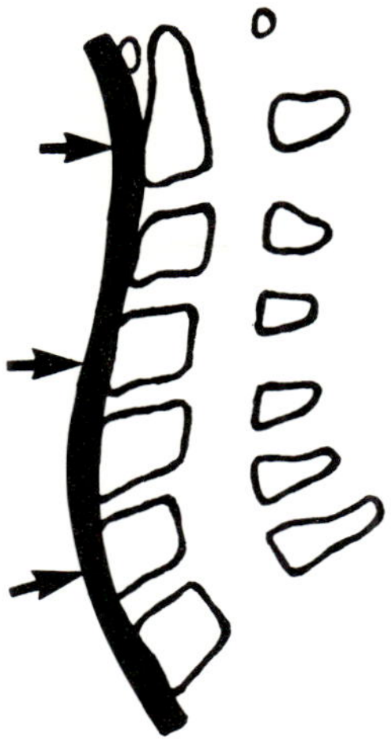

1200 C
350 C
250 T

Predicts Upper Cervical Fracture

Figure 3c.

Clevis Fixed, Anterior Loading, Initially Straight Spine (Simulates Distributed Impact Which Prevents Head Nodding).

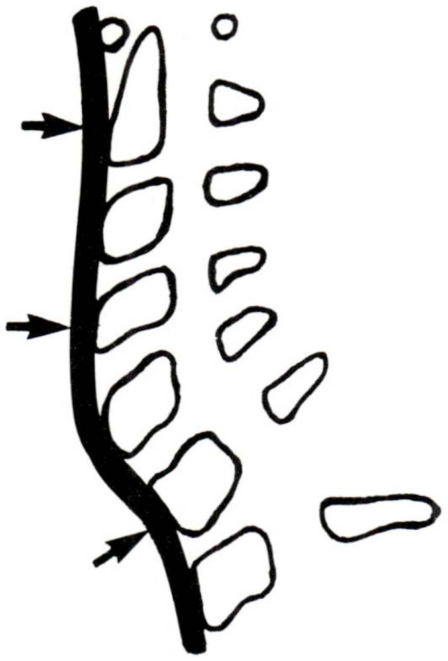

860 C
310 T
1200 C

Predicts Lower Cervical Fracture/Dislocation

Figure 3d.

(Figure 5). Shown superimposed on the data is the best estimate of axial compression tolerance for young (high school and college) football players, and a lower curve for the adult population. The peak load of 1500 lb (6.67 kN) is in good agreement with the findings of Roaf (7) who loaded 18 spinal units* in compression and achieved uniform results of 1400 lb (6.23 kN) at which point the load fell off slightly, coincident with end plate bulging, and 1600 lb (7.12 kN) ultimate strength due to disc failure. A live injury film study by Torg, et al., estimated a peak range of 790–1390 lb (3.5 kN-6.2 kN) was involved in a crown impact which produced quadriplegia due to unilateral dislocation of C3–C4. It should be observed that the neck in the Hybrid III dummy has only been calibrated for flexion and extension movements in the sagittal plane and not for axial loading. However, it was and is the only physical model available and was used to begin getting a handle on the problem. Bauze and Ardran (8) experimenting statistically with an entire cervical spine subject to axial compression, flexion and horizontal shear forces, produced bilateral dislocation with only 319 lb (1.42 kN) applied force.

2.2.2.2 Distributed Crown Loading in the Cadaver—In the tests with the Hybrid III dummy it appeared that axial neck loads could be attenuated by interspersing energy absorbing material between the crown of the dummy and the impacting surface. However, this was found not to be the case in the cadaver as can be observed by studying the data in Table 1. Several thicknesses and types of resilient foams that varied in degree of stiffness did not have a significant effect on the strain in the cadaver neck for what was considered to be crown axial loading. One reason for this difference was that the dummy was relatively much stiffer in the axial direction than the cadaver. The dummy neck, which has a slenderness ration ($1/r \simeq 15$)* does not even qualify as a column, i.e., would fail in compression before buckling. On the other hand, the cadaver neck is usually in some state of curvature at impact, which curvature is further exaggerated by axial compression loading.

Other reasons for the lack of attenuation with crown padding in the cadaver are that the effects of an impact are very sensitive to the line of action (Figure 6) and blow location (Figure 7). It can be seen in Figure 6 that minimum strain was recorded for force alignment with the relatively straight cervical spine, and maximum strain was recorded when the cervical spine was in flexion for impacts to the same location on the head. In Figure 7 the minimum strain was recorded for blows to the forehead as compared to blows on the crown of the head for any location. As will be noted from the peak force data (shown on the head), the minimum force on the head was also recorded for the forehead impacts. Consequently, the strain in the neck was less for the forehead impacts because less body mass was involved in inertia loading the neck caudally.

For any blow location or line of action in the sagittal plane the only method found to be effective in relieving the strain in the neck of the cadaver wearing a protective helmet was by means of a silicon putty collar (silly putty), in which the putty was stuffed like a sausage inside a clear flexible vinyl tube. The collar was interposed between the helmet and shoulder pads and stiffened upon impact, partially transferring some of the load around the neck into the shoulders as the neck would otherwise be compressed (Table 1). Culver, et al., have found that a peak force of 1280 lb (5.7 kN) is a level above which cervical spine fractures will begin to occur in fresh cadavers subject to their crown loading conditions (12).

*Spinal Unit: Two vertebral, an intervertebral disc, two posterior articulations and a number of ligaments.

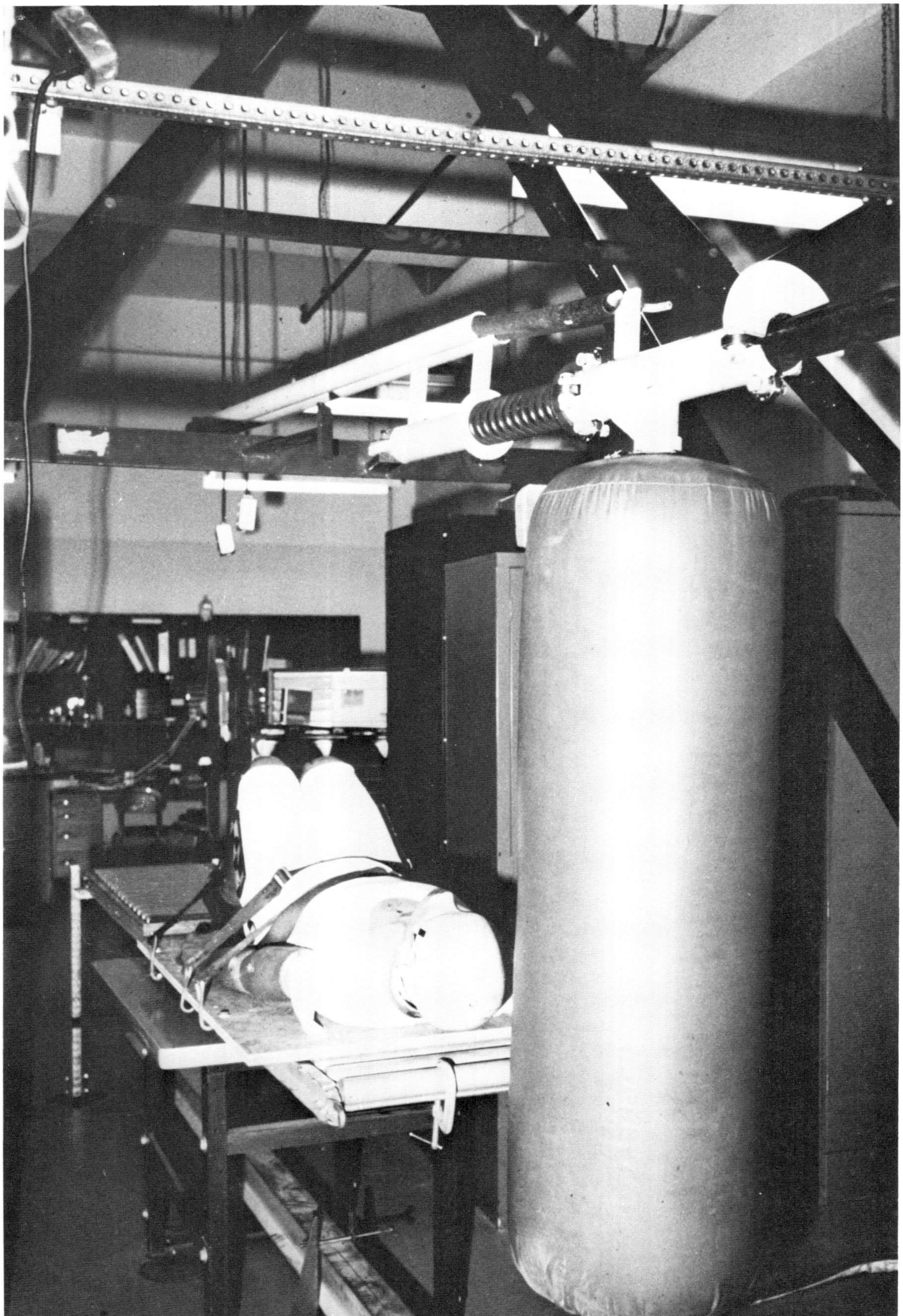

Figure 4.

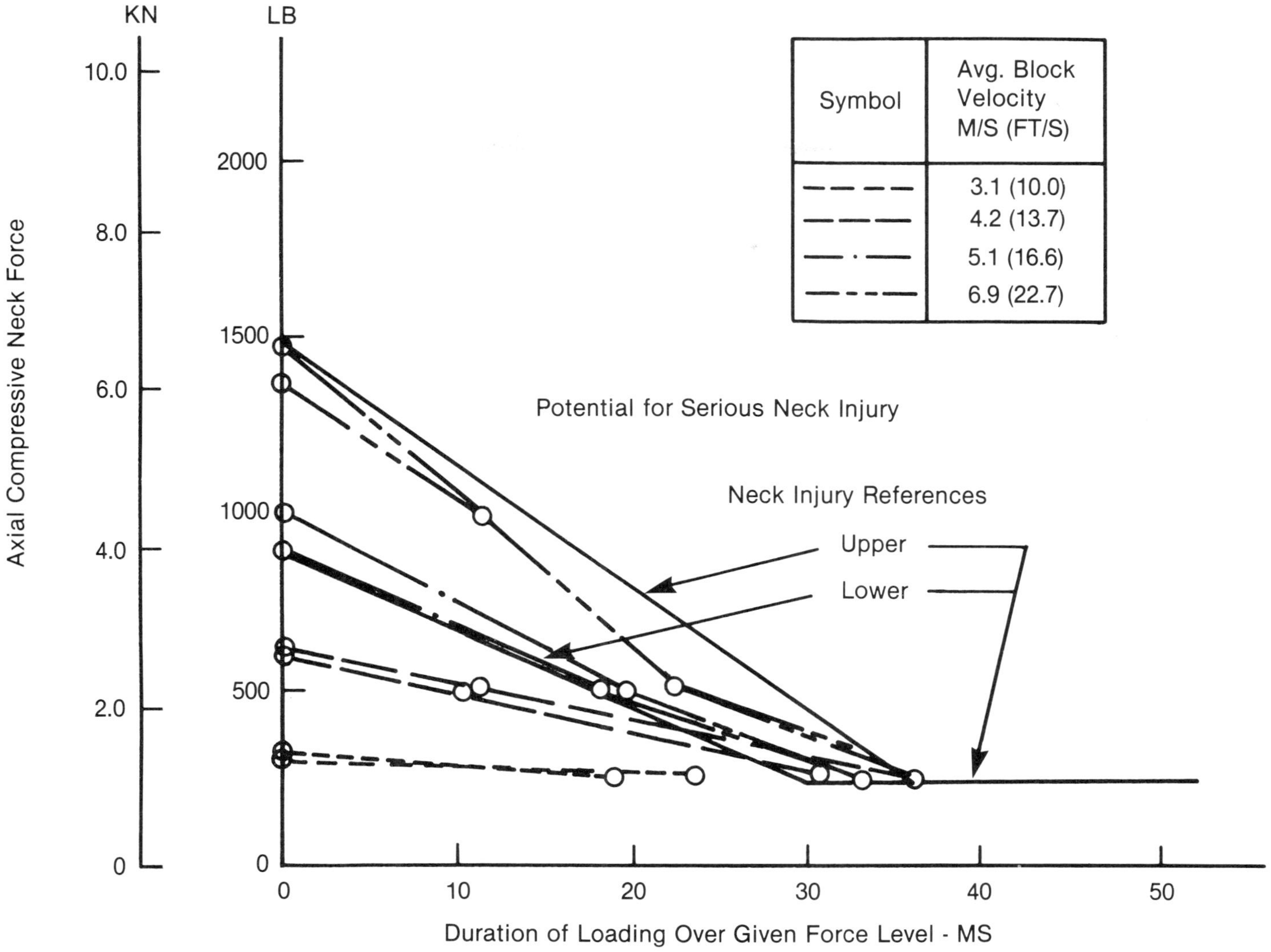

Figure 5.

2.2.2.3 Concentrated Loading — Compression-Flexion With Torsion—Roaf (7) has shown that, using a cervical spine unit, the spine is very strong in compression and flexion but very weak in torsion. After studying the problem of neck injury with segments, he predicted that a unilateral dislocation could occur only with torsion. Shown in Figure 8 are excerpts taken at a film speed of 500 fps during an impact with a dummy knee to a helmeted head, approximately in the sagittal plane and anterior to the crown. The concentrated load allowed nodding at the atlanto-occipital axis and at an energy level of 164 ft-lb (222 N.m) compression, and high cervical flexion occurred with no failure. Increasing the energy of impact of the knee to 263 ft-lb (357 N.m) produced the unilateral dislocation of the left C2–C3 facets as shown on film. When filming perpendicular to the plane of motion, which was essentially in the sagittal plane, it is difficult to detect when torsion occurred, and it appeared at first that the primary motion prior to dislocation was compression-flexion. However, further study has shown that as the motion continued, a considerable amount of tor-

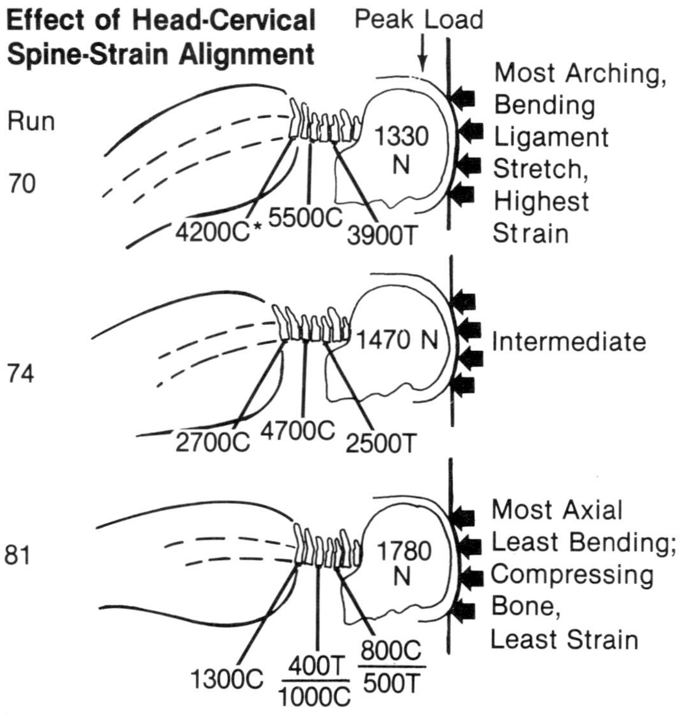

Figure 6.

*Units of Strain

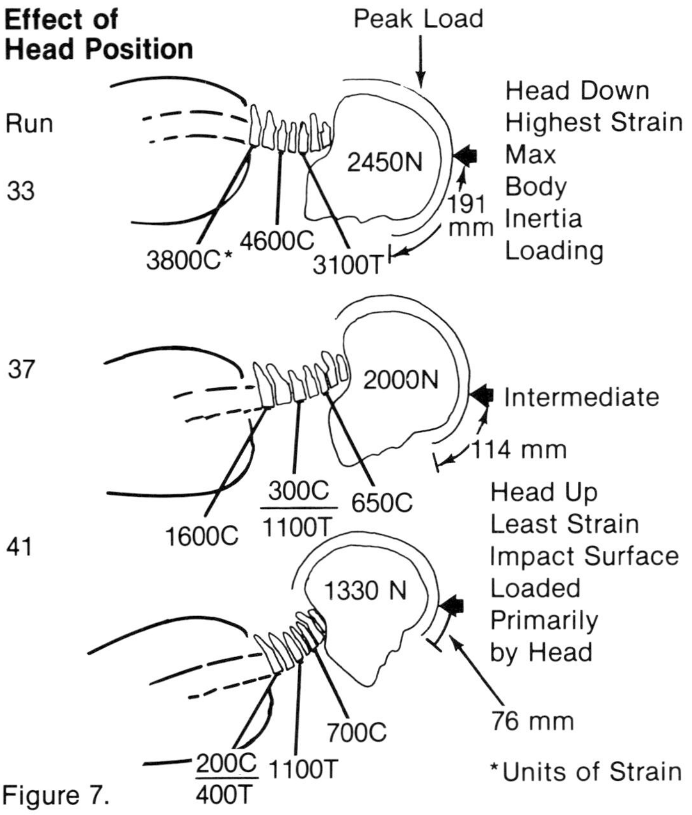

Figure 7.

sion was apparent as the jaw swung in the direction of the dislocated left side, and very likely started well before and contributed to the dislocation as predicted by Roaf (7).

2.2.2.4 Extension Due to Direct Impact of the Head Through a Lever—The neck is probably more amenable to prediction of the mechanics of injury, tolerable levels of injury and mathematical modeling in flexion or extension loading modes than it is in the axial compression mode. Mertz and Patrick were among the first to investigate the situation of extension and flexion due to inertial head loading in cadavers and volunteers and have published load limits in terms of forward flexion at the occipital condyles of 140 ft-lb (47–57 N.m) for rearward extension (9).

Carter and Frankel (10) have recently made a biomechanical analysis of the situation in which the neck is extended due to a force with a-p and caudocephalad components applied to a face guard attached to a helmet. The purpose of the Carter-Frankel model was to test the "guillotine" mechanism suggested by Schneider and co-workers (11). Schneider had urged that helmets be cut higher posteriorly so that they would not impact the cervical spine in hyperextension,

Table 1. Crown 'Energy Absorption Inadequate' Theory:
Effect of Energy Absorber (EA) Material on Cervical Spine Strain Due to Crown Impacts by 49 Kg MASS

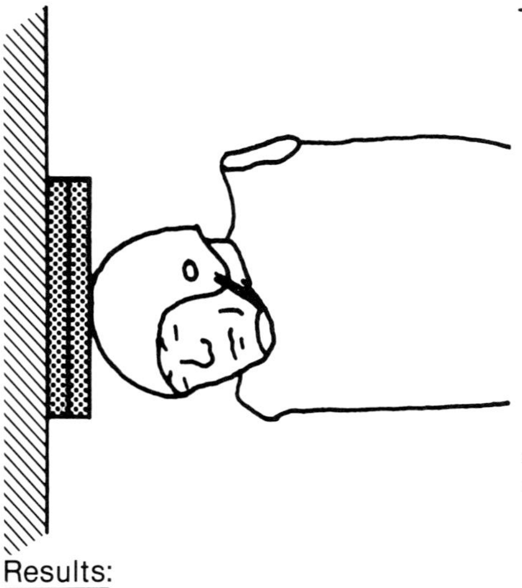

Run	Pad Type	Pad Thickness mm	Helmet	Peak Force kN	Tension C_3	Compression C_5	C_7
61	No	—	No	2.0	3700	5200	4400
68	Firm	76	No	1.8	3700	5500	4700
69	Firm	76	Yes	1.3	3700	5200	4000
72	Soft	76	Yes	1.3	3800	5200	3840
'Silly Putty' Collar							
102	No	—	Yes	2.0	700	1600	960

Results:

Practical Amounts of Padding Did Not Significantly Reduce Strain Because:

1. Axial Loading of a Straight Spine Is Usually Distributed Over a Large Head Area (~ 129 cm^2). Therefore Padding Is Relatively Stiff, Doesn't Dissipate Much Energy by Deformation, and

2. In Case of Off-Axis Impact with a Curved Spine the Padding Is in Series with a Softer Ligament Stretching System Over which it Has Little Control.

3. Energy Available Is Much Greater than Can Be Asorbed by Practical Amounts of Padding Worn on the Helmet Crown.

4. A 'Silly Putty' Collar Was Very Effective in Reducing Cervical Spine Strain. It Is Assumed to Act by Stiffening Under Impact to Transfer Loads from Helmet to Shoulder Pads and Provide a Simulated Tensed Muscle Lateral Stability.

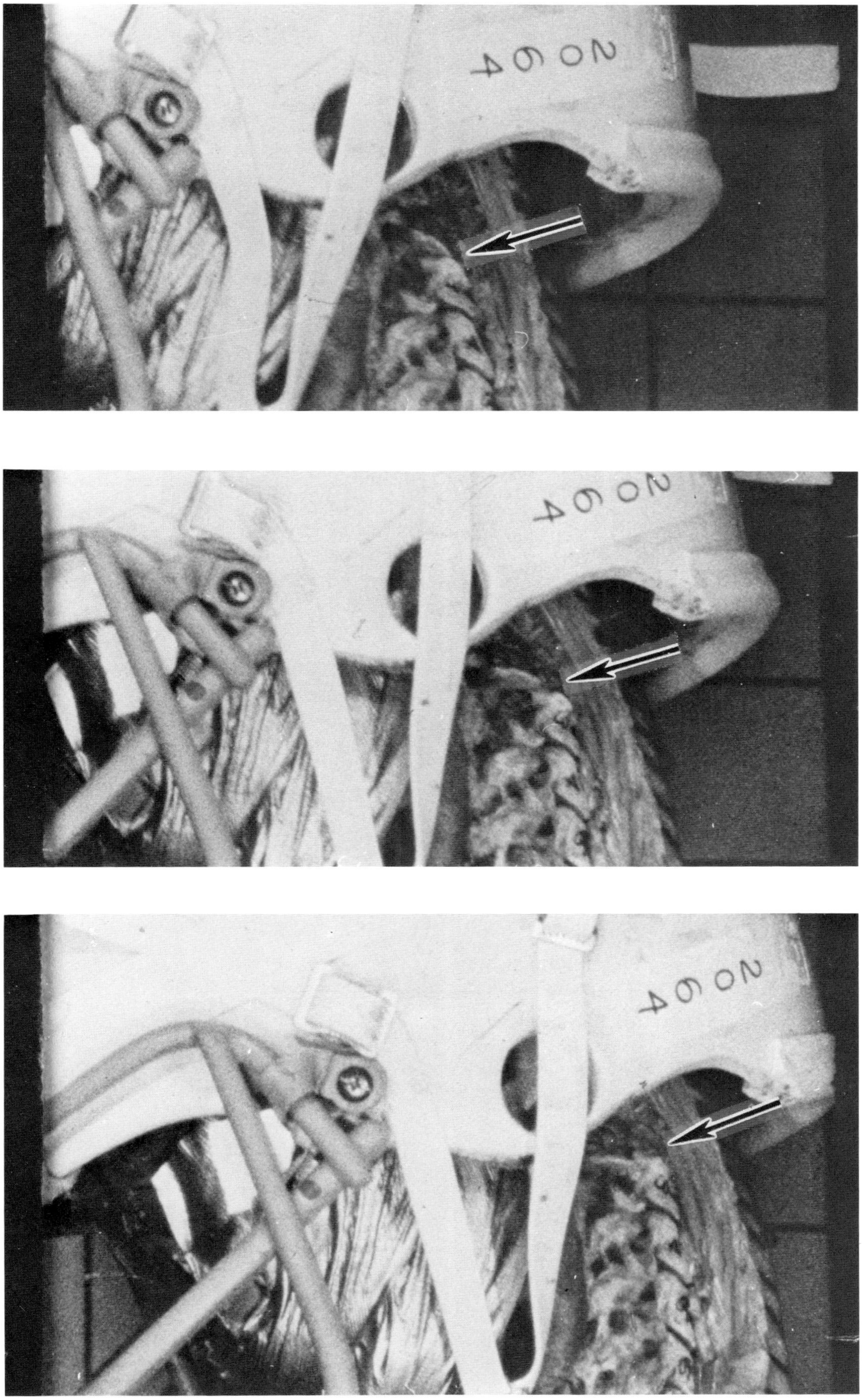

Figure 8.

thus theoretically preventing serious injuries to the spine at the point of impact (10). Several manufacturers of football helmets and crash helmets have been influenced enough to raise the rear rim of their helmets to avoid this alleged injury mechanism. The two dimensional model of Carter and Frankel assumed a hinge at C1–C2 allowing only shear to act and a bending moment with shear acting at the C7–T1 juncture. They then considered the effects of impingement of the posterior rim of the foramen magnum in the skull striking C1, and comparing this to the rim of the helmet striking C4, or the rear of the helmet striking the shoulder pads. They concluded that the worst case was when the helmet did not strike the back of the neck and that both shear strain and bending moment were relieved when the helmet contacted either the neck at midcervical or the shoulder pads. They concluded that when the helmet did impinge midcervical, maximum shear was directed posteriorly at the atlanto-occipital junction which would tend to cause posterior displacements of vertebrae superior to the vertebra level of impingement by the rear rim of the helmet. Their findings were that Schneider's theory is untenable and that the helmet impinging on either the neck or shoulder pads of the wearer helped limit extension and thereby reduced the shear and bending in cervical spine compared to the case of no helmet impingement. Their findings also refuted abuses of Schneider's hypothesis in the courts. Frequent charges have been made and continue to be made on behalf of injured plaintiffs that injuries which appear on x-rays to have occurred from compression-flexion loading with forward displacement of the superior over the injured vertebra, have been caused by Schneider's extension-guillotine mechanism, thereby sometimes indicting the helmet for improper design.

A static guillotine of a cadaver neck was conducted for the purpose of examining the mechanics of failure in this mode of loading. The guillotine blade of steel had a $^{3}/_{16}$ in. (4.8 mm) round rod welded across its 6 in. (152 mm) length, simulating the rear rim of a helmet. Load was applied to the back of the neck with the forehead resting on a load cell and from chest to feet the body was supported by a rigid table. Figures 9a-d show the successive x-rays as the spine was flexed and broken by the load. Initial failure is shown in Figure 9c. Tension in the anterior longitudinal ligament developed as the neck was forced into increased extension, finally resulting in an avulsion fracture of C2 body which is the cranial attachment of the ligament. Subsequent separation of the C2–C3 intervertebral disc occurred and the head and neck above C3 were forced posteriorly and superiorly, hinged by ligaments attached to C2–C3 spinous processes. This high cervical failure agreed with the predication by Frankel and Carter (10) on the bases of their analysis.

Further experimental evidence against the guillotine mechanism and its effect on the design of helmets was determined dynamically, by comparing the effect on the neck of high and low cut helmets when subjected to impact forces acting through the face guard as shown in Table 2. The high cut helmet allowed 13 degrees more extension and produced significantly

Table 2. 'Guillotine' Theory:

Effect of Knee to Faceguard Impact Standard vs High Cut Rear Shell RIM-610 mm Drop

	Strain[1] in/in							of Ext. Rotation- Deg.
	Facets			Anterior Body				
Helmet	C2	C3	C5	C2	C3	C4	C5	
Standard Suspension	-1030	550	-300	-480 150	1100	1140	270	28
High Cut[2] (Padded)	-1320	900	-320	-260 260	1380	1330	500	41
% Change	28	64	7	—	24	16	85	46

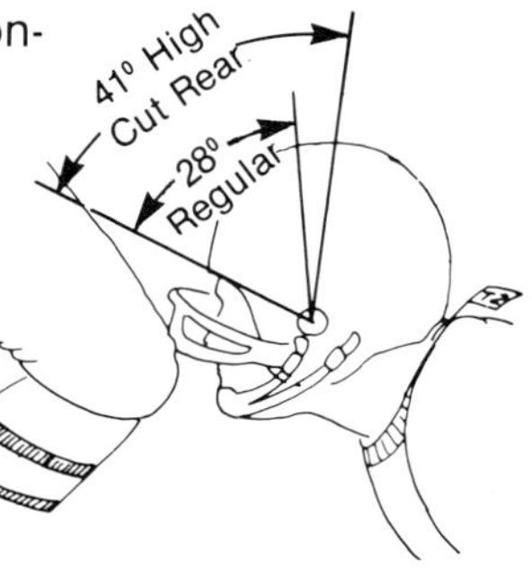

[1] (-) Indicates Compression
[2] Done First

Results:

No Injury Was Produced
Rear Rim Impinged in C7-T2 Area
Higher Cutout Caused More Extension and Larger Strains

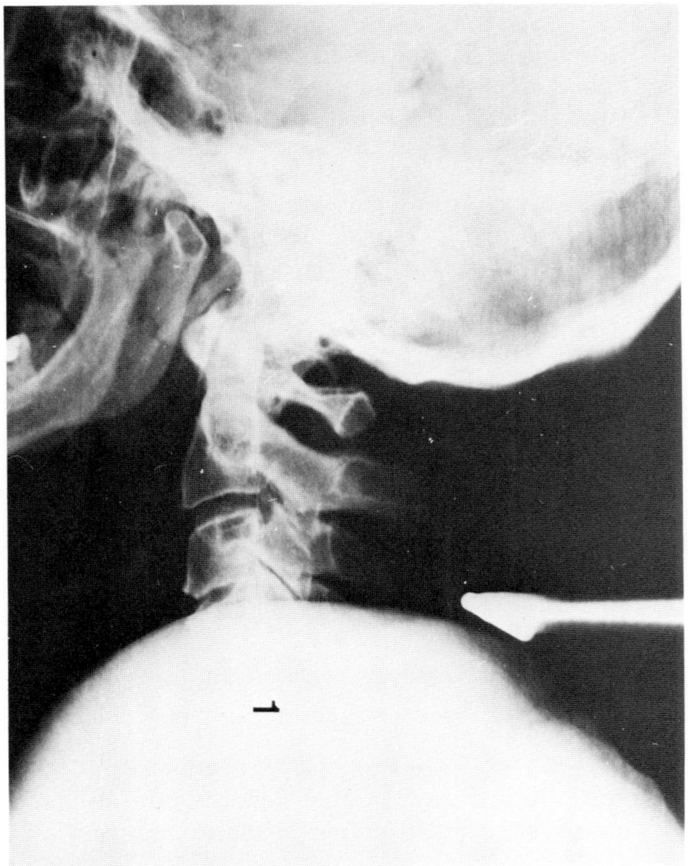

Figure 9a.

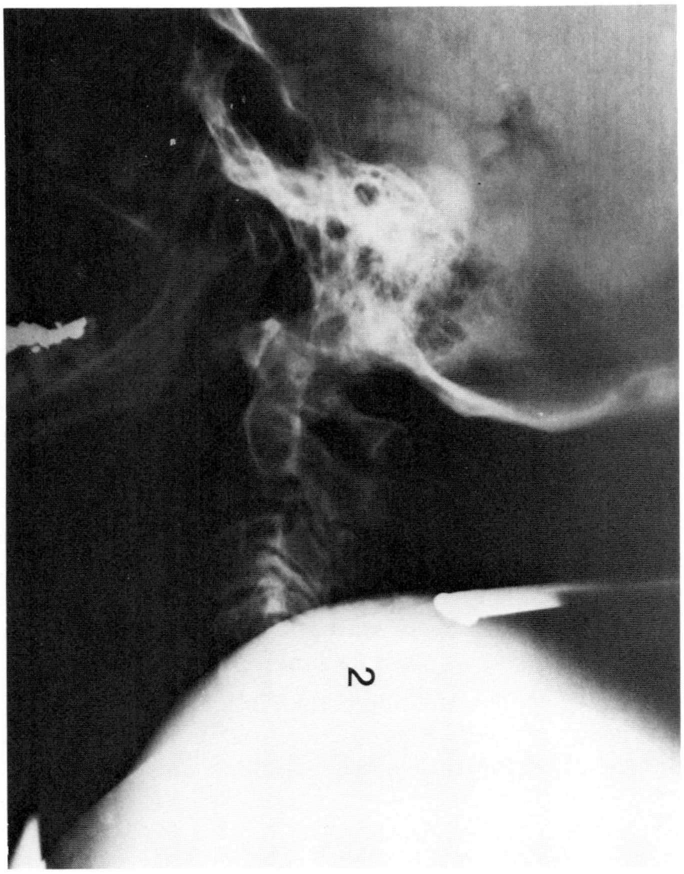

Figure 9 b.

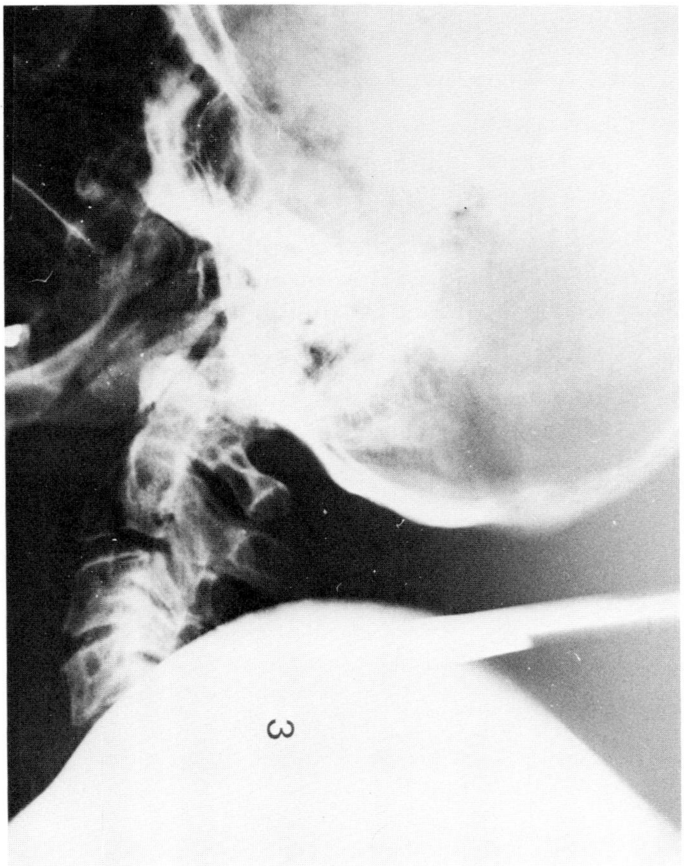

Figure 9c.

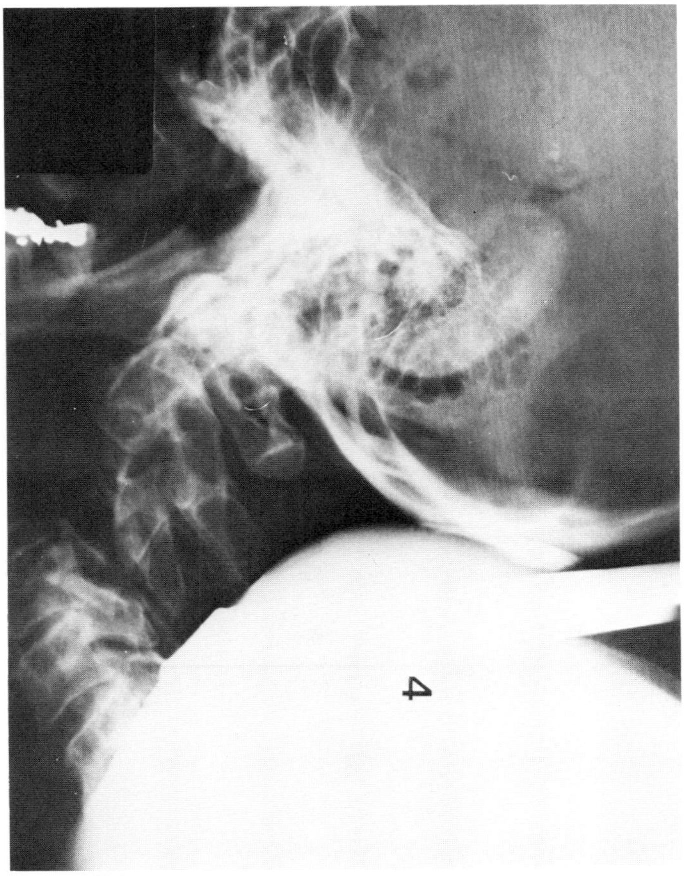

Figure 9d.

higher strains in six out of seven strain locations on the anterior bodies of the vertebra and near the superior facets at locations on the cervical spine between C2 and C5.

3. Conclusions

1. The mechanics of cervical spine injury are more clearly understood with the help of neck cutdowns and high speed photography, standard and cineradiography as well as strain gages, in conjunction with accelerometer and force transducer measurements.

2. Specific neck loading conditions such as extension and flexion resulting from torso acceleration, as well as axial compression loading in cadavers and dummies have been investigated by several groups and tolerable limits under these conditions have been published (9).

3. For compression loading in general there are too many variables affecting cervical spine injury to publish suggested tolerable limits presently.

4. The potential for establishing tolerable limits, devising methods of protection and improving the fidelity of mathematical models, depends upon further understanding of the mechanics of cervical spine injury due to head impact.

4. Recommendation

It is recommended that cadaver and dummy static and dynamic head loading experiments be conducted to investigate separately and later in combinations, the effects of axial, off-axis, torsional and transverse shear loading.

References

1. Hodgson VR and Thomas LM: Mechanisms of cervical spine injury during impact to the protected head. *24th STAPP Car Crash Conference.* 1980 Society of Automotive Engineers, Inc.
2. Mueller F and Blyth C: Catastrophic and neck football injuries. *Physician and Sportsmedicine* 8:10. 1980
3. Torg JS, Truex Jr RC, Marshall J, Hodgson VR, Quedenfeld M, Spealman AD and Nichols III CE: Spinal injury at the level of the 3rd and 4th cervical vertebrae from football. *J of Bone and Joint Surg:59A*:8. Dec 1977
4. Nachemson A: Lumbar interdiscal pressure. *Acta Orthop Scand 43 (suppl).* 1960. In book *Sports injuries—the unthwarted epidemic,* ed. Vinger PF and Hoerner EF. PSG Publishing Co., Littleton MA. 1981
5. Torg JS, Truex Jr R, Wuendenfeld TC, Burstein A, Spealman AD and Nichols III C: National football head and neck injury registry: report and conclusion 1978. *JAMA 241:*14. Apr 1979
6. Mertz HJ, Hodgson VR, Thomas LM and Nyquist GW: An assessment of compressive neck loads under injury-producing conditions. *The Physician and Sportsmedicine* 6:11. Nov 1978. McGraw-Hill
7. Roaf R: A study of the mechanics of spinal injury. *J of Bone and Joint Surg 60B(2)*:95–106. 1978
8. Bauze RJ and Ardran MA: Experimental production of forward dislocation in the human cervical spine. *J of Bone and Joint Surg 42B(4)*:810–823. 1960
9. Human tolerance to impact conditions as related to motor vehicle design—SAE J855. Soc of Automotive Engrs, Inc. Apr 1980
10. Carter DR and Frankel VH: Biomechanics of hyperextension injuries to the cervical spine in football. *Am J of Sports Med 8*:5. 1980
11. Schneider RC: *Head and neck injuries in football—mechanisms, treatment, and prevention.* Williams & Wilkins Co. (Balto). 1973
12. Culver RH, Bender M and Melvin JW: Mechanisms, tolerance and responses obtained under dynamic superior-inferior head impact. OSHA Final Report. May 1978

Comments on Soft Tissue Injuries of the Neck

Victor H. Frankel, M.D.

The soft tissues of the cervical spine consist of the named ligaments of the neck, ligamentum annulus, nucleus pulposis and the muscles. The ligaments act as kinematic restraints controlling, limiting and guiding motion of the spinal segments. The disc structures act as shock absorbers modifying the stresses from impact loading and also perform kinematic functions. The muscles, in addition to their motor activity, are a major source of energy dissipation and shock absorption. In order to allow for motion, the ligaments must be extensible. Their basic characteristics are indicated in Figure 1, a force elongation curve. Zone 1, the toe portion, allows for motion with very little internal force; Zone 2 is a physiological range in which the ligaments become stiffer with elongation; Zone 3 starts the failure region in which cartilage fibers are disrupted and finally at Zone 5 there is complete ligamentous failure. This is illustrated in Figure 2 correlating motion with ligamentous function and trauma. Ligaments exhibit viscoelastic properties so that the rate of loading is very important in predicting whether or not ligament failure will result.

Muscles as they function follow the well-known Blix curve for length-tension characteristics. There is an optimum tension for each muscle length. If the muscle is contracted, and the length changed, reflex relaxation of the muscle must take place or else muscle ruptures will result. This is important when one considers hyperextension of the neck as occurs in deceleration injury of the neck. If the sternocleidomastoid muscles are contracted, and the head accelerated backwards rapidly, a rupture may result. Since muscle

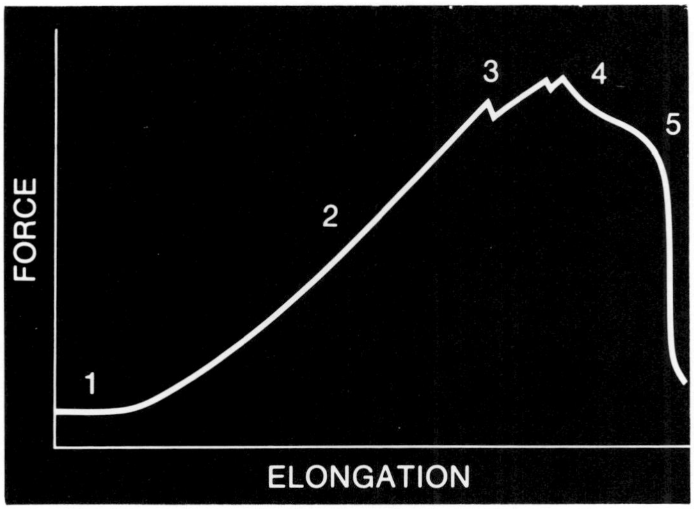

Figure 1.

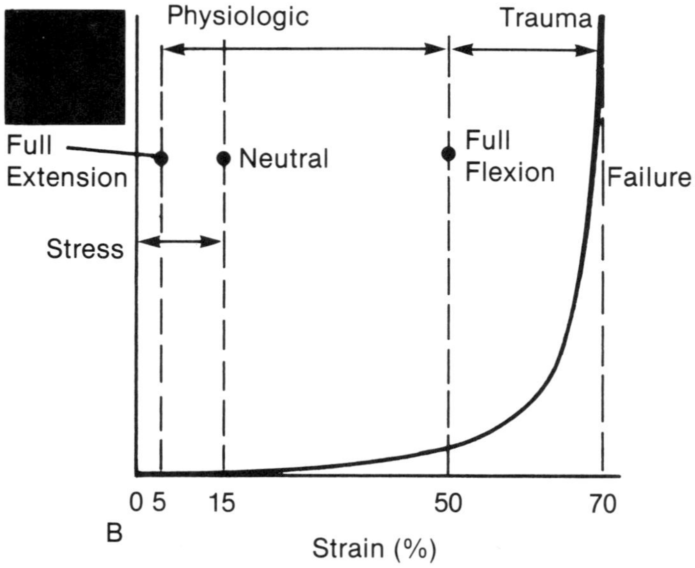

tension for the same length is higher in an eccentric (muscle contraction while the muscle is being extended) than during a concentric contraction, higher internal stresses may result in muscle rupture.

The nerves in the neck may also be damaged by rapid and forced neck motion. Roots may be evulsed or nerve trunks damaged as they course through the thick investing fascia of the neck to attain their cutaneous distribution. Trauma to ligaments and muscles surrounding the nerves may lead to hemorrhage and nerve compression. In addition to the lower cervical roots supplying the arm and easily identifiable clinically, the nerves emanating from the cervical plexus whose distribution is to scalp, neck and upper shoulders may also be damaged and overlooked.

Motion of the cervical spine in the important flexion and extension ranges occurs about an instantaneous center of rotation (Figure 3). This instantaneous center of rotation bears a relationship to the facet joints so that when flexion and extension occur, sliding of the facet joint also occurs. If uncontrolled motion of the neck occurs during trauma, or altered motion of the neck results from ligamentous or muscular damage, and the neck is forced to rotate about an abnormal instantaneous center of rotation, pain can result from abnormal motion of the joints. There will be an abnormal stress and strain distribution in the ligaments and disc mechanism. This may lead, if chronic, to degenerative changes in the cervical spine. Figure 3 (left) illustrates normal motion about a normal instantaneous center of rotation and Figure 3

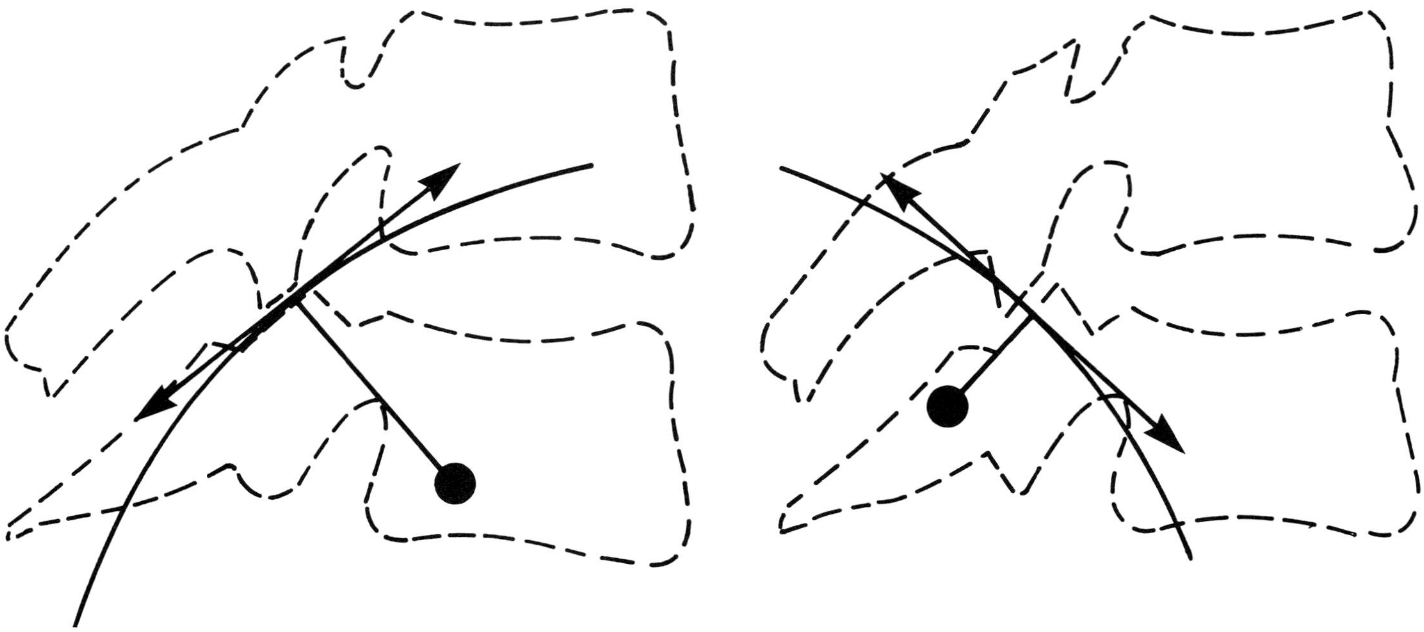

Figure 3.

(right) abnormal motion about a displaced instantaneous center of rotation. Alternate compression and distraction of the joint surfaces occur with flexion-extension in the latter.

In impact loading of the head or inertial loading of the neck, the soft tissues may be loaded past their failure levels resulting in dangerous cervical spine dislocations due to the loss of soft tissue integrity. Fracture-dislocations may also result from rupture of ligaments and evulsion of their bony attachments due to similar loading mechanisms.

The behavior of the cervical spine and its constituent substructure is well understood in a qualitative manner. It is necessary to develop qualitative data drawing upon the disciplines of biomechanics, orthopaedic and neurological surgery and muscle physiology in order to develop a qualitative understanding of the injury mechanism and load tolerances of the cervical spine.

References

1. Frankel, V.H., and Nordin, Margareta: *Basic Biomechanics of the Skeleton System,* Lea & Febiger, Philadelphia, 1980.
2. Noyes, F.R. and Grood, E.S.: "The Strength of the Anterior Cruciate Ligament in Humans, and Rhesus Monkeys." *J. Bone and J. Surgery,* 58A; pp. 1704–1082, 1976 (1&2)
3. White, A.A., and Panjabi, M.M.: *Clinical Biomechanics of the Spine,* J.B. Lippincott Company, Philadelphia, 1978.

SESSION 2, PART 3:

Closing Comments on Head and Neck Injury

Session 2, Part 3

Theoretical and Physical Models for Head and Neck Injuries

Closing Comments on Head and Neck Injury Criteria Discussions

A. K. Ommaya, M.D.

It would appear from our discussions that much further work remains to be done. In the interim, it may be useful to suggest sources for some improvements which could be made in criteria based on available data for injuries in these two body areas. For the head it seems necessary to suggest at least **two** criteria; firstly for the contact phenomena of head impacts which primarily address the lesions related to skull fracture. The HIC and other criteria such as the Michigan Strain criterion could be used with suitable adjustment for tolerances at varying AIS levels. Secondly, because of the overwhelming importance of inertial loading effects, particularly those related to rotation of the head, there should be separate provisions for a head injury criterion based on measurement of angular acceleration as indicated in our previous work on three sub-human primate species suitably scaled for extrapolation to the human. It would also be necessary to include in such criteria the important variable of **rate of onset** of the inertial loading.

Turning to the neck, it would also appear to be necessary to suggest at least two sets of criteria, i.e., to define levels of axial compressive, tensile and shear loading as well as torques sustainable by the neck, e.g., at the occipito-cervical junction as defined by the moment-envelopes of Mertz and Patrick. Work aimed at improved quantification of such criteria coupled with validation studies on human accident data is urgently required.

Problems in the Mathematical and Physical Modeling of Head and Neck Injury

Y. King Liu

The use of theoretical and physical models towards the establishment of human head and neck injury criterion is valid for the same reasons that models are valid in other branches of science. They systematize thinking and provide the framework for the retrospective delineation of the relative importance of the existing experimental evidence. Prospectively, these models make predictions and as such suggest experiments which otherwise might not have come to mind. Furthermore, mathematical models have the advantage of absolute repeatability. It is ideal from the point of view of control. Sensitivity studies involving the effects of system parameter variations are easily done. Once developed, theoretical models are perhaps the most compact and economical of all research methodologies available. In concert with experimental animal and cadaveric data, math-

One of the most difficult parts in the mathematical simulation process occurs during the idealization and problem formulation stage. It is at this stage where the knowledge and understanding of the investigator are brought to bear on the problem. The first order of business is to delineate what questions are to be answered. It is worth repeating the cliché: A well-posed problem is half the solution. Having posed the question, what methodologies are available to provide the solution? The mathematical solutions, once obtained, must be translated back to the physical domain and either viewed in the light of available experimental data or become the basis for experimental validation studies.

The critiques of the three papers presented in this section of the workshop should be viewed against the above backdrop. More importantly, these critiques are undertaken to identify the areas of possible improvement and not to detract from the original contributions already made by these authors. The format of these critiques is in question form.

I. Are stress waves important for the direct contact close-head impact problem?

Implicit in the past and current criteria, such as the Wayne State Curve (WSC), Gadd Severity Index (GSI) and the Head Injury Criterion (HIC) and their variants, is that stress waves are **not** relevant. As pointed out in Prof. Goldsmith's present paper and many times previously, e.g., von Gierke (1964) and Liu (1970a, 1970b), these "dose-response" type curves are based on the impact sensitivity procedure of Kornhauser (1962) associated with a linear spring-mass-dashpot system analysis.

The system response can be divided into approximately two regions at a critical pulse duration, t_c. For $t<t_c$, only the pulse area, which is equal to the imposed velocity change, is important. For $t>t_c$, the pulse shape is **the** important factor. If one were to assume that the elastic element always breaks at a given peak force level, the so-called **equal tissue strain assumption**, it is then possible to relate the damage or injury, through the system response, to the parameters of the input pulse. Typically, the result is plot of the maximum, or average, applied acceleration versus the duration of the pulse. In this tolerance graph, e.g., Figure 1 in Prof. Goldsmith's paper, the "knee" represents the critical duration, t_c. To its left, the region is sensitive to velocity-change and to its right, the peak acceleration of the pulse.

If one attempts to experimentally identify the system parameters, an immediate difficulty arises. Because the human body parts consist of **distributed** masses, generally no point can be picked where the displacements of the effective mass can be measured. Coermann (1961) circumvented this difficulty by adopting the concept of mechanical impedance. Specifically, mechanical, or driving point, impedance is defined as the ratio of the transmitted force to the velocity of that point where the force is transmitted. For such an elementary analysis, no stress wave propagation is possible since waves have infinite speeds in a **rigid** body.

If the head impact problem is modelled by deformable bodies, then stress waves do occur. The pertinent question is: To what extent do stress transients contribute to the field variables of interest in head injury? The simplest mathematical model consistent with explaining the physical phenomenon is the model proposed by Hayashi (1969) and improved by Liu and Chandran (1975). The system consists of a rigid but massless vessel (skull) containing elastic fluid (brain and cerebrospinal fluid). The vessel is attached to a linear spring k and dashpot c, which represent the composite elastic and damping properties of the helmet, skull, hair and elasticity of the wall. Thus, the problem can be simplified to that of a fluid "rod" enclosed in a rigid vessel with an attached spring and dashpot striking a rigid wall (Figure 1).

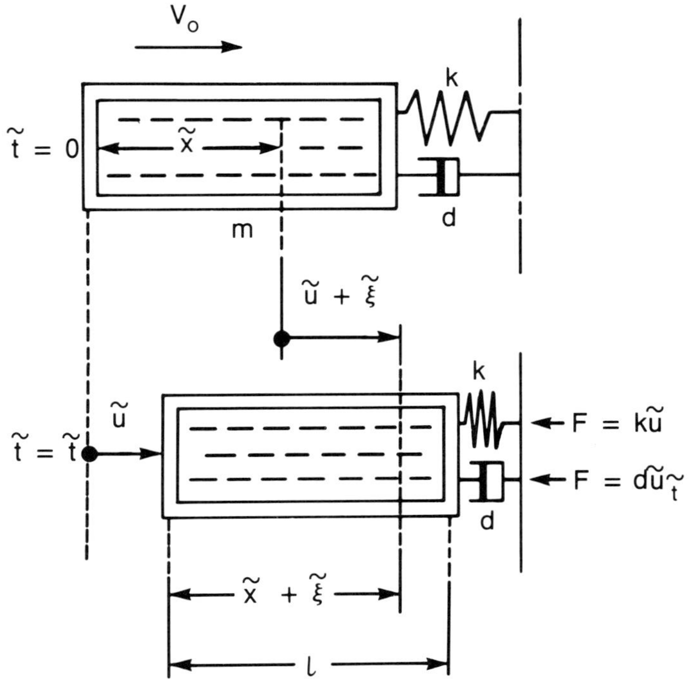

Figure 1. One-Dimensional Continuum Model of Head Impact, Liu and Chandran (1975)

The system response was obtained **exactly** and found to be dependent on four dimensionless ratios: (a) The brain to skull (and jaw) mass, μ; (b) the skull to closed brain stiffness, K; (c) the damping factor of the skull, Z; and (d) the impact velocity to the brain wave speed, V. The above parameters for the human head are: $\mu \leqslant 0.5$, $K \leqslant 0.01$, and $Z \leqslant 0.5$. Two typical dimensionless solutions are represented by Figures 2 and 3, where a, P and t are the dimensionless acceleration, pressure and time. The dimensionless pressure is a function of the normalized coordinate, x, i.e., $0 \leqslant x \leqslant 1$ and t. Note that the pressure and acceleration due to an incompressible fluid in the container are given by smooth curves, whereas the pressure and acceleration variations due to the compressible fluid are fluctuations about the smooth curves. In fact, the smooth curves appear to be the **mean** of the variations. Thus, for head impacts against a theoretically **rigid** barrier, the head acceleration and intracranial pressure are determined solely by the constituent stiffness and damping properties of the head. Experimental results have shown that contact impact duration on the skull with an almost rigid impactor is of the order of 1 to 4 ms. Thus, this contact time is at least an order of magnitude greater than the stress wave transit time through the closed intracranial fluid space, i.e., the cer-

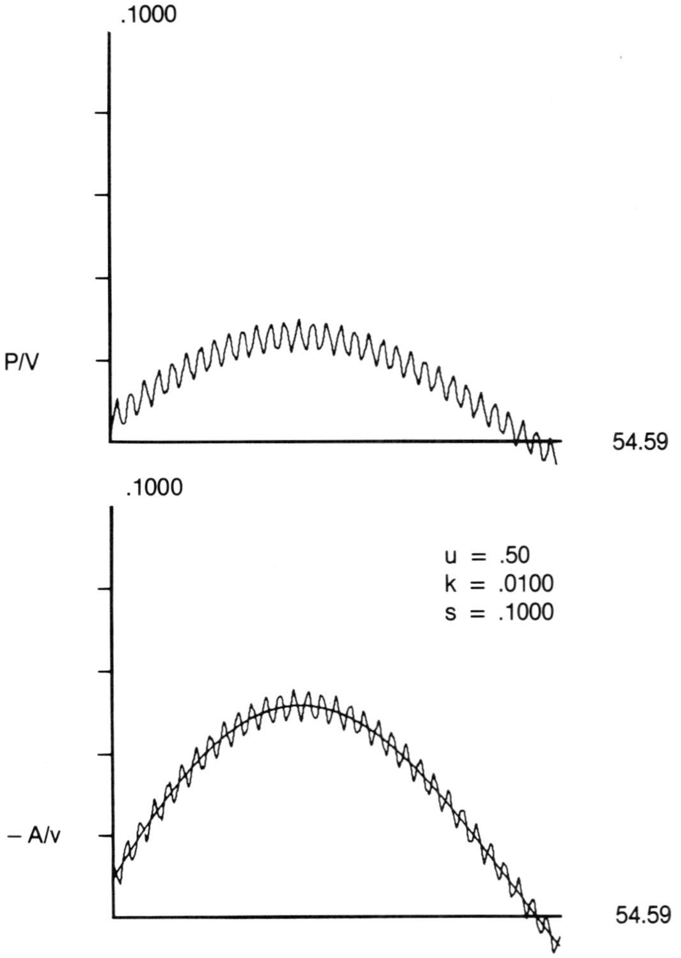

Figure 2. Contrecoup Pressure and Container Acceleration for the Parameter Values Shown. Note that the Mean Pressure Corresponds to the Result for Incompressible Fluid and the Pressure Fluctuations About the Mean Are the Results when the Fluid Compressibility Is Accounted for. From Liu and Chandran (1975).

ebrospinal fluid (CSF) and brain. In view of the vast differences between these time ratios, wave propagation effects are **not** expected to be important in such closed models of direct impact head injury, except perhaps in the coup region. Similar conclusions were given in Ripperger (1975).

II. When will the impact effects to the head be felt in the cervical spine?

The answer to this question depends on the contact duration and the direction of impact. Hosey and Liu (1982) recently synthesized a finite element model of the head and neck from the brain model of Ward and Thompson (1975), skull model of Hardy and Marcal (1971) and the neck model of Pontius and Liu (1975). Figure 4 illustrates a sagittal view of the model. Note in particular the continuity of the CSF space, brain and spinal cord materials was maintained throughout the intracranial spaces in order that the proper flow of "fluid-like" materials between the brain and spinal cord cavities can take place during the excitation of the model. Furthermore, the model mass distribution has been optimized with respect to the known experimental mass, center of mass and mass moment of inertia of the head and neck, making it an **anthropo-dynamic** model.

When this model was given an occipital half-sine impact of 6,000 N for 4-ms duration over an area of 26.7 cm^2, the solution indicated that the neck displacements were negligible until about 6 ms. Thus, an occipital contact impact of 4 ms affected the neck only marginally during the contact period, i.e., the material and geometrical properties of the neck are almost irrelevant since its displacements are small. After 6 ms, however, the displacements of the head will begin to substantially interact with the neck structures.

Using the same model, Hosey et al. (1982) studied the consequences of crown, or supero-inferior, impact.

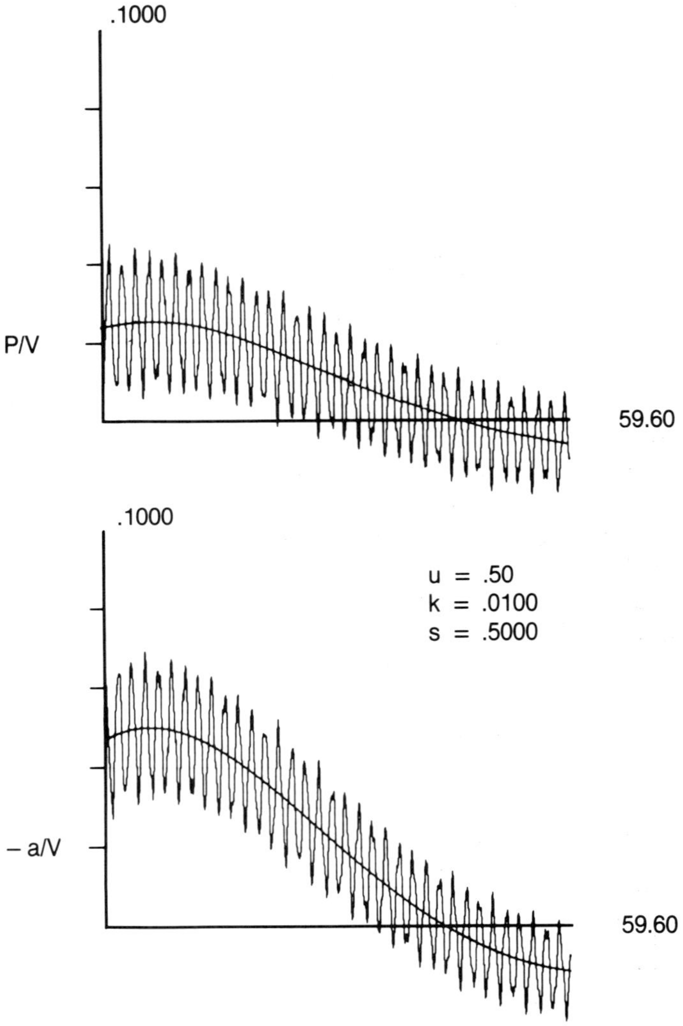

Figure 3. Contrecoup Pressure and Container Acceleration When the Damping Factor ζ Is Increased to 0.5 as Compared to Figure 2. From Liu and Chandran (1975).

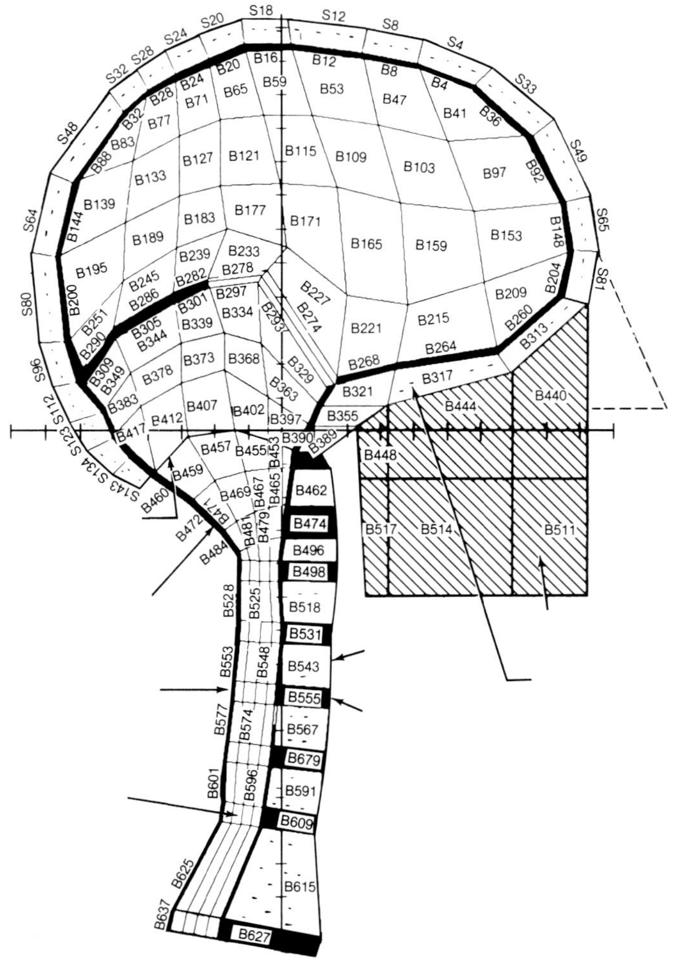

Figure 4. Sagittal View of the Homeomorphic Finite Element Model of the Human Head and Neck. From Hosey and Liu (1982).

For impact in the supero-inferior direction, the material and geometrical properties become extremely important. The average compressive stiffness of six young (aged 18–40) male cadavers, as well as some critical geometric dimensions, have been experimentally determined by Liu et al. (1981) and are reproduced below:

Location of disc	Stiffness (dynes/cm² x 10⁶)	Disc area (cm²)	Disc height (cm)	Equivalent Young's modulus (KPa)
H-C1	529.5	2.93	0.91	16,340
C1-C2	2,293.0	3.17	0.96	69,270
C2-C3	1,980.0	3.16	0.61	38,200
C3-C4	3,180.0	3.16	0.61	61,300
C4-C5	871.7	3.71	0.61	14,320
C5-C6	3,582.0	3.71	0.61	58,860
C6-C7	937.5	3.81	0.61	15,000
C7-T1	3,376.0	6.32	0.61	32,560

We note that the weakest disc locations are at H-C1, C4–C5, C6–C7, which correlates with the sites of fracture dislocation or subluxation in traumatic injuries to the cervical spine. With the above geometry, the total neck length, measured from the occipital condyles to the superior endplate of the T1 vertebra, is approximately 15 cm. The loading function is of the form: $F(t)=F_o \sin \omega t[H(t)-H(t-0.004)]$, where F_o=peak value of the loading time history, $H(t-\tau)$=Heaviside function starting at $t=0$ and ending at $t=\tau$, ω=circular frequency$=2\pi/0.008=2\pi(125)$.

For $F_o=1500$ N applied over 21 cm² (3.25 in.²) of the crown, the responses are:

(1) Maximum horizontal displacement of the cervical column nodes occurs at the C4 vertebra with a maximum anterior displacement of 2.8 mm at 6.0 ms. The vertical motion of the column is complicated. The maximum vertical displacements of the nodal points occur at various times (from 3.8 ms to 6.0 ms), indicating small vertebral rotations. Maximum vertical deflection occurs at the superior C1 vertebral posterior node with a maximum value of 1.4 mm at 5.0 ms. The maximum vertical displacement of the C4 vertebra occurs at the superior, anterior node with a value of −0.67 mm at 5.2 ms. To compare the displacement time-history of the cervical spine, we have plotted the initial configuration (Figure 5(a)), the configurations at t=6 ms for $F_o=1500$ N, Figure 5(b) and for $F_o=6000$ N, Figure 5(c).

(2) The cervical discs remain in compression throughout the 6-ms run. The maximum normal stress σ_z of the cervical discs and vertebrae occur at 4.4 ms. The average of all disc elements as well as the maximum values are:

Location of disc	Average σ_z(MPa)	Maximum σ_z(MPa)
C1–C2	−5.19	−5.90
C2–C3	−5.23	−5.01
C3–C4	−5.24	−5.40
C4–C5	−4.62	−4.79
C5–C6	−4.61	−4.63
C6–C7	−4.55	−4.62
C7–T1	−2.76	−2.72

(3) The maximum tangential stress in the skull (thin shell) elements does not exceed 0.86 MPa. These values occur in the crown region of impact between 1.8–2.2 ms, i.e., during the time of peak load (2.0 ms). Hence, the maximum tangential stress is far below the ultimate strength of 43.4 MPa for skull bone in tension.

(4) The normal stresses in a cord element at the C3 vertebral level remained positive throughout the 6-ms duration, i.e., the cord element was in a state of tension. The maximum normal stress σ_z was 0.028 MPa, which occurred at 4.2–4.4 ms (the same time as the disc and vertebral elements). The same behavior was observed in a cord element at the C3/C4 disc level with a maximum σ_z=0.039 MPa at 4.4–4.6 ms.

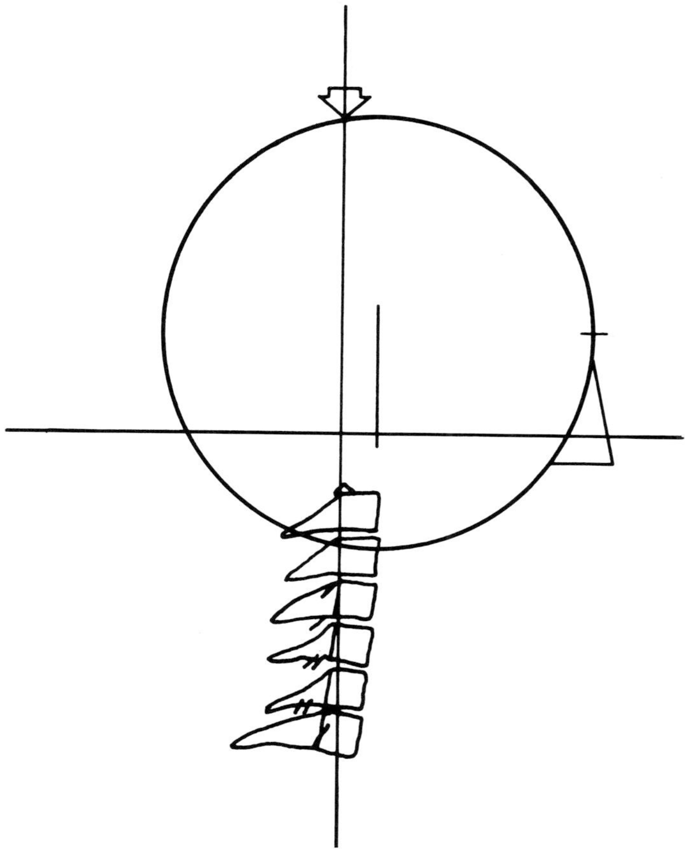

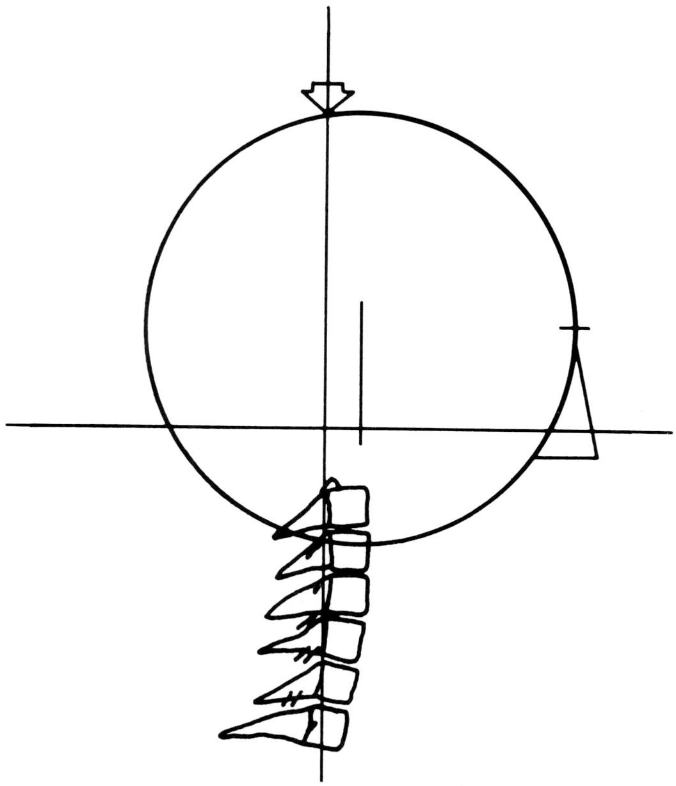

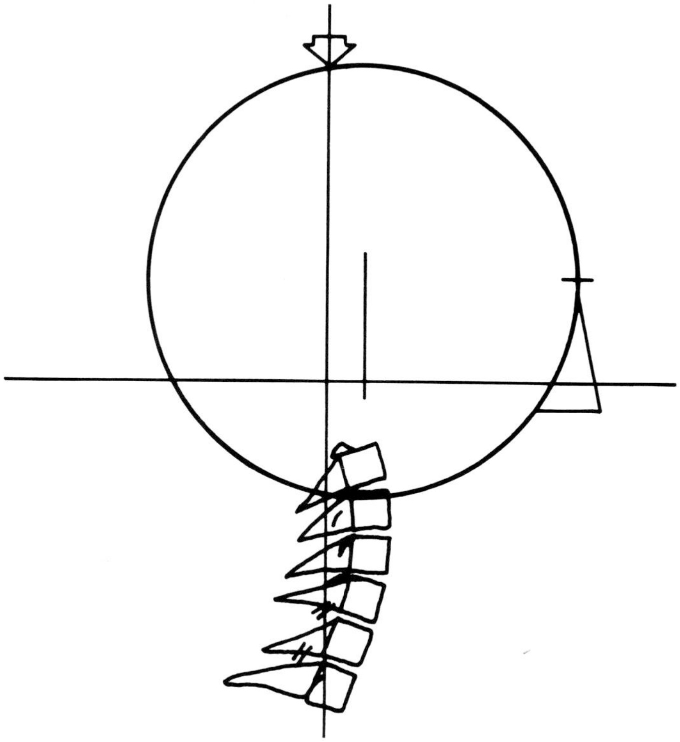

Figure 5. (a) Initial Sagittal Plane Configuration of the Human Head and Neck Prior to Crown Impact Shown Near the Vertex. (b) Configuration of Head and Neck at 6 ms for $F_0 = 1{,}500$ N Over a Contact Area of 21 cm^2 for an Impact Duration of 4 ms. (c) Configuration at 6 ms for $F_0 = 6000$ N Over a Contact Area of 21 cm^2 for an Impact Duration of 4 ms. From Hosey et al. (1982).

(5) Maximum compressive stress in a typical brain (brick) element (B53 near the center of the crown-load is −0.019 MPa at 1.8 ms. All normal stresses of this element become tensile at 3.4 ms, which is near the end of the contact (4 ms). The maximum tensile stress is 0.024 MPa at 5.0 ms.

The horizontal and vertical displacements computed for F_o=1500 N can be scaled linearly up or down since SAP IV is a linear code. For example, a maximum horizontal displacement of 2.8 mm occurred at the anterior node of C4 for F_o=1500 N at 6 ms. The maximum horizontal displacement for the same mode at the same time for F_o=6000 N is 11.2 mm.

Bauze and Ardan (1978) "compressively" loaded the entire cervical spine with the lower part fixed and the upper part free to move. Bilateral dislocation of the apophyseal joints without fracture was attained at 1420 N (332 lb). According to Liu et al. (1981), a maximum horizontal displacement of 2.8 mm at C4 is unlikely to cause fracture either. Since our present model does not account specifically for the apophyseal joints, we are not in a position to comment on the bilateral dislocations found experimentally. Culver et al. (1978) experimentally studied impact to the crown of fresh cadavers, which were placed in a supine position with the impactor axis aligned along the cervical spine. Their data showed that, for the "average" cadaver, a peak impact force of 5700 N (1293 lb) will result in cervical spine fractures. Post-experimental dissection revealed spinous process fractures predominate. The residual deformation is hyperextension of the normal lordosis which the authors characterized as "compressive arching." These experimental results are in qualitative agreement with the displacements shown in Figure 5(c) where an impact force of 6000 N was simulated. Nusholtz et al. (1981) extended the data base established by Culver et al. (1978) by additionally measuring the responses of the thoracic spine and torso. Of the 12 fresh cadavers tested, 10 sustained extension-compression type injury of the neck—further testimony to the qualitative agreement with our simulation results for $F_o = 6000$ N.

For a 6000-N crown impact load the maximum pressure in the brain is 0.097 MPa, which is below the cavitation pressure. Hence, the effect of the crown load in the brain region is not quite as severe as that observed from occipital impact where the pressure rose to 0.100 MPa. More of the impact energy from the crown load is absorbed by the spinal column as evidenced from the disc and vertebral body normal stresses shown in Hosey et al. (1982). These disc and vertebral body stress values are 2 orders of magnitude larger than the normal stresses in the brain, and 5 to 6 times larger than in the skull.

A simulation of crown impact to the human head, using the finite-element model of Hosey and Liu (1982), yielded the following insights:

(a) If the impact does not result in a skull fracture, most of the load is transferred to the cervical spine.

(b) For an impact load vector aligned along the C1–C2 axis, the most likely bony injury will be to the posterior elements of the cervical spine.

(c) The stresses are relatively uniform for different regions in the cervical spine as a result of crown impact.

(d) By enlarging (almost doubling) the contact area of the impact the stresses did not change appreciably.

(e) For crown impact, cavitation is unlikely to occur in the brain stem.

III. Can equal protection be provided the head and neck simultaneously?

The preliminary data of King et al., presented at this Workshop, on neck injuries in $-G_x$ impact is interesting in that it is an example of protecting one part of the human body at the expense of another, i.e., an impact with an air bag protected the chest and the head but increased the load on the neck to the point of injury. Increasing the available crush distance for the chest and/or the head, the magnitude of the contact forces is lowered but the contact duration is prolonged. According to the air bag pressure time histories given in the authors' Figures 6, 11 and 22, the contact durations for the 3 cadaveric impacts are roughly 120, 130 and 190 ms, respectively. The corresponding knee contact durations as shown in the authors' Figures 7, 12 and 23 are all approximately 80 ms. If one were to accept 4 ms as the contact duration between the chest and a relatively rigid object like the steering wheel, we note that the air bag prolonged the impact by an order of magnitude. During these additional times, the head may undergo hyperflexion and hyperextension while the chest is, relatively speaking, held in place (colloquially expressed as "pocketed"). Since the cadaveric heads were all appropriately instrumented, it is surprising that the authors did **not** compute the corresponding angular accelerations and velocities, which would have **quantitatively** characterized "the whipping of the head," which they believe to be the reason for the observed neck injury.

In what specific ways the model of Prasad and King (1974) was used "to resolve the paradox" of the severe neck injuries observed as a result of air bag restraint is not clear from their report. Presumably, the scenario goes as follows:

1) The cadaveric results showed neck injuries as a result of the impact parameters (given in Figures 3–12 and Figures 19–23);
2) These same, or similar, parameters, in addition to certain neck loads, were measured in a physical model (Hybrid III ATD) and presented in Figures 13–18;
3) Based on the "similarity" of responses between the cadaveric and Hybrid III results, the Hybrid III data are compared with a mathematical model output;
4) Having thus "validated" the mathematical model, the authors use it alone to compare the differences between air bag and seat belt restraints.

If indeed a belt system is "twice as stiff as the air bag," and there is no reason to doubt their assertion, the contact period between the chest and the belt system should be shortened. Presumably, with a belt system there will be no head contact at all. Finally, was the belt system a 3-point shoulder-lap type restraint? If so, the contact area would be very different as compared to the air bag system. Were these differences between the air bag and the belt restraint simulated in their model studies? If not, then the results given in the authors' Figures 24–33 should only be considered as interesting pilot data. To conclude that "If belts were used in place of the air bag, equally severe injuries could be expected to occur" based on the model studies alone, is premature. Assuming all the boundary conditions for the seat belt restraint were reasonably simulated, the predictions of the model should be checked by further cadaveric experiments.

A cursory comparison between the data for the cadavers and the Hybrid III–ATD show the following discrepancies:

1) If one were to compare the wave shapes for the head accelerations of the 3 cadavers with the Hybrid III–ATD, i.e., the authors' Figures 3, 4, 8, 9, 19 and 20 with Figure 13, there is a sharp spike at 300 ms which is absent in the cadaveric data;
2) At 200 ms, Figure 13 shows a negative acceleration of about 50 g's in the X-direction, whereas all cadaveric data show a positive acceleration varying from 40 to 150 g's;
3) The head acceleration in the Z-direction at 200 ms shows a positive peak value of 40 g's, whereas the range for the cadaveric data goes from 60 to 170 g's.

Thus, from the standpoint of dynamic similitude, the response of the Hybrid III–ATD is a far cry from the cadaveric results. The discrepancies are certainly understandable since the Hybrid III–ATD mimic neither the inertial properties of the cadaveric head and neck nor its material (or the stiffness) properties. Of the two properties, the inertial properties have been shown to be the more important. This is rightfully so, since we are dealing with an impact problem. Some inertial property data for the head and neck have been reported by Becker (1972) and Walker et al. (1973). Both builders of mathematical and physical models should, at least, account for these data. Material properties and some failure data for the cervical spine have been obtained by Liu et al. (1982). Without accounting for these two data sets, any model of the head and neck is incomplete.

A couple of examples from the papers presented at this Workshop will suffice to further illustrate these points. In the models of Ward and colleagues, the inertial property data is not part of the model formulation. Instead of using the impact force as input, they selected the head acceleration, which is acceptable. However, once a model is thus completed, it must meet the test of self-consistency, i.e., for a given set of initial and/or boundary conditions, the solutions should have validity on their own. If these solutions agree with one set of experimental data, one can be pleased. If its predictions for a different set of input conditions once again is validated by a new set of experiments, one has reasons to be moderately excited. However, if the isotropic material properties had to be changed in order to get the new agreement with the experimental data, then the model has failed its test for self-consistency. For example, for high rates of onset of the acceleration pulse, the viscoelasticity of the brain material should perhaps be included to account for the strain-rate sensitivity. If one wishes to quantify the material properties more precisely, the experimental data base can be compared with the outputs of the finite element model and these parameters optimally obtained. Such a systems identification procedure has been given in Lin et al. (1978).

The second example is drawn from the cavitation investigations reported by Goldsmith. In his Figure 5, the fluid-filled skull is without the jaws, decreasing the effective mass considerably. Furthermore, to what extent did the GM artificial neck replicate the inertial and material properties of the human cadaveric neck is unclear. To simulate the spinal cord cavity by a rubber tube, of unknown compliance (or elastance), attached to a hole on the fluid-filled skull is too simplistic a simulation. According to the dog studies of Lofgren and Zwetnow (1973), the spinal cord cavity has an extremely low elastance in the order of 1 mm Hg/ml for pressures between 0 and 15 mm Hg. They attributed this low elastance to the existence of **potential** spaces in the spinal cord cavity in the form of partially collapsed **dura mater** and venous vasculature. The previous simulation by Roberts et al. (1966), using a thin latex membrane of low elastance to close off the foramen magnum, was probably better. A fluid-filled latex tube of low elastance would have been more appropriate.

Conclusions

(1) Stress waves are not expected to be important in closed models of direct head impact except perhaps in the coup region.

(2) For short-duration (< 4 ms) contact impacts to the frontal, occipital or temporal skull, the role of the neck is relatively unimportant until after 6 ms, after contact is broken.

(3) For crown impact to the vertex, the inertial and material properties of the neck are important to the outcome almost immediately upon contact.

(4) Further studies of the fracture characteristics and behavior of the cervical spine are urgently needed.

(5) One must not protect one part of the body, e.g., the head, at the expense of another, e.g., the neck.

(6) In constructing mathematical or physical models to simulate impact trauma, the inertial properties are of primary importance, followed by the material properties.

References

Bauze, J. R. and Ardan, M.A. (1978) "Experimental Production of Forward Dislocation in the Human Cervical Spine," *J. of Bone & Joint Surg.*, 60B, pp. 95–106.

Becker, E. G. (1972) "Measurement of Mass Distribution of Anatomical Segments," *Proc. Sixteenth Stapp Car Crash Conf.*, Soc. Auto Eng., Warrendale, PA, 15096, pp. 160–185.

Coermann, R. R. (1961) "Comparison of the Dynamic Characteristics of Dummies, Animals and Man, "*Proc.* National Academy of Sciences Symposium on *Impact Acceleration Stress,* Brooks AFB, San Antonio, Texas, November.

Culver, R. H., Bender, M. and Melvin, J. W. (1978) "Mechanisms, Tolerances, and Responses Obtained Under Dynamic Superior-Inferior Head Impact," Final Report, UM–HSRI–78–21, Highway Safety Research Institute, University of Michigan, Ann Arbor, MI 48009, USA.

Hardy, C. H., and Marcal, P. V. (1971) "Elastic Analysis of a Skull," ONR Report No. N00014–0007/8, Nov.

Hayashi, T. (1969) "Study of Intracranial Pressure Caused by Head Impact," *Journal of the Faculty of Engineering,* University of Tokyo, 30, p. 59.

Hosey, R. R. and Liu, Y. K. (1982) "A Homeomorphic Finite Element Model of the Human Head and Neck." *Finite Elements in Biomechanics,* (Eds: R. H. Gallagher, B. R. Simon, T. C. Johnson and J. F. Gross), John Wiley & Sons, Ltd., Chap. 18, pp. 379–401.

Hosey, R. R., Liu, Y. King and Ryerson, J. E. (1982) "A Finite Element Model of the Human Head and Neck During Crown Impact," Proceedings of the International Conference on Finite Element Methods, Shanghai, China.

Kornhauser, M. (1962) *Structural Effects of Impact,* Spartan, Cleaver-Baltimore.

Lin, H. S., Liu, Y. K., Ray, G. and Nikravesh, P. (1978) "Systems Identification for Material Properties of the Intervertebral Joint," *J. of Biomechanics,* Vol. 11, pp. 1–14.

Liu, Y. King, (1970a) "The Biomechanics of Spinal and Head Impact: Problems of Mathematical Simulation," *Proc. of Symposium on Biodynamic Modelling and Its Applications,* Dayton, OH, pp. 701–736.

Liu, Y. King (1970b) "Distributed-parameter Dynamic Models of the Spine," *Proc.* NIH Workshop on *Bioengineering Approaches to the Problems of the Spine,* Bethesda, MD, September.

Liu, Y. King, and Chandran, K. B. (1975) "Package Cushioning for the Human Head: I. Analytical Considerations," *J. Applied Mechanics,* Vol. 42, No. 3, pp. 541–546.

Liu, Y. K., Krieger, K. W., Njus, G., Ueno, K., Conners, M. P., Wakano, K., Thies, D. (1981) "Cervical Spine Stiffness and Geometry of the Young Human Male," Report No. AFAMRL–TR–80–138, Air Force Aerospace Medical Research Laboratory, Wright Patterson Air Force Base, Ohio, USA.

Lofgren, J., and Zwetnow, N. N. (1973) "Cranial and Spinal Components of the Cerebrospinal Fluid Pressure-volume Curve, *Acta Neurol. Scand., 49,* pp. 557–574.

Nusholtz, G. S., Melvin, J. W., Huelke, D. F., Alem, N. J. and Blank, J. G. (1981) "Response of the Cervical Spine to Superior-Inferior Head Impact," *25th Stapp Car Crash Conference,* SAE, Warrendale, PA 15096, pp. 197–237.

Pontius, U. R. and Liu, Y. K. (1975) "Neuromuscular Effects in a Dynamic Model of the Cervical Spine," Proceedings of the NSF Workshop of the Biomechanics of Volitional Effort, University of Florida, Gainesville, FL, pp. 147–175.

Prasad, P. and King, A. I. (1974) "An Experimentally Validated Dynamic Model of the Spine," *J. Applied Mechanics,* 41, pp. 546–550.

Ripperger, E. A. (1975) "The Mechanics of Brain Injuries," Vinken, P. J. et al. (Eds.): Injuries of the Brain and Skull, *Handbook of Clinical Neurology.* New York: Ame. Elsevier Publ. Co., pp. 91–109.

Roberts, V. L., Hodgson, V., and Thomas, L. M. (1966) "Fluid Pressure Gradient Caused by Impact to the Human Skull," *Biomechanics Monograph,* Ame. Soc. Mech. Eng., pp. 223–235.

Von Gierke, H. E., (1964) "Biodynamic Response of the Human Body," *Applied Mechanics Reviews,* 17, pp. 961–968.

Walker, L. B., Harris, E. H.. and Pontius, U. R. (1973) "Mass, Volume, Centre of Mass, and Mass Moment of Inertia of Head and Head and Neck of the Human Body," *Proc. 17th Annual Stapp Car Crash Conference,* Soc. Auto. Eng., pp. 525–537.

Ward, C. C., and Thompson, R. B. (1975) "The Development of a Detailed Finite Element Brain Model," *Proc. Nineteenth Stapp Car Crash Conf.,* Soc. Auto. Eng., pp. 641–0674.

Acknowledgements

The generous support of the National Institute for General Medical Sciences (NIGMS), NIH, (Grant No. 2 R01 GM 26608–03) and the U.S. Army Aeromedical Research Lab, Ft. Rucker, AL, (Contract DAMD 17–81–C–1186) is very much appreciated.

Some Aspects of the Physical and Mathematical Modeling of Loading to Head/ Neck Systems and Implications of Current DOT Injury Criteria

Werner Goldsmith

Introduction

Experimental generation of cerebral concussion in biological systems was initiated by E. S. Gurdjian in the United States, later in collaboration with H. R. Lissner, L. Patrick and numerous associates (1), as well as Denny-Brown and Russell (2), involving primarily methods of production of such trauma and some measurements of mechanical parameters such as intracranial pressure or acceleration of the injury-producing device including free falls. Substantial emphasis was placed on a qualitative explanation of the observed phenomena, with postulated mechanisms of brain damage and exhibition of a variety of skull fractures predominating. This activity was initiated in the early 1930's and propagated fruitfully until the retirement of Dr. Gurdjian around 1970 when the work was carried on by others. One of the most widely quoted, if not the best-known results of these investigations, is the Wayne State Tolerance Curve, shown in Figure 1, (albeit subsequently frequently revised in terms of its long-duration tolerance limit) which has served as the basis for all subsequent head injury criteria that were derived from its representation by some type of mathematical manipulation, highly simplified physical model or even by empirical techniques. Basically, the curve was developed from the measured intracranial pressure changes and accelerations generated in an adult cadaver skull by a frontal impact combined with corresponding data from anesthetized animals subjected to similar blows, using a cross combination of observed linear skull fracture in the cadavers and concussive effects in the animals as a measure of brain tolerance.

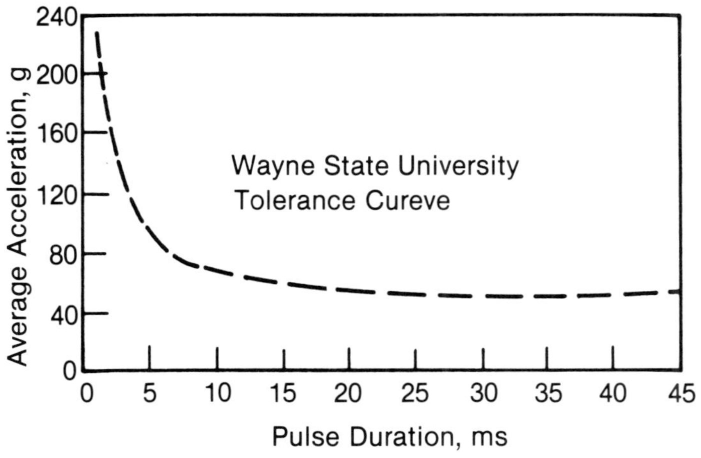

Figure 1. Wayne State Tolerance Curve

The curve was based on an extremely limited set of data involving only linear accelerations with durations in the range from 3–5 ms and extrapolated in both directions using an impact sensitivity procedure based on a linear spring-mass system. In addition, no clear description is given of the scaling of the data from cadaver and animal to the living human. In spite of these and many other possible criticisms, the curve even today represents the only reasonably acceptable measure of head injury, even though it is widely recognized that skull fracture can occur without brain injury, and vice versa, as well as simultaneous production of both deficits. However, one of the major criticisms of this and any other criteria enunciated subsequently is their failure to address the question of variability of the results with respect to living humans, i.e., their levels of confidence. Thus, the stipulation of such a curve or of various official or unofficial criteria derived from this type of data would tend to lead the uninitiated, unsophisticated or predisposed to consider the results as inviolate, whereas the vast majority of the continuum mechanics and material behavior community is aware of the huge variations in both properties and tolerance levels of human beings, where the value of the standard deviation of a mechanical parameter is not infrequently uncomfortably close to the mean. Furthermore, no information is currently available for tolerance and mechanical limits at the cellular level, although this question is currently being addressed.

It is imperative to recognize that any such no-go criterion is truly too simplistic for the description of human behavior under dynamic load and that all efforts should be directed toward (a) Refining our knowledge of tolerance involving at a minimum a differentiation between skull and brain failure, with the latter even further subdivided (as should be the case for any soft tissue) between physiological and physical failure, the former obviously being achieved at lower input levels, perhaps very substantially so, (b) Recognition of the difference between head impacts and impulsive loading through the torso and (c) Incorporation of the enormous variability in the physical characteristics of human beings by delineating the differences in failure characteristics at some selected population index. Although the latter will represent an enormous challenge, it is the opinion of the writer that this point must be addressed and recognized regardless of potential legal implications which, regrettably have already been misapplied relative to the intended use of any such established criterion. The importance of this subject has been recognized in a recent literature review (3).

Head injury modelling may have been developed earlier, but surely one of the outstanding champions of this procedure was Holbourn (4), who postulated that the principal causes of head injury were due tc the simultaneous effects of skull deformation resulting from local indentation or structural deformation or vibration of the entire shell; later, he also added the concept of angular motion as a significant potential cause of such injury. Other mechanisms proposed as the cause of head trauma included the establishment of pressure gradients in the brain, perhaps generated by propagation of stress waves that could produce damage as the result of linear acceleration responsible for both absolute motion of the brain components and their relative displacement with respect to the skull. Such a phenomenon could evoke both brain stem shear and production of hematoma as a result of the collapse of cavitation bubbles induced by tensile states in the brain caused by wave reflection, both mechanisms generating deficits leading to anything from temporary impairment to death. A third postulated event provoking brain damage concerned the flexion-extension and/or bending of the upper cervical cord in the process of abrupt motion of the head-neck junction, although this theory did not find as many adherents as the other mechanisms (5).

Substantially later, the present author suggested the analysis of head injury by means of the methods of continuum mechanics involving an investigation of the effect of a concentrated, time-dependent load on a fluid-filled spherical shell representing surely the crudest possible model of a head impact (6). This prompted a slate of analytical efforts in which modifications of the system in all possible manners were attempted, including the distortion of the shell,addition of the neck, various numerical techniques for the evaluation of the field variables, etc.; a survey of some of these results is presented in references (7), (8) and (9). Concomitantly, a national effort was launched to measure the mechanical properties of the various components of the head, suggested and directed for four years by the present writer, which resulted not only in the first definitive data ever generated for many of the local and global mechanical and structural properties of the head elements, but also propagated into numerous individual continuations at a variety of institutions after cessation of support for this program through a central agency. Very little information of this type has been produced outside of this umbrella to the present day.

Substantially less information concerning the neck is available, although proposed tolerance levels for the neck in extension and flexion, (Figure 2) have been developed by Mertz and Patrick (10). These and other data for the neck, including mechanisms of failure for particular loading conditions, are catalogued in the encyclopedic reference on trauma for the entire body and its constituent parts (11). A composite of the impact experience from falls is presented in Figure 3 (12) recently supplemented by an extensive case study (13), and purported tolerance curve for sled tests, cadaver and human falls is indicated in Figure 4 (12), studied more completely by Snyder at the University of Michigan. A discussion of the principles involved in accidents to the head and neck in sports is given in reference (14).

An encyclopedic data bank for the response of human volunteers to indirect loading of the head-neck

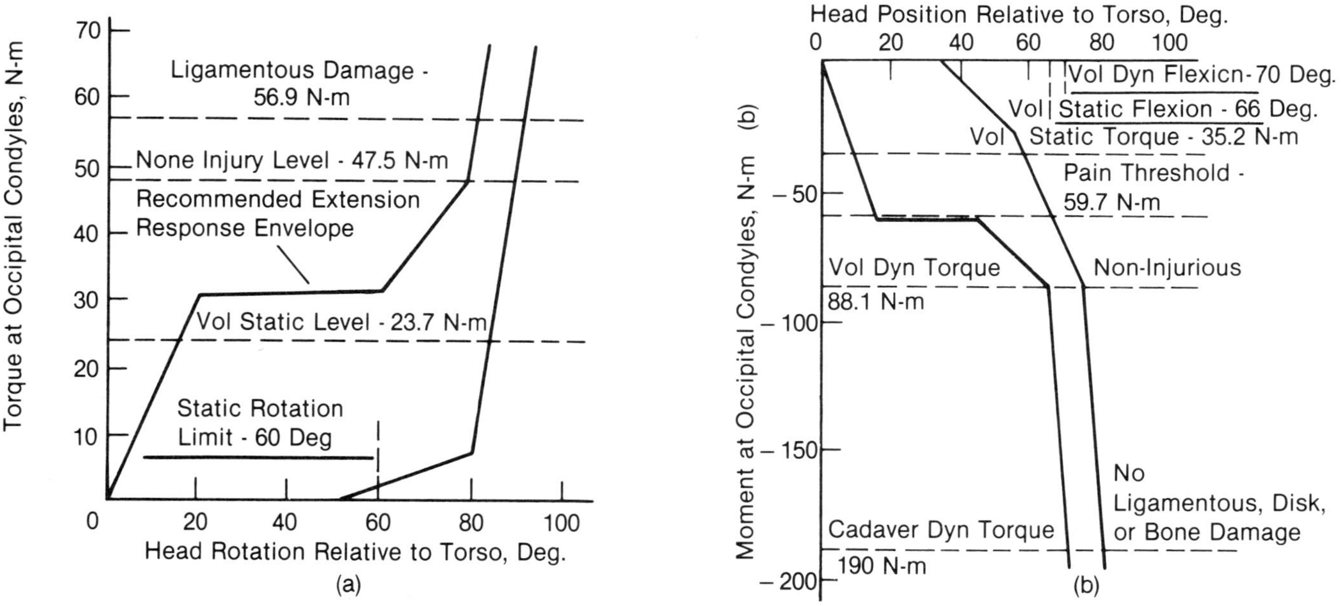

Figure 2. Head-Neck Response Evenlope and Tolerance Levels for (a) Extension and (b) Flexion (Ref. 10)

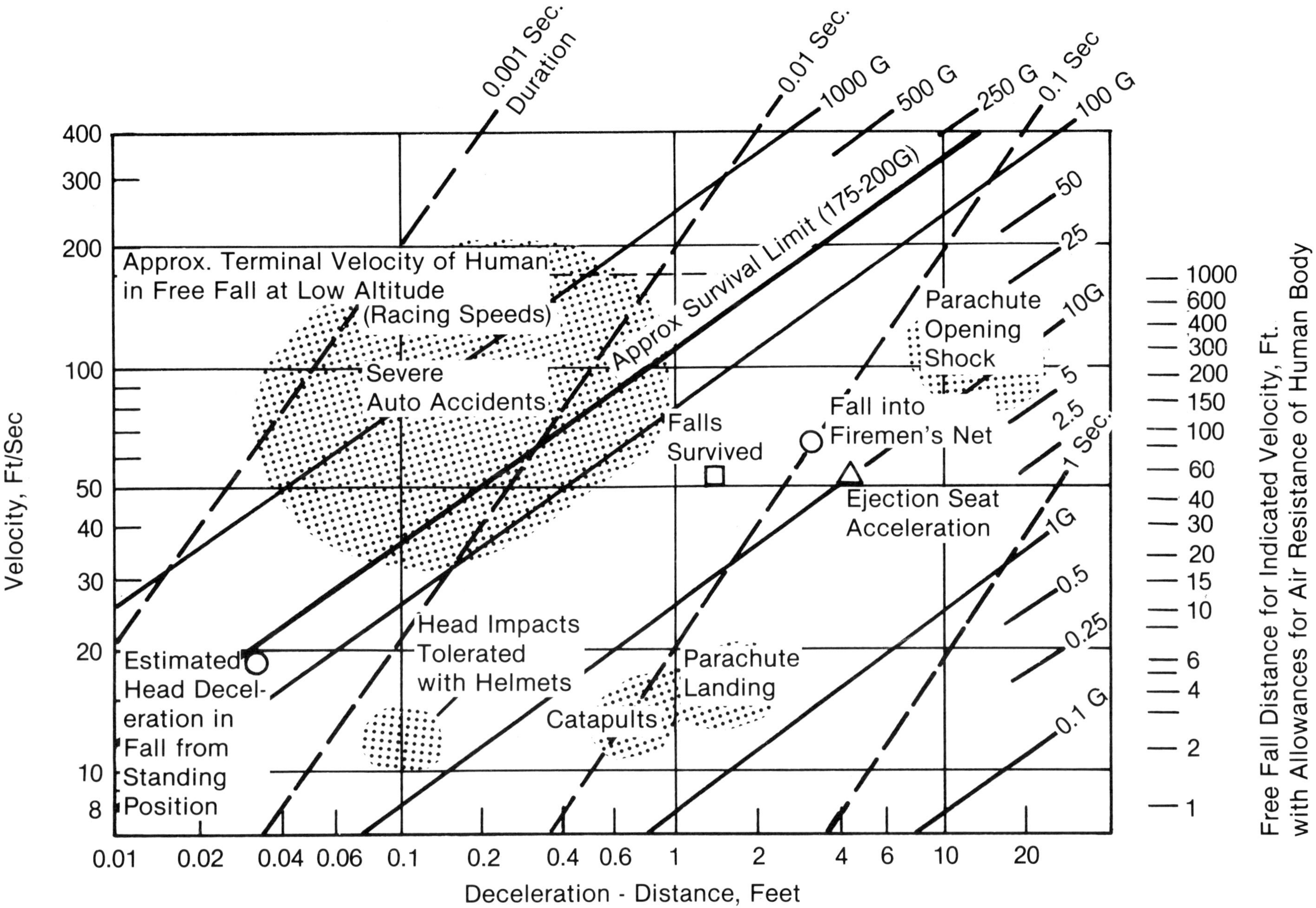

Figure 3. Composite of Impact Experience from Falls (12)

system by means of controlled acceleration histories applied to sleds with the subject seated in various orientations to the acceleration vector has been compiled by C. Ewing and associates at the Naval Biodynamics Laboratory, Michaud Station, New Orleans. The scope of the available information is so enormous that it cannot conceivably be reported here. The overall conclusion of the analyzed data, involving both mechanical and physiological response, is that it does not currently correlate directly with corresponding tests on cadavers or anthropometric dummies, primarily because of the enormous difference in mechanical properties between the three classes of targets, and also because of the absence of voluntary or involuntary muscular and reflex effects. This thesis has been supported by numerous other researchers, including a late comprehensive publication addressing the adequacy of dummies to replicate human mechanical response under identical dynamic loading conditions (15).

The present manuscript will report some work involving the question of the existence of cavitation in the human head as the result of a direct blow, previously published in the literature (16), the response of dummy head proposed for the testing of protective baseball caps under loading by a projected baseball directly on the head form and when covered with a cap, with direct implications of the results concerning the present state of official head injury criteria—a condensation of a paper appear in the American Journal of Sports Medicine (17), as well as some acceleration records for other helmeted impacts that do not fit the standard patterns and hence present substantial questions of interpretations with respect to these criteria, and a very short exposition of the construction and testing of two successive head-neck models replicating the human (18)(19). Correlations with existing theories and other data, as well as the results of both unembalmed and embalmed cadaver tests, will also be described in abbreviated form.

Finally, this paper will address itself to the question of the adequacy of current head injury criteria with particular reference to a recent legal case where, in the opinion of the writer, statements concerning these criteria were made that are grossly misleading, and, further, the laws of mechanics were both violated and incorrectly applied.

Cavitation Investigations in Two Head/Neck Models

The only previous work specifically directed towards the examination of the cavitation theory of brain damage (20)(21) employed water-filled ellipsoidal glass vessels whose bubble behavior under impact was examined by a framing camera and a large-sized

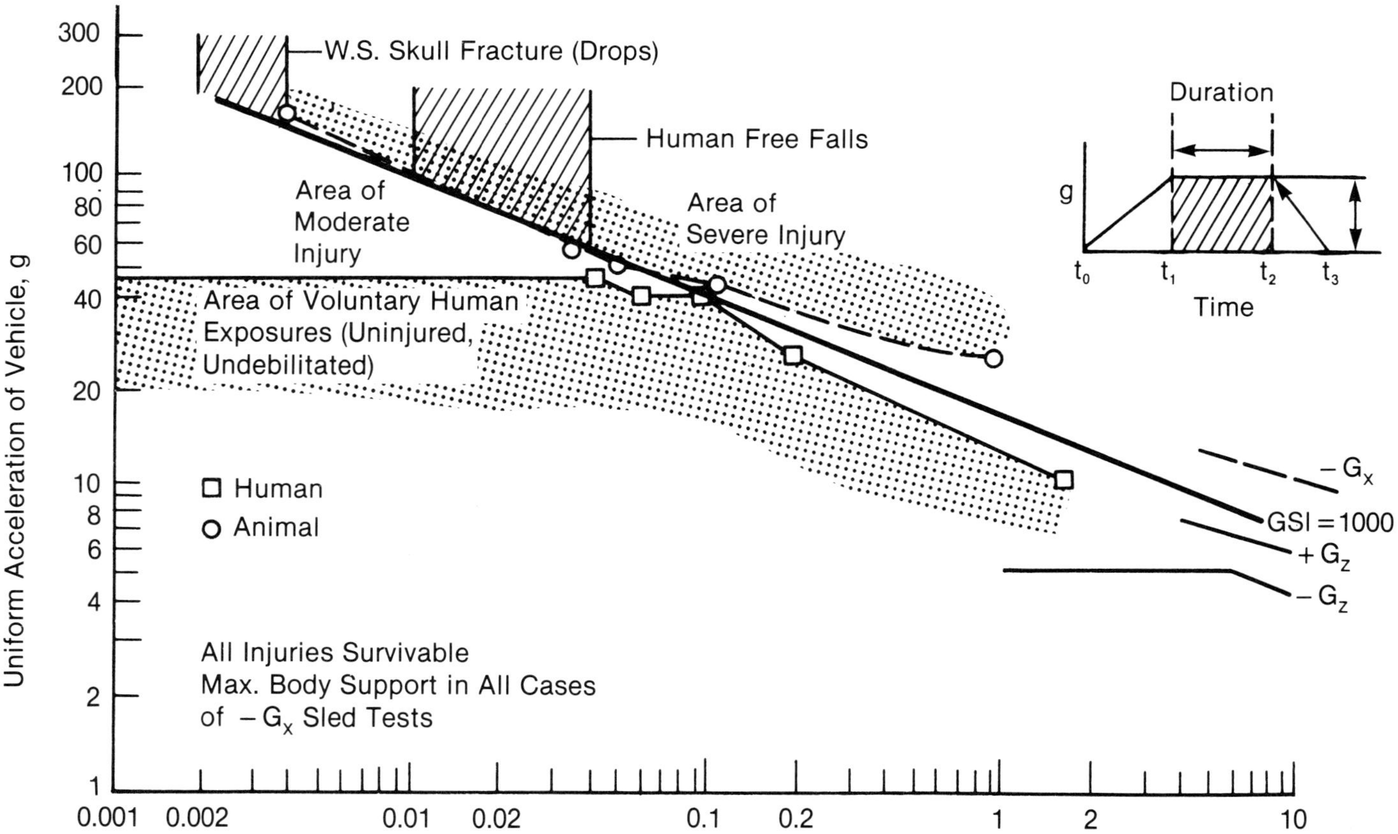

Figure 4. Tolerance Curve for Sled Tests, Cadaver and Human Falls (12)

single pressure transducer inserted into the vessel. The theoretical outline was based on a steady-state pressure profile due to a constant acceleration for the entire head and proposed contrecoup, coup and resonance cavitation, observed experimentally, as the cause of the petechial hemorrhages at the two positions and the punch-drunk syndrome, respectively. The present investigation was designed to investigate the possibility of damage in the brain due to cavitation employing more realistic replications, a variety of media simulating the brain, and more modern instrumentation.

Two head models were attached through an aluminum coupling to the top of a 1.41 kg, 0.14 m long General Motors artificial neck (22)(23) whose bottom was attached to a heavy plate delineating an essentially rigid torso relative to the neck. The first model consisted of an acrylic shell with a mean mid-surface radius and a thickness of 3.71 mm and a port providing fluid communication to a rubber tube simulating the spinal canal. The second model consisted of a cadaver skull whose occiput and a portion of the parietal area were removed and replaced by a transparent polyester resin to permit contrecoup region photography and the directing of adequate light to this area by means of a high-powered beam, respectively. A port at the top of the skull and a second one leading for the foramen magnum through the aluminum coupling to a plastic tube permitted fluid entry and removal to the system as well as replicating again the spinal canal. The acrylic shell was tested using four fluids: distilled water, glycerin, a high-density capacitor-type liquid (Fluorinert) and artificial CSF; the skull was only filled with distilled water and Jello. Pressure histories were measured by means of minute, thin tourmaline disks suspended at the center near the coup and contrecoup positions in the two models (16).

Impact was produced either by propelling 21 g, 12.57 mm, 21.6 long steel projectiles with flat faces from an air gun or by the drop of 3 kg, 188 mm outer diameter aluminum shell, suspended ballistically, from a height of 25.4 mm. A strain gage transducer arrangement at the impact point permitted the monitoring of the input history. The cavitation processes were filmed by a 16 mm framing camera with a 90-mm macrolens placed approximately 1.37 m from the occipital regions of both models and operating in the range from 4000–8000 pps. The displacement of the shell/neck joint was measured by the filming at the rate of 3500 pps of the reading of a dial gage positioned against the coupling. The experimental arrangement for the skull model is shown in Figure 5.

The presence of the scalp was simulated in some of the experiments by the placement of a layer of 6.53-mm thick silicone rubber between input transducer and head model. The effect of fluid communication

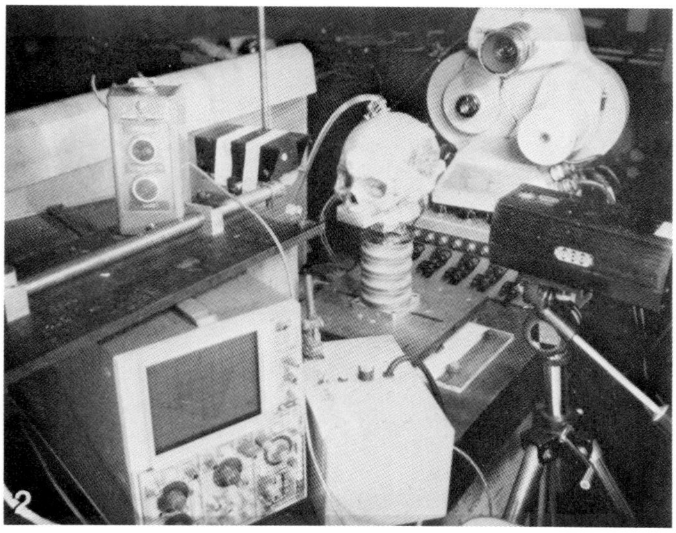

Figure 5. Experimental Arrangement for Impact on a Skull-Neck System (16)

was examined by permitting such flow or by preventing it upon clamping the appropriate tube shut. Pierced polyethylene sheets were also placed in the spherical shell model in an attempt to crudely simulate some neural structure; further, the shell was clamped directly to a rigid support to assess the function of the neck relative to bubble formation.

Figure 6 portrays the pressure records at the three positions in the water-filled skull head-neck model due to a nearly triangular input pulse of approximately 129 MPa and a duration of about 22.7μs. The compressive pulse propagates with a speed of 1.53 km/s compared to a theoretical value of 1.48 km/s determined from the mass density and bulk modulus of water, initiating contrecoup response after 170μs. Initial peak skull pressure is substantially lower and smoother due to the attenuating characteristics of the three-layered skull than for the corresponding loading on the shell system; the largest negative pressures occur at the contrecoup position for both models.

Figures 7–9 portray observed cavitation bubbles at the coup and contrecoup position, resonating contrecoup bubbles, and a ring pattern in the water-filled shell struck by the spherical projectile at a speed of 16.5 m/s with a framing rate of 4000 pps, whose occurrence coincided temporally with the peak negative pressures. Such bubbles were found for all fluids employed here. Figure 10 portrays contrecoup cavitation in the water-filled skull head system with the same loading but at a framing rate of 500 s^{-1}; other cavitation phenomena are presumed to be present, but cannot be observed with the present model. Maximum diameters and durations of existence of coup and contrecoup cavitation bubbles in all fluids were essentially the same ranging from 0.3–0.42 mm and 0.75–1.5 ms

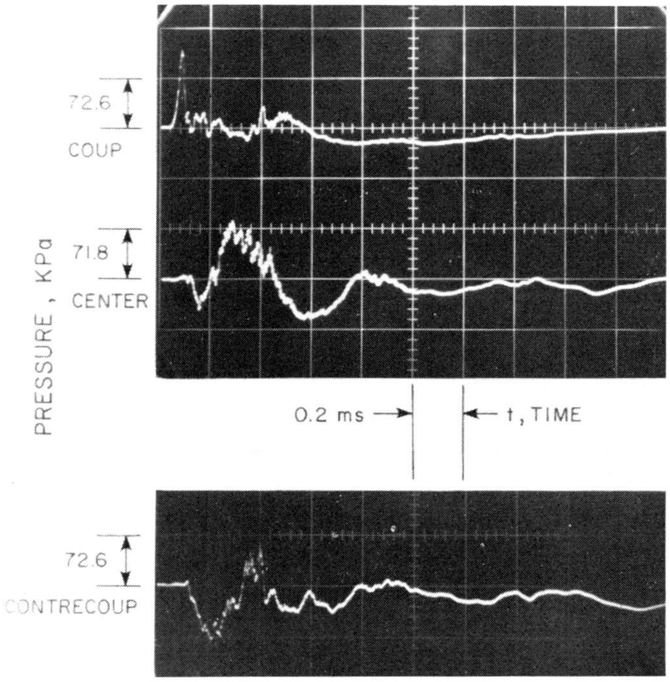

Figure 6. Pressure Histories at the Coup, Center and Contrecoup Location in a Water-Filled Skull Head-Neck Model Struck by a 21 g, 12.6 mm Dia Cylindrical Flat-Faced Steel Projectile at a Speed of 16.5 m/s on the Forehead (16)

respectively, for the shell model; for the skull, the corresponding values for water were 0.69–1.38 mm and 0.4–0.6 ms, respectively. No cavitation was noted when the skull was filled with gelatin.

A comparison of the pressure and bubble radii measurement with the predictions of the Rayleigh theory of cavitation (24) which neglects the effects of surface tension, viscosity, compressibility and finite extent of the medium indicates that the analysis evaluates a bubble radius more than one order of magnitude greater than that observed. Of course, incorporation of each of the neglected effects would tend to reduce the calculated value; thus, an improved analytical model of the cavitation process that would indicate these terms appears to be urgently needed.

The significant differences in pressure profiles and cavitation processes noted between the shell and skull models imply that the geometric and especially the material properties of the cranial vessel dominate the system response in model impacts. Cavitation was found in all fluids except gelatin; this suggests that the likelihood of cavitation in the brain matter is substantially reduced, since both gelatin and neural tissue are colloidal suspensions; however, such cavitation may very well occur in both blood and CSF. The presence of a model spinal canal did not noticeably affect the process of bubble formation. Similarly, rigid

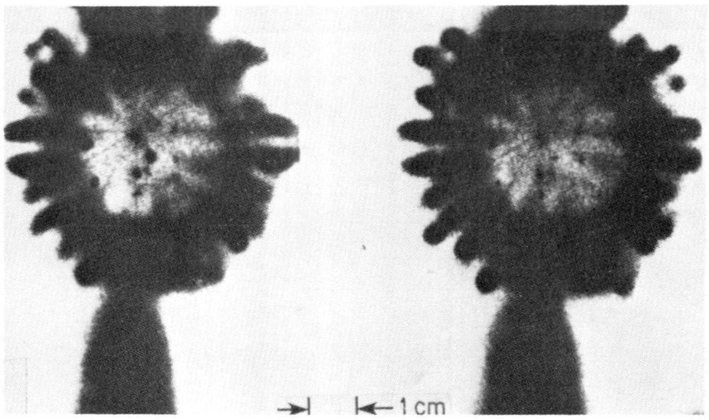

Figure 7. Coup and Contrecoup Cavitation Bubbles in a Water-Filled Acrylic Shell Head-Neck Model Struck by a 21 g, 12.6 mm Dia Cylindrical Flat-Faced Steel Projectile at a Speed of 16.5 m/s on the Forehead (16)

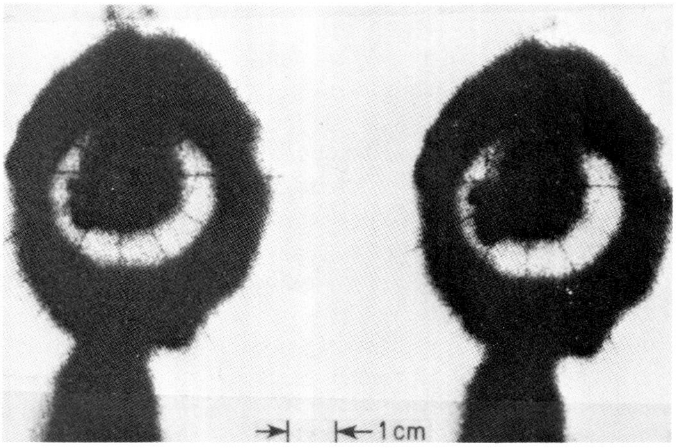

Figure 8. Resonating Contrecoup Cavitation Bubbles for the Case of Figure 7 (16)

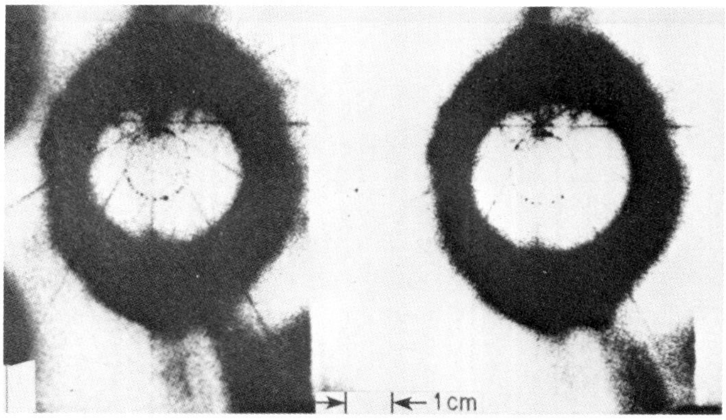

Figure 9. Ring Pattern of Bubbles for the Case of Figure 7 (16)

clamping of the water-filled shell did not inhibit coup and contrecoup cavitation, but suppressed resonating contrecoup cavitation and the long-duration ring-like bubble pattern (which was not reported by Gross). The

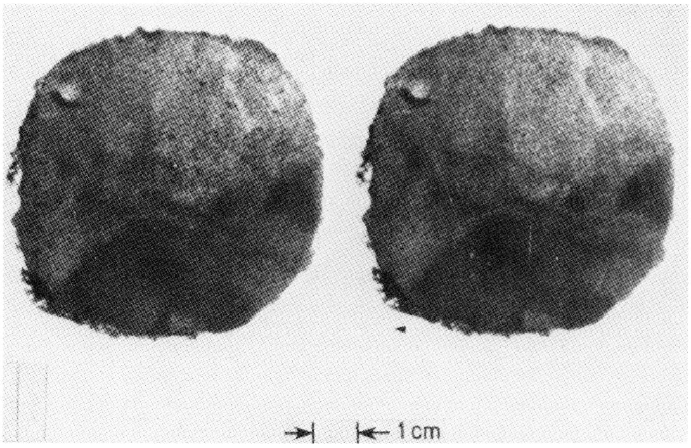

Figure 10. Contrecoup Cavitation in a Water-Filled Skull Head-Neck Model Struck by a 21 g, 12.6 mm Dia Cylindrical Flat-Faced Steel Projectile at a Speed of 16.5 m/s on the Forehead (16)

major conclusion derivable from this investigation is the probability that cavitation damage in the brain due to a blow certainly can exist in the fluid components, but is unlikely to occur in the neural tissue proper.

Results of Helmeted Head Model Impact Studies and Implications Concerning Official Injury Criteria

A series of approximately 200 tests have been executed on a headform* specifically recommended for use in assessing the efficacy of baseball caps both in the unprotected state and covered with various commercial caps of this type (17). Impact was produced at a variety of locations in the frontal and temporal areas, using a specially designed baseball gun capable of producing an impact at a predetermined location on the target within a few hundredths of an inch and pneumatically propelling Little League balls at speeds ranging from 50 to 120 mph (80.5–193 km/hr) with the upper limit substantially in excess of recorded major league pitching speeds. The initial and rebound velocity of the ball were ascertained from the signals produced by the interruption of a laser net emplaced across the ball trajectory and observation of the rebound path. A uniaxial accelerometer was placed at the center of mass of the head form with the sensing axis along the direction of impact (which consists of an oil-filled ceramic structure covered by a plastic rubber-like material) which recorded the history of the parameter at this position; the suggested tri-axial sensor exhibited severe ringing obviating its employment here. For most runs, a carbon paper placed across the impact position recorded the maximum contact area of the ball; furthermore, for a number of runs, a framing camera operating at a speed of approximately 1000 pps recorded the duration of contact and the initial velocity of the model head after the collision.

Typical records of the accelerometer traces are presented in Figure 11. It may be noted that the traces exhibit excursions in both the positive and negative directions, corresponding to tensile and compressive waves generated successively at the free opposite surfaces of the unit after initial traverse as a compressive transient. The periods of these signals correspond to the transit time of the model; however, the camera record indicated a duration of contact of the ball and cap (or headform) of a nearly constant duration of 2.5 ms, approximately five times greater than the signal period for the initial traverse. This raises the immediate question how an oscillatory phenomenon such as shown here can be interpreted in terms of the Head Injury Criterion (HIC) defined as

$$\text{Supremum } [(t_2 - t_1)^{-1} \int_{t_1}^{t_2} a\, dt]^{2.5} (t_2 - t_1)$$

where the supremum indicates the maximizing of the function for any arbitrary times t_1 and t_2 occurring during the action of the pulse. Clearly, acceleration, which is a vector quantity, exhibits at least positive and negative values, even if it is unidirectional. Thus, the application of an oscillatory record to the criterion expressed by Eq. (1) is meaningless unless one adopts the concept that it is the absolute value of this quantity that governs—a concept not envisioned in the original development of this criterion and just as uncertain in its implication today as when this criterion was first suggested.

An explanation of Eq. (1) proffered at the Consensus Workshop that it represents a weighted energy criterion is not convincing to this author. Obviously, competent specialists may properly differ in their interpretation of the meaning of quantity as complicated as a stipulation for skull fracture or brain damage, but from a fundamental viewpoint, the only mechanically acceptable manner in which a vector quantity can be converted to a scalar is by the use of an operator involving a scalar product. This has not been delineated and, in consequence, this writer is not persuaded—nor has he ever concurred in the desirability of a simplistic representation of one of the more complicated processes encountered in the field of continuum mechanics—that it is even possible to stipulate a single numerical value, particularly of acceleration as a time function, to provide a limit of tolerance for the brain; however, skull fracture may well be properly described by an ultimate strength. At the moment, and probably for the foreseeable future, the knowledge developed and the state of the art appear to preclude the specification of a ritualistic expression that could define whether a mortal insult is delivered to a living

*Manufactured by Valjem Corp., East Detroit, Michigan

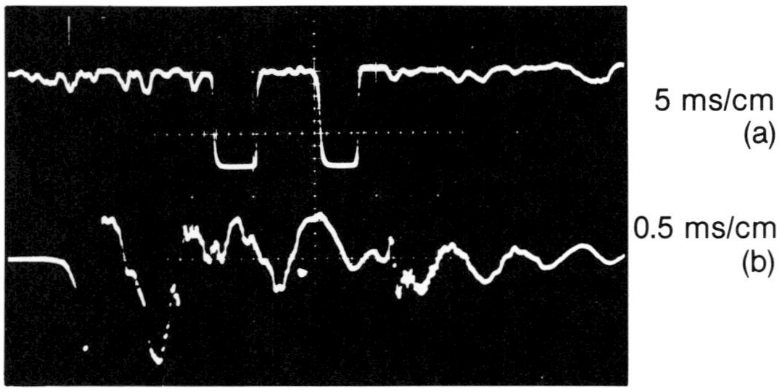

(i) Temporal Impact on a Capped Headform at an Initial Velocity of 113.6 mph (50.8 m/s). Acceleration Ordinate 500 g/cm (Ref. 17)

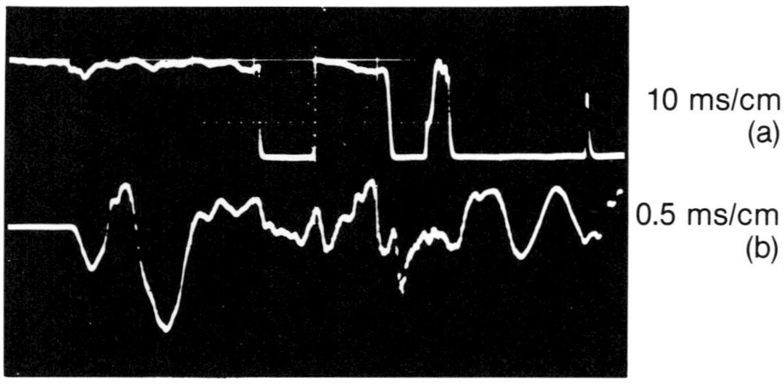

(ii) Temporal Impact on a Bare Headform at an Initial Velocity of 63.1 mph (28.2 m/s). Acceleration Ordinate: 200 g/cm (Ref. 17)

Figure 11. Rebound Histories (a) and Acceleration Traces (b) for Baseballs Striking Headforms.

human or whether a given blow, if even traumatic, might not result in reversible damage. This viewpoint is even far more emphatically supported by the known and widely documented enormous variability of human response to direct or indirect loading applied to the head-neck system.

Furthermore, an evaluation of this supremum is not a simple matter for an irregularly shaped acceleration curve; computer programs must be developed for this purpose (and have been by the writer), and these require substantial cost for their proper evaluation. Only when the force history can be approximated by a trapezoid—as is a reasonable step in the case of acceleration histories derived for vehicular helmets placed on magnesium headforms (which bear no resemblance to the properties of a human head) when dropped onto surfaces in accordance with ANSI (American National Standards Institute) codes—can the Head Injury Criterion be evaluated in a relatively simple fashion.

Lest it be suggested that baseball caps mounted on the headform described represent a unique situation with regard to the head injury criterion, Figures 12 and 13 represent qualitative force and quantitative mass center acceleration histories for a skull-neck head model covered by a jockey helmet striking a massive steel barrier at a velocity of about 7.5 ft/s with the target bare or protectively padded, respectively. Aside from circuit ringing, it may be observed that the acceleration record also exhibits oscillatory characteristics, and that in the case of the padded impact, the head injury criterion would be virtually impossible to apply. A human cadaver skull covered with a suitable plastic to represent the scalp and stuffed with a substance similar in properties to brain and further weighted to bring its mass up to that of a living human served as the head replica.

Thus, these experiments which clearly show a wave phenomenon leading to oscillatory acceleration responses appear sufficiently persuasive to strongly suggest the urgent need for the improvement in the current brain injury criterion, since it cannot handle a history involving excursions above and below the base line unless additional stipulations are invoked. In that case, however, the entire criterion should be reevaluated, including at the very minimum a differentiation between skull fracture and brain damage, and a recognition that various types of brain damage may require different tolerance criteria, as nearly unani-

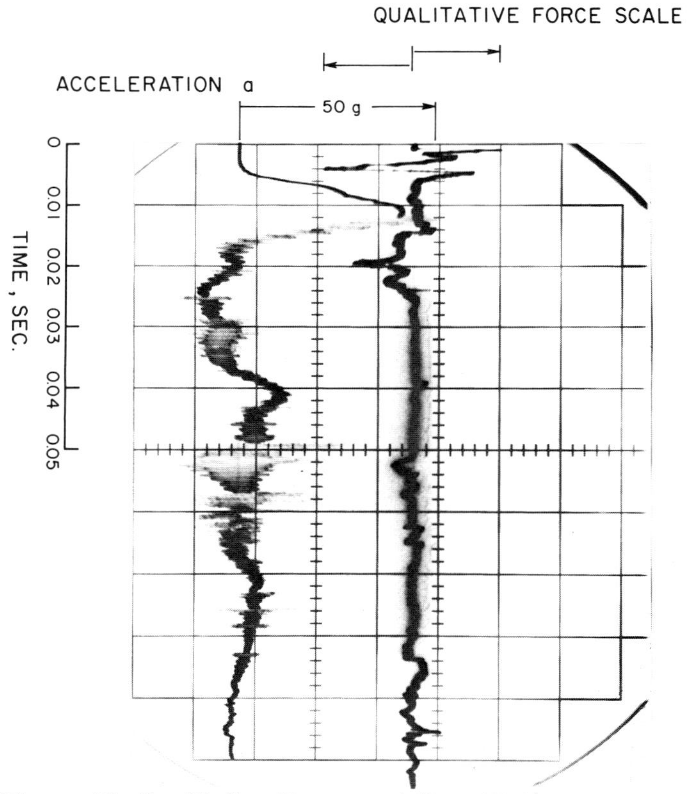

Figure 12. Qualitative Force and Quantitative Acceleration Histories for the Impact of a Skull Covered by a Jockey Helmet Against an Unpadded Massive Steel Barrier at a Velocity of 7.5 ft/s

mously suggested by the Workshop participants. Furthermore, such revamping will necessarily require a distinct separation of tolerance criteria for adults and for children, the latter perhaps even by age groups, as has been published for the skull stiffness parameter (25) and for general head tolerance (26), the latter differing sharply from the values currently mandated by the Department of Transportation.

Construction and Impact Testing of Physical Head-Neck Models of the Human

An initial attempt to construct a head-neck system replicating that in the living human so as to permit a reasonable duplication of the kinematic and other field variable histories when the unit was subjected to both front and rear loading of the skull and similar loading at the base of the structure, all in a sagittal plane, resulted in the model shown in Figure 14 (18). This consisted of a human cadaver skull filled with water and covered with an artificial rubber-like material, RTV, emplaced on a series of vertebrae, duplicating a human cadaver spine down to the level of T2; these vertebrae consisted of a fiberglass-reinforced resin and were separated by fluid-filled disk elements. The unit was supported by passive silicone rubber muscle and ligament replications that were connected

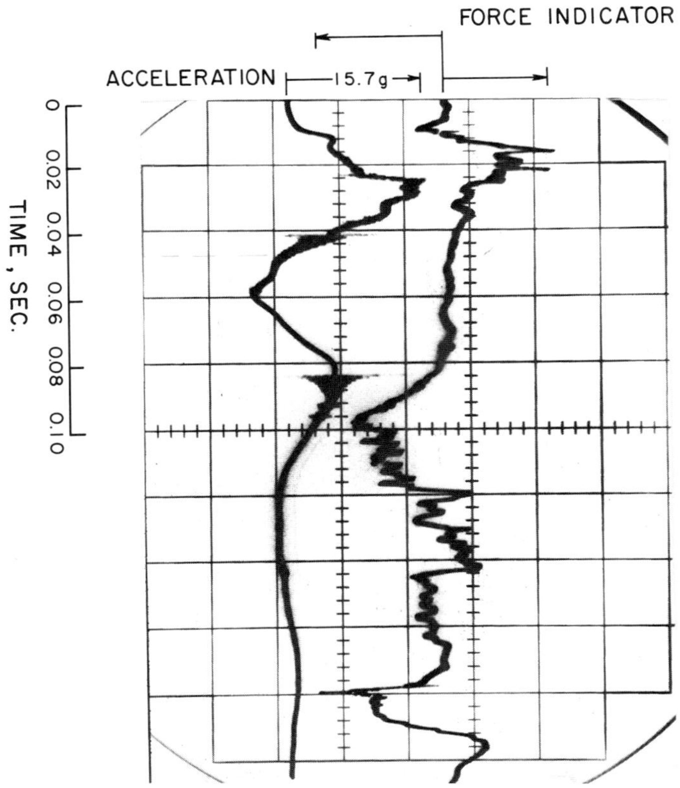

Figure 13. Qualitative Force and Quantitative Acceleration Histories for the Impact of a Skull Covered by a Jockey Helmet Against the Padded Side of a Massive Steel Barrier at a Velocity of 7.5 ft/s

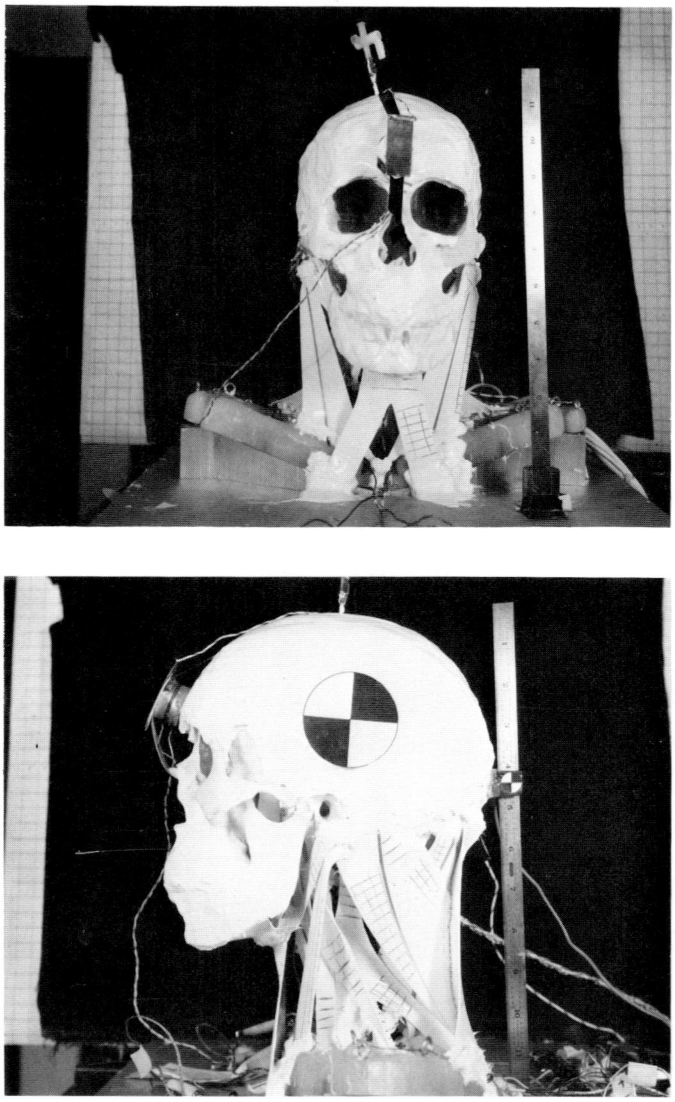

Figure 14. Zero-Order Head-Neck Replica of a Human

to an aluminum base simulating a rigid torso below T2. Instrumentation was developed to measure contact force, head accelerations, disk pressures and intracranial pressures for inputs ranging from 0.009–4.63 N-m, resulting in head accelerations up to about 170 g. The excursion of the unit was photographed with a framing camera operating at about 1000 pps.

The loading effects produced were non-traumatic according to the Wayne State Tolerance curve, as shown in Figure 15 and posttraumatic x-ray examination. A peak acceleration of 169 g with a duration of 1.93 ms for an occipital impact was observed which falls uncomfortably close to the original tolerance curve as presented in reference (1), resulting in values of the Gadd Severity Index and the HIC of 244 and 220, respectively, while the most severe frontal blow with an input energy of 4.9 N-m resulted in a peak value of 104 g and a duration of 4 ms, either at or just above this limit. Although the tolerance curve of

Figure 15 is considered to be conservative and the tolerance limit of the two indices cited were adjusted accordingly, the result is another demonstration of the state of flux or the subject which precludes the specification of tolerance limits except for the possible ad hoc guidance of manufacturers of protective equipment, where the test conditions do not replicate real accidents.

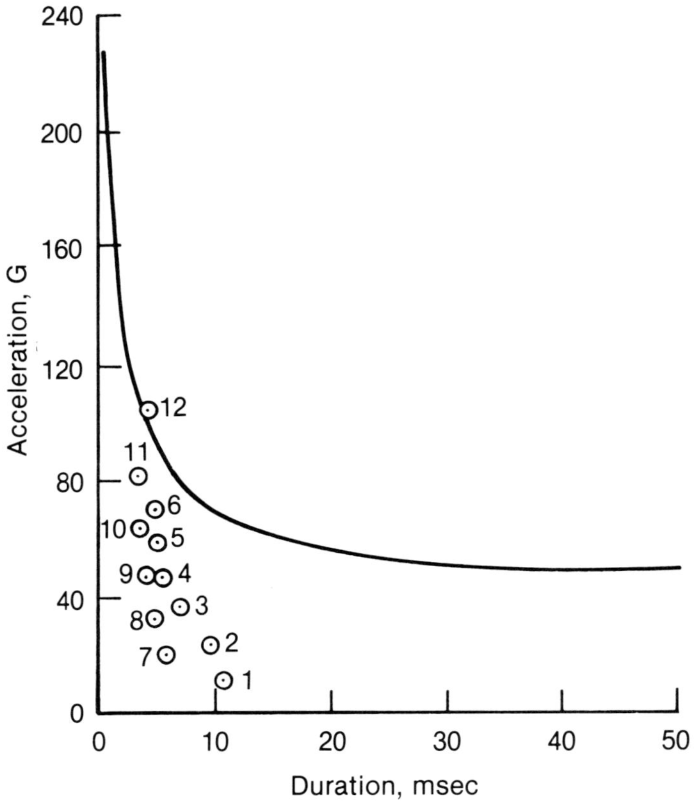

Figure 15. Response of Sagittal Plane Dynamic Leading of a Zero-Order Human Head-Neck Model in Relation to the Wayne State Tolerance Curve

The observed kinematic results were compared with the excursions observed in both unembalmed and embalmed cadaver models and with several theoretical approaches; moderate success can be claimed in the correlation between these three methodologies. Analytical results were based upon lumped parameter and discretized continuum systems. Occipital skull accelerations and disk pressures measured in the cadaver studies were in good correspondence with those from corresponding tests on artificial head-neck replicas. A priori and posteriori x-ray examination of the cadaver system did not evidence any skull or vertebral fractures, but the loading was considered to have been sufficiently severe so as to have caused significant soft tissue damage in a living human.

A second-generation human head-neck replica (Figure 16) was constructed, instrumented and tested in a manner similar to the earlier model, with, however, the addition of lateral impacts (19). Improvements relative to the previous structure consisted of the addition of an upper torso bony configuration which permitted constrained motion relative to a rigid base, rather than immobility. Furthermore, this allowed a more realistic attachment of the neck musculature to its lower termini; an additional feature to portray a more lifelike response was a stiffening of the ligaments which were modelled as orthotropic materials, and incorporation of nonlinearities in muscle response. Furthermore, a special effort was directed toward the placement of the spinal tissues in their appropriate *in vivo* rest condition.

The maximum value of the linear acceleration and velocity of the head were found to occur either during or immediately after the impact, with corresponding peak rotational values appearing subsequently, but well before the peak displacement of the skull. In the case of rear head or frontal base impact, two modes of loading that are similar, the head experienced a significant period of translation without rotation immediately after loading, and the system appears to respond more violently to side impact indicating greater vulnerability of the neck to this type of loading. The muscle comportment demonstrates its influence in limiting the excursion of the head, yielding strain values of up to 40 percent. The disk pressure histories were similar to those found in the previous model, with the largest values found in the region between T2 and C4, whereas the intracranial pressure exceeded that in the previous model by about an order of magnitude which appeared to be realistic. It is interesting to note that when the improved model was further refined by the insertion of filler material between the replicated soft tissue to resemble the fascia and eliminate the interstitial spaces and the unit was then covered by a cloth representing the skin, the

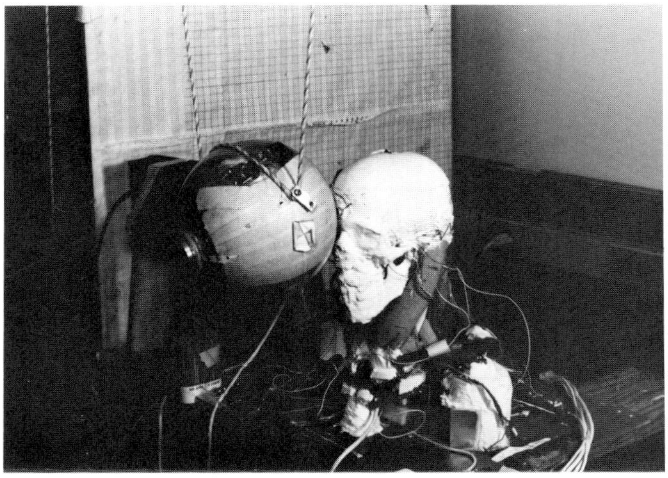

Figure 16. Impact on a Second-Generation Human Head-Neck Model

head acceleration for identical impacts on this unit without these improvements exhibited a lower peak value. This effect can only be attributed to the increase in mass of the system.

A detailed description of the construction, instrumentation, test results and correlations for these models can be found in references (18) (19) and will be published shortly in archive journals.

Commentary on Some DOT Head/Neck Injury Workshop Presentations and Head Injury Criteria

The writer considers it to be fortunate that he had the opportunity to attend the 1981 DOT-sponsored Workshop on Head and Neck Injury to evaluate some of the presentations at this meeting before the composition of his contribution to its Proceedings. In particular, he would like to address the question of modeling of the head impact phenomena suggested by some of the participants, using finite element methods, and the concomitant proposal for the establishment of a head injury criterion.

The writer and virtually the entire audience trained in continuum mechanics were appalled to be confronted with the proposal of "inertia waves" which presumably consist of the sequential motion of entire segments of the central nervous system, each of which separately executes states of uniform motion. It must be emphatically reiterated, and without any qualification whatever, that such a representation violates the fundamental law of mechanics. Impact between two objects can be modelled in two totally different ways: (a) The objects can be regarded as rigid, in which case there are no waves and the bodies move by a combination of rigid-body translation and rotation; the dynamics of the impact are controlled by the linear and angular impulse-momentum laws, that can be supplemented by a specification of an energy loss (which always occurs) for the component of the motion along the normal to the colliding surfaces and a knowledge of frictional effects for the corresponding tangential motion component. Representation of a system in this fashion includes lumped parameter models and has the obvious advantage of greater simplification and the enormous deficit of obfuscating some of the most crucial effects resulting from the impact, including the contact phenomenon which, almost invariably, controls the maximum stress state and thus determines the occurrence of failure of the material when its fracture limit is exceeded.

Alternatively, (b) the phenomenon can be modelled in terms of a description of the objects as deformable media, in which case there are always **waves**, internationally recognized and appelled as **stress waves**, although they could be characterized in terms of any other field variable such as displacement, velocity, acceleration (or strain for objects characterized as solid). Here, the effects of the contact phenomenon, which must be analyzed as a time-dependent pressure event occurring over a variable area of contact, are communicated to distant parts of the two objects by a continuous signal called a stress transient, which can be measured by any competent procedure employing instrumentation with an adequate frequency response at the required locations, and which can be mathematically delineated by well-recognized analytical and/or numerical methods. Whenever the existence of stress waves due to an impact in an actual object are not reported, then (i) either the instrumentation lacks adequate sensitivity or (ii) the numerical method utilizes a time increment much too large to capture the effect of the waves, or both.

As an example, in the human head, the transit time of a wave either through the brain or the skull from pole to contrecoup point is of the order of 100μs. Clearly, a finite-element network with a time discretization of say, 500μs, will be totally unable to consider the effects of such a wave, but when a mesh of such size is employed (for reasons of economy or whatever) and the results fail to indicate wave propagation, the conclusion that the phenomenon is absent can only indict the approach of the perpetrator. The writer apologizes for the repetition of these statements that are obvious, but there are apparently still those attempting to propose a phenomena unknown in rational mechanics and incapable of being described by accepted analytical methods.

As disturbing as the previous contravention of the laws of mechanics and physics is, an even more incorrect procedure, in the opinion of the writer, is the attempt to persuade the biomechanical community interested in head and neck injury to accept a criterion of brain damage that is based on an arbitrary variation of mechanical moduli of the brain as a function of, not of strain rate, but of the duration of the load ranging from zero up to about 10 ms, proclaimed as a way to permit the stipulation of a continuous curve of acceleration as a function of time purporting to delineate tolerance levels. The writer also was informed by a Workshop attendee in a position to know that "the worst available data" was employed for this correlation. This type of artificial curve-fitting for the purpose of achieving a predetermined result, i.e., a single rather than a series of brain tolerance criteria, has no precedent in accepted scientific procedure. No material known exhibits this type of behavior; certain solids are characterized by a constitutive relation where stress is described in terms of strain and strain rate, but, by definition, this can never occur for an elastic material, especially a linear one, which is the only material description that the numerical code employed is capable of handling. Furthermore, fluid bulk moduli do not possess such a rate-dependent characteristic, although their viscous characteristics may be slighty influenced by loading rates. Since viscosity is not involved here, as manifested by the linearly elastic limitation of the operative computer program, the procedure employed is totally unacceptable, entirely contrary to scientific principles and procedures established over centuries, and it, and the results obtained by such methods, should be accordingly rejected. The proffered explanation that a variation of the modulus is permitted because a flow processes into and out of the brain further contravenes accepted methods because a flow process, by definition, cannot affect a fundamental material property, but is, in turn, controlled by such property. Yet, this curve is urged upon the community as the epitome of head injury tolerance criteria. The writer has received strong unsolicited support, both verbal and written, from Workshop participants with regard to his criticisms of the procedures described by the comment that such exposure is long overdue.

The dangers inherent in this completely unsound representation or, for that matter, any explicit level of dosage as an absolute tolerance criterion is tragically demonstrated by a recent legal case involving the question of accidental death or murder of a 2-year-old girl. An individual was indicted and convicted of first-degree homicide solely on the basis of totally incorrect biomechanical "evidence," presumably proving that a fall down a set of stairs could not possibly have been accidental. A dummy was pushed or thrown down the steps in what was described as an attempt to locate the possible landing sites for various initial conditions; a pressure indicator consisting of an aluminum material deforming on impact was also used in some of the tests. The videotapes taken indicated to the writer that the fall of the dummy was equivalent to that of a sack of potatoes, with no basic reproducibility, and certainly no resemblance to the fall of a living child. Furthermore, no attempt was made to specifically produce impact on the edge of the carpeted steps, or to consider the possibility of the fall of the child from a 3-ft-high railing above the landing after losing her balance and travelling through a vertical distance of 8 ft.

A set of totally inapplicable, wrong and unscientific calculations were performed to show that "the peak head acceleration was below established head injury tolerance levels" (the analysis will be described in more detail subsequently). The criteria for the acceleration comparison were the unacceptable model just described and also an HIC value of 1000, employed as substantive "proof" that the child could not have sustained a fatal injury accidentally, the trauma consisting of a 7-cm long irregular linear skull fracture in the occipital region adjacent to an approximately 1-in.-diameter contusion on the back of the scalp with no apparent marks on the outer scalp surface. Death was declared as being due to cerebral edema and fungi.

Of course, skull fracture is produced by stresses exceeding a critical limit, not by accelerations. Proper stress analysis requires examination of the contact problem involving the interaction of two deformable objects, and this was not done here. Furthermore, there is no basis of comparison with experimental values even if this procedure had been followed.

The criteria utilized for brain damage are known to apply only to adults and were primarily developed for the purpose of evaluating protective head gear; they are known universally not to apply to children whose tolerance is substantially less (27) (26). In fact, the exhaustive compilation of reference (26) which, is as indicated by court records, was known to the author of these procedures, shows a value of 83 g for the critical biomechanical loading limit in children due to frontal or dorsal loading beyond which irreversible damage ensues. This magnitude is less than any of the values calculated—no matter how incorrectly—in contradiction to the crucial statement on tolerance that prompted the change of opinion of the coroner from accidental death to homicide in this case. Deliberate deletion of mention of this critical value of 83 g, which is the **only** composite tolerance magnitude (the values of reference (27) are even lower) in a case involving the entire future of a human being, in such a report or court testimony is contrary to scientific procedure and thus, in the opinion of the writer, indefensible.

The writer attempted to ascertain by international correspondence and other communication whether any data exist on the fracture strength of children's skulls; none such appears to have been obtained. However, it is obvious that the limit for fracture in radial compression will be substantially less than that quoted for adults, approximately $10{,}000 \pm 5{,}000$ psi for cadaver skulls (28). A contact impact finite element program could have evaluated the crucial question of stress variation in the contact region (29); this was not done. The finite element program purporting to represent skull and brain stresses suffers from a multitude of deficiencies, as documented, by a finite element expert; minimally, the program is capable of handling only linear elasticity, the skull is not described by a three-layer element, nor is the input properly represented.

The inapplicability, fallacy and internal inconsistency of the rigid-body calculations representing the primary basis for conclusions can be summarized as follows: (1) An energy equation was used to represent the rigid-body impact instead of an impulse-momentum relation, as demanded in every elementary text-book on mechanics; the argument that such an approach yields a maximum force value is valid only if all the energies are properly accounted for; (b) The kinetic energy of the impact was attributed only to the head, whereas if, in the worst case, the body was not in contact with the staircase upon skull impact, the mass of the body should most definitely have been included; (c) Most scientifically reprehensible, the kinetic energy was equated to potential energy in the form of a force-deformation curve initially represented as trapezoidal, as shown in Figure 16, with a value of the maximum deformation picked arbitrarily as 1 in. (including a compression of the scalp to something larger than its total thickness); no material acts that way unless it undergoes plastic deformation or fracture, and since the stair step certainly exhibited neither, such a final deformation must have occurred solely in the skull—according to the curve—yet the possibility of fracture was categorically denied; (d) This curve was not sufficiently simple for the author who had conducted tests on the stair step and was aware of the concave-upward comportment of such material and should have certainly been aware that such behavior is universally observed in virtually all biological tissue as well; consequently, the curve was replaced by a rectangular force-deformation curve shown dashed in Figure 17 with an overall deformation reduced to 0.75 in. Now an evaluation of the force required was performed, Newton's law applied to the mass of the head, and the resultant accelerations tabulated, ranging from 84–156 g's for various conditions.

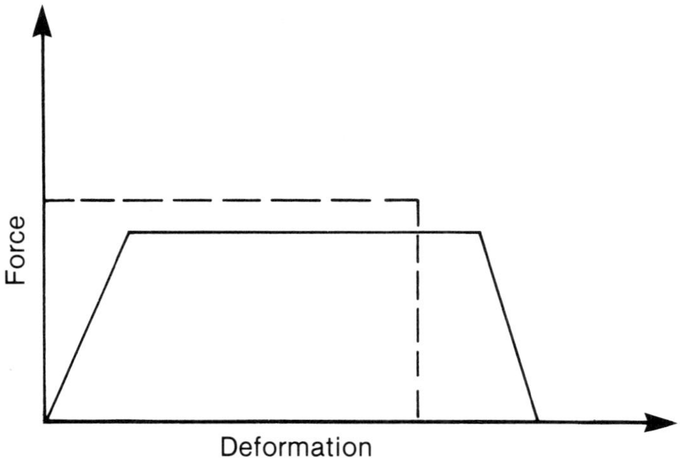

Figure 17. Stipulated Force-Deformation Curve Behavior for the Impact of a Child's Skull on a Padded Stair (Solid Line) and its Approximation (Dashed Line)

The author of these calculations obviously does not realize that the performance of these calculations is purely kinematic, in that substitution in the work energy equation of Newton's law for this case leads to the relation $v^2=2$ as, with v as the initial velocity, s as the travel distance and a as the constant acceleration, a formula known to high-school physics students. Thus, if v and s are specified, a is predetermined, and this means that even if the value of the velocity v is obtained correctly—disputed by at least one senior colleague—that the specification of s predetermines the value of the acceleration to anything desired. Finally, for this case of constant acceleration, the duration is also predetermined from $t=(v/a)$, yielding a value of 6.7 to 5 ms for the range of calculated accelerations, instead of the value of 8 ms (obviously also assumed) exhibited on the curve delineating the previously mentioned invalid model, representing an internal contradiction of the most elementary possible equation of motion. It is also astounding that the same constant value of deformation should have been assumed for all velocities; it appears to be obvious that the maximum deformation of any system would depend on the value of the relative impact speed.

All of the above material is in the public domain and will be furnished upon request.

The writer has shown these calculations to over 20 professors on many campuses in California and one Engineering Dean, all recognized as authorities in the fields of mechanics, a half dozen professors and respected scientists attending the Workshop and numerous other experts throughout the country. The universal reaction was an incredulity that this approach could ever be perpetrated by someone formally trained in mechanics to some extent, much less be the critical factor deciding a person's life in a court case, with appropriate comments concerning the inadequacy of this work. In addition, one of the leading experimental head injury neurosurgeons and his medical colleagues were emphatic that, in their opinion, a skull fracture of the type described could have occurred from a height of 5 or perhaps 8 ft onto a padded stair step of 1 in. thickness, especially if the head hit the edge without the body first supported by a portion of the stairs.

No one can duplicate the event because the physical information required is unknown, and an adequate substitute for the decedent's body is not available. However, the writer has conducted impact tests both against both the flat and the edge of padded stair steps using both a 14-lb dummy head (also employed in the baseball cap tests) and a cadaver skull stuffed with clay, resembling the bulk modulus of brain, to a total weight of 7 lb, stipulated as the head weight of the decedent. The models were suspended ballistically, dropped from a predetermined height, and rebound velocity was noted. An accelerometer was placed at the mass center of both models and the acceleration history recorded; Figure 18 shows results both against the flat and the edge of the stair steps. The former exhibits several peaks, resulting from the multiple impact of the clamped board, whereas the latter were triangular. The records were used in first line only to obtain the duration of the contact; the measured initial and rebound velocity, the impulse momentum relation and a force history either triangular or of sine-squared shape (which has been nearly universally found to be a reasonable approximation in almost any impact test not involving perforation and which, if slightly skewed, would still represent the final result to an excellent level of approximation) permitted the calculation of the peak force.

Since impact tests were conducted only up to a speed of 9.6 ft/s to avoid the fracture of the skull model and, if this had occurred, then would require consideration of the unknown variations inherent in a second biological model, the results were extrapolated linearly on the basis of the change of momentum, a conservative estimate since the contact duration of 3 ms, measured for the tests at maximum velocity, was retained; in actuality, such duration probably would decrease slightly, increasing the peak force value. For the cadaver skull and edge impact, the peak force so obtained was about 3,850 lb assuming an impact speed of 20 ft/s and only the effect of the mass of the head—both regarded as conservative. This is more than five times greater than that found in the previously described unacceptable calculation. Flat-sided impact reduced this force, and so did the use of a headform relative to the cadaver. Realistically, the skull employed was substantially stiffer than what would be the case for a child's skull; approximating the contact duration as the inverse ratio of stiffness cited in reference (25) yields half the peak force cited, but still leads to a value of 275 g, substantially in excess even of the tolerance levels cited in both the unacceptable model and the HIC standard at a duration of 6 ms for adults.

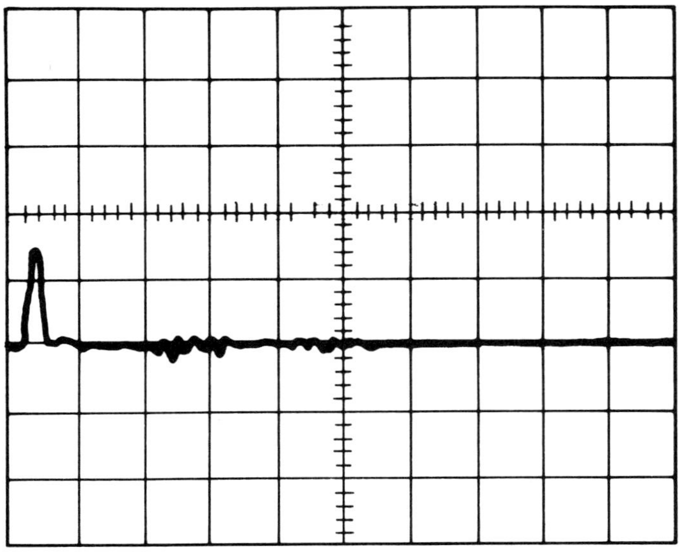

(a) 7 lb Skull Acceleration Trace for an Impact on the Round Edge of a Carpeted Stair Step at a Velocity of 9.55 ft/s. Time Scale: 10 ms/cm; Peak Acceleration, 139.5 g

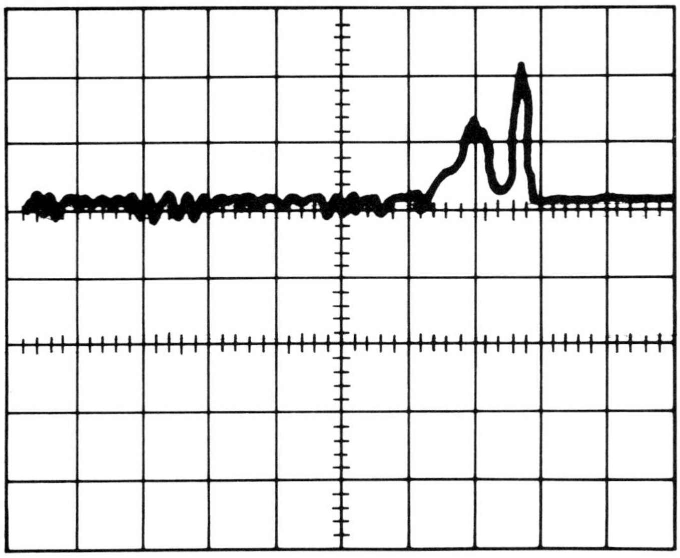

(b) 7 lb Skull Acceleration Trace for an Impact on the Flat Side of a Padded Stair Step at a Velocity of 4.33 ft/s. Time Scale: 10 ms/cm; Peak Acceleration, 43.3 g

Figure 18. Acceleration Traces for Skull Impacts on a Padded Stair Step

Conclusions

The writer strongly believes that a national responsibility exists to publicize methodologies that contravene the long established and accepted precepts of science and mechanics, with particular reference to the completely arbitrary stipulation of mechanical properties to either permit curve-fitting of disjointed data representations or to satisfy erroneous notions of material behavior. He also wishes most emphatically to go on record that the variability of human systems and our relative ignorance concerning their behavoir under dynamic loading does not currently permit anything more than the techniques for establishing effectiveness of protective components, but certainly not an absolute stipulation of bounds below which no injury could ever conceivably occur. While the latter admission may pose certain legal problems for the enforcement of test criteria for helmet manufacture or other types of protective environment, it may also prevent the use of such criteria in situation for never so intended, such as the case cited, under guise of the authoritative voice of the Federal Government. Responsible officials are undoubtedly cognizant of this problem, but require support from the scientific community to insist on better delineation of tolerance criteria. The general public is not receptive to the process of rational mechanics, so that any one in the field can convince random groups that tolerance levels are either exceeded or not, as the occasion demands, by using procedures soundly rejected by most recognized experts, but not understood by laymen, together with arbitrarily chosen physical parameters that might suit particular needs. A general statement to the effect that the maturity of the field of head injury is not sufficient to permit the establishment of absolutes is urgently required by competent authority and would be supported by the vast majority of the respected engineering and medical community. Clearly, this area is in dire need of further substantive investigation and more rational efforts to define tolerance in terms of both individual head components and/or specific damage manifestations as well as some sampling to provide an idea of the variation of any of these limiting dosages relative to age, locale, occupation and other important parameters controlling the structural development of human beings.

References

1. Gurdjian, E.S., *Impact Head Injury.* C.C. Thomas, Springfield, Ill., 1975.
2. Denny-Brown, D., and Russell, W.R., "Experimental Cerebral Concussion," *Brain,* vol. 64, pp. 93–164, 1941.
3. Hess, R.L., Weber, K., and Melvin, J.W., Review of Literature and Regulations Relating to Head Impact Tolerance and Injury Criteria, Univ. of Michigan, Highway Safety Research Institute, Report UM-HSTI-80-52-1, July 1980.
4. Holbourn, A.H.S., "Mechanics of Head Injury," *Lancet,* vol. 2, pp. 438–441, 1943.
5. Goldsmith, W., "Biomechanics of Head Injury," In: *Biomechanics, Its Foundations and Objectives,* ed. by Y.C. Fung, N. Peroone, and M. Anliker. Prentice-Hall, Englewood Cliffs, N.J., pp. 585–634, 1972.
6. Goldsmith, W., "The Physical Processes Producing Head Injuries," In: *Head Injury Conference Proceedings,* ed. by W.F. Caveness and A.E. Walker. J.B. Lippincott, Philadelphia, pp. 350–382, 1966.
7. Goldsmith, W., "Some Aspects of Head and Neck Injury and Protection," In: *Progress in Biomechanics,* ed. by N. Akkas. Sijthoff & Noordhoff, Alphen aan den Rijn (The Netherlands) pp. 333–377, 1979.
8. King, A.I., and Chou, C.C., "Mathematical Modeling, Simulation and Experimental Testing of Biomechanical System Crash Response," *J. Biomechanics,* vol. 9, 301–317, 1976.
9. Liu, Y.K., "Biomechanics of Closed Head Impacts," *J. Engineering Mechanics Division,* ASCE, vol. 104, EM 1, pp. 131–152, 1978.
10. Mertz, H.J., and Patrick, L.M., "Strength and Response of the Human Neck," In: *Proceedings of the 15th Stapp Car Crash Conference,* pp. 207–255 (SAE Paper No. 710955), 1971.
11. McElhaney, J., Roberts, V.L., and Hilyard, J., *Biomechanics of Trauma.* Duke University Press, Durham, N.C., 1976.
12. Eiband, A.M., *Human Tolerance to Rapidly Applied Accelerations: A Summary of the Literature,* NASA Memo 5–19–59E, 1959.
13. Snyder, R.G., Foust, D., and Bowman, Bruce W., "Study of Impact Tolerance Through Free Fall Investigations," Final Report December 1977, University of Michigan, HSRI UM-HSRI-77-8.
14. Hodgson, V.R., "Biomechanics of Head and Neck Injury and Principles of Protection in Sports," In: *Sports Medicine*—the Unthwarted Epidemic, ed. by P.F. Vinger, and E.F. Hoerner, Littleton, Mass., PSG Publications Co., 1980.
15. Newman, J.A., "Head Injury Criteria in Automotive Crash Testing," Proc. of the 24th Stapp Car Crash Conference, pp. 701–747, 1980.
16. Lubock, P., and Goldsmith, W., "Experimental Cavitation Studies in a Model Head-Neck System," *J. Biomechanics,* vol. 13, pp. 1041–1052, 1980.
17. Goldsmith, W., and Kabo, J.M., "Performance of Baseball Caps," *American Journal of Sports Medicine,* vol. 10, pp. 31-37, 1982.
18. Kabo, J.M., "Response of a Head-Neck System to Transient Sagittal Place Loading," Dissertation (Ph. D.), University of California, Berkeley, 1980.
19. Winters, J., "Response of an Advanced Head-Neck Model to Transient Loading," Thesis (M.S.), University of California, Berkeley, 1980.
20. Gross, A.G., "A New Theory on the Dynamics of Brain Concussion and Brain Injury," *J. Neurosurgery,* vol. 15, pp. 548-561, 1958.
21. Gross, A.G., "Impact Thresholds of Brain Concussion," *J. Aviation Medicine,* vol. 29, pp. 725–732, 1958.
22. Landkof, B., Goldsmith, W., and Sackman, J.L., "Impact on a Head-Neck Structure," *J. Biomechanics,* vol. 9, pp. 141–151, 1976.
23. Landkof, B., and DiStefano, N., "Identification of the Viscoelastic Characteristics of an Artificial Neck," *Mathematical Biosciences,* vol. 26, p. 109, 1975.
24. Rayleigh, Lord, "On the Pressure Developed in a Liquid During the Collapse of a Spherical Cavity," *Phil. Mag.,* vol. 34, pp. 94–98, 1917.
25. Mohan, D., Bowman, B.M., Snyder, R.G., and Foust, D.R., "A Biomechanical Analysis of Head Impact Injuries to Children," *Journal of Biomechanical Engineering,* vol. 101, pp. 109–118, 1979.

26. Stürtz, G., "Biomechanical Data of Children," Proc. of the 24th Stapp Car Crash Conference, pp. 511-599, 1980.

27. Fayon, A., and Tarrière, C., Essai de definition de la tolerance de la tete de jeunes enfants aux chocs, In: *Proc. 2nd IRCOBI Meeting on Biomechanics of Trauma in Children,* Lyon, France, pp. 252-259, 1974.

28. McElhaney, J.H., Fogle, J.L., Melvin, J.W., Haynes, R.R., Roberts, V.L., and Alem, N.M., "Mechanical Properties of Cranial Bone," *J. Biomechanics,* vol. 3, pp. 495-512, 1970.

29. Taylor, R.L. and Sackman, J.L. *Contact Impact Problems,* Department of Transportation, NHTSA, DOT Reports Nos. HS805-629 and 805-630. Washington, D.C., August 1980.

Modeling of Human Surrogate Neck Response to −Gx Impact Acceleration

A. I. King
R. S. Levine
R. Cheng
S. S. Nakhla
K. H. Yang

Abstract

In the process of evolving a standardized test for driver air bag restraints, serious neck injuries were observed in two of the three cadavers tested. The impact severity was at the limits of FMVSS 208 as measured in a Part 572 ATD. Axial neck loads as measured in a Hybrid III ATD averaged 3kN. A spine model was used to compute head acceleration and neck loads. If belts were used in place of the air bag, equally severe injuries could be expected to occur. Head impact with an air bag does not increase neck loads which are a function of the whipping of the head.

Introduction

Severe neck injuries are rarely reported in frontal automotive collisions, particularly for restrained occupants. In a carefully documented study by Patrick et al. (1), only one cervical fracture was reported out of 128 cases of frontal collisions involving belted occupants of Volvo cars. In another study by Ewing et al. (2), fully restrained rhesus monkeys were subjected to high levels of −Gx impacts (over 100 g), resulting in severe cervical injuries. Heulke et al. (3) surveyed the literature and case histories from the files of the Highway Safety Research Institute of the University of Michigan. The objective was to locate cases in which cervical fractures and fracture dislocations occurred without head impact. For automotive occupants involved in the frontal collisons cervical injuries were rare, but the serious ones that were reported involved the upper cervical area—hangman's fracture and atlanto-occipital separation.

In an ongoing project at Wayne State involving the use of a driver air bag system, severe neck injuries were observed in two of the three cadavers tested to date. The air bag system was not representative of any known system in production and the experiment was designed to evolve a standard test methodology involving a driver air bag rather than the solicitation of human surrogate response to such a system.

These results prompted a modelling effort designed to elicit response parameters which could be responsible for the observed injuries. The specific aims of this paper are:

1. To compute neck forces and moments during a severe −Gx impact.
2. To look for possible injury mechanisms.
3. To study the effect of head impact and torso restraint stiffness on neck forces.

Model Description

A two-dimensional spinal model developed by Prasad and King (4) was used for this study. This model was modified by Tennyson and King (5) to include the capability of stimulating involuntary muscular response to extend the spine. The ability of the articular facets to bear compressive as well as tensile loads is one of the unique features.

This model has been subjected to validation against cadaveric as well as volunteer response data (4)(5). Relatively good correlation of model predictions with experimental data was achieved in both cases without making changes to most of the material constants used in the model. Since this is a discrete parameter model involving the head, the 24 vertebrae

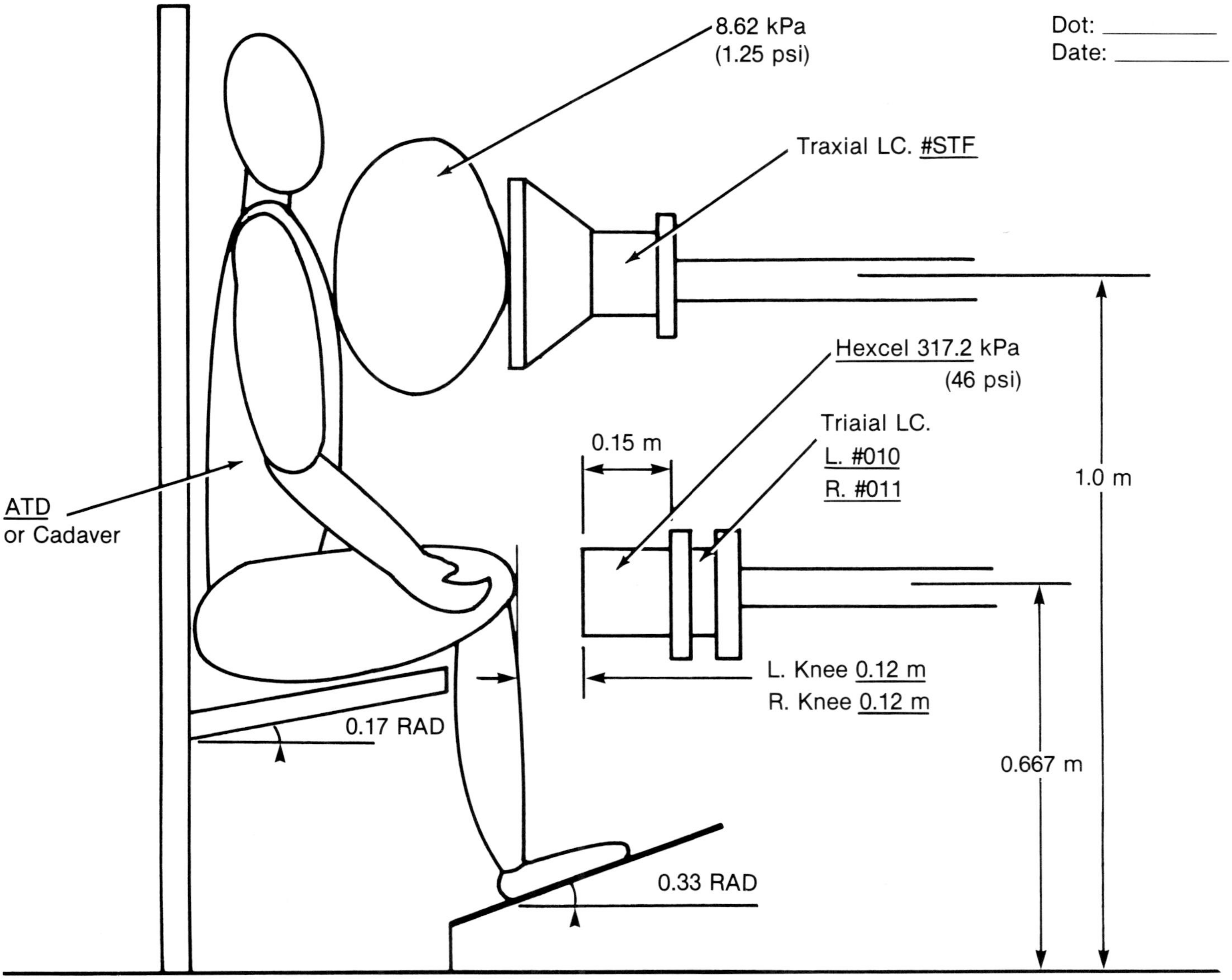

Figure 1.

and the pelvis, the input to the model is seat acceleration. A large number of output variables can be requested. These include linear and angular kinematics of any of the 26 elements, the forces and moments at any level of the spine and restraint system forces which come into play at the pelvic or thoracic level.

Experimental Test Conditions

The series of experiments designed to evolve a standardized test for driver air bags was carried out at a sled deceleration level which resulted in a 60 g, 3-ms chest acceleration response from a Part 572 anthropomorphic test device (ATD). The set up is shown schematically in Figure 1. The steering wheel plane was vertical and the steering column was rigid (non-collapsible). The air bag and steering wheel were purchased from an Oldsmobile dealer, as the bag was a production item for 1973–1975 GM cars. The gas generator unit was removed and the bag was pre-inflated to a pressure of 8.6 kPa (1.25 psi). The hard seat pan was tilted upward 0.175 rad (10°). Many adjustments were made to the seating arrangements to obtain the specified chest g-level as well as to keep the Head Injury Criterion (HIC) and the knee loads at or below the limits set by Federal Motor Vehicle Safety Standard (FMVSS) 208. The hexcell used as knee restraints had a stiffness of 317 kPa (46 psi).

The pulse which satisfied all of the FMVSS 208 limiting conditions for a Part 572 ATD is shown in Figure 2. It has a 38-g peak, is approximately triangular in shape and has a duration of 100 ms. This corresponded to a 48-km/h (30-mph) impact speed with a 0.47 m (18.5 in.) stopping distance. The center of the air bag was located at mid-sternum barely touching the anterior surface of the ATD chest. The hexcell was placed 127 mm (5 in.) from each knee and targeted to pocket the knee during impact. The center of the knees were 292 m (11.5 in.) apart. An automotive seat back equipped with a pair of shock absorbers was used to attenuate rebound from this unvented bag.

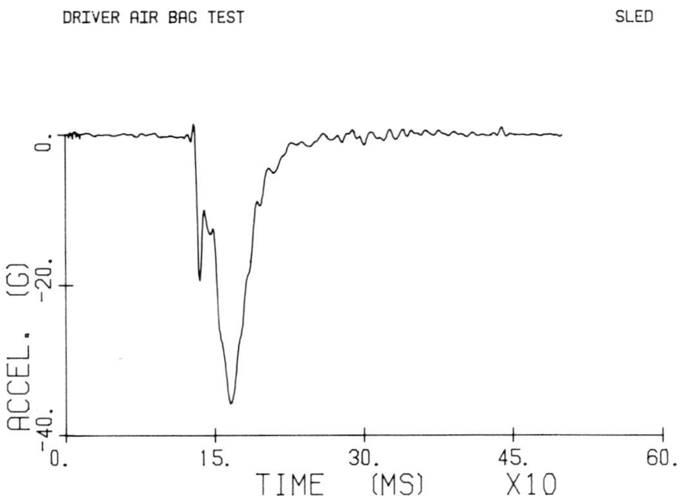

Figure 2.

Test Subjects and Instrumentation

The primary test subjects were unembalmed cadavers. Pertinent data regarding the three subjects used are listed in Table 1. Anthropometric data revealed that they were approximately representative of a 5th percentile female, a 50th and a 95th percentile male. All were victims of cardiovascular disease.

The role of the Part 572 ATD was to obtain the desired pulse shape and seating conditions. It was not used for any other purpose. A Hybrid III ATD was also used to measure neck loads after severe neck injuries were sustained by two of the three cadavers.

The cadavers were instrumented with a full array of 12 chest accelerometers, a configuration first used by Eppinger et al. (6). There were nine head accelerometers in the configuration proposed by Padgaonkar et al. (7). The thoracic aorta was pressurized to 13.8 kPa (2 psi) and the vascular pressure was monitored by a pressure transducer. The lungs were inflated to a pressure of 3.45 kPa (0.5 psi) and bronchial pressure was also measured. Air bag pressure and steering column load were recorded along with triaxial knee loads of both knees.

For the ATDs, triaxial accelerations of the head and chest were measured instead of the 21 channels monitored during cadaveric runs. Of course, there were no vascular or bronchial pressure data, but the air bag parameters and knee loads were measured. In the Hybrid III, neck loads were also measured. In fact, the principal purpose for using the Hybrid III was to obtain axial and shear loads at the atlanto-occipital junction.

Experimental Results

1. Cadaver 1

This 50th percentile 66-year-old male subject sustained a complete fracture separation of the first and second cervical vertebrae. The odontoid process was completely avulsed from the anterior arch. There was partial transection of the cord.

The head accelerations along the x- and z-axis associated with this run are shown in Figures 3 and 4, respectively. The accelerations at T1 are shown in Figure 5. The air bag pressure time history is shown in Figure 6. Steering column and knee loads are shown in Figure 7.

2. Cadaver 2

This 5th percentile 54-year-old female subject sustained a basilar ring fracture of the skull, approxi-

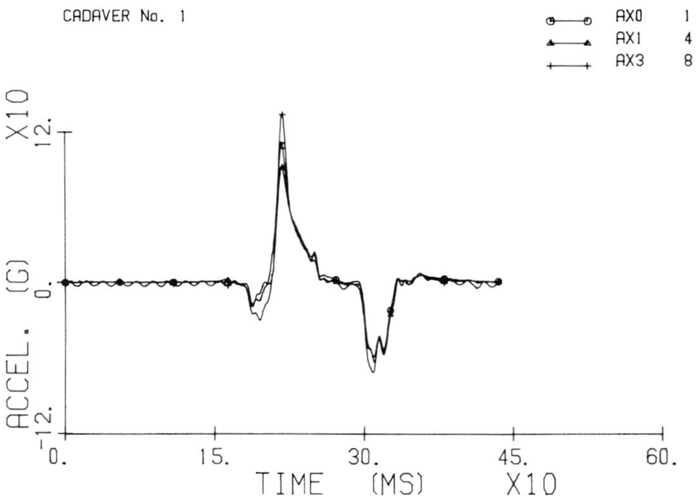

Figure 3.

Table 1.

Cadaver No.	Age	Sex	Weight	Height	Cause of Death
1	66	M	711 N	1.70 m	Myocardial Infarction Metastatic Cancer of the Prostate
2	54	F	491 N	1.51 m	Myocardial Infarction Arteriosclerosis
3	56	M	942 N	1.85 m	Hypertensive Cardiovascular Heart Disease, Diabetes Mellitus

mately 50 mm in diameter. The cervical cord at the level of the inferior portion of the medulla oblongata was completely severed.

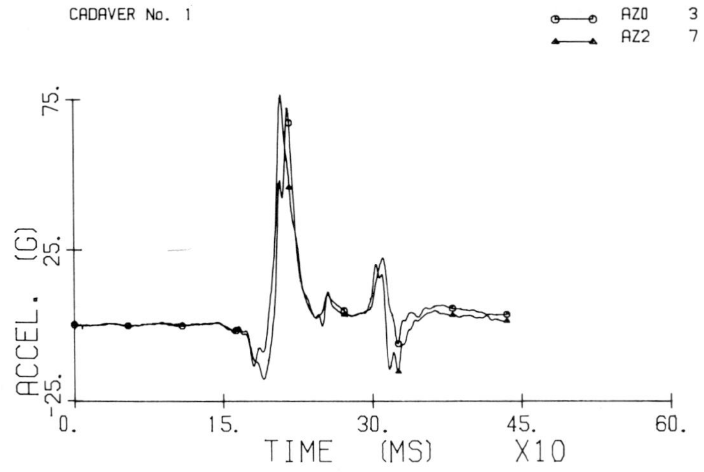

Figure 4.

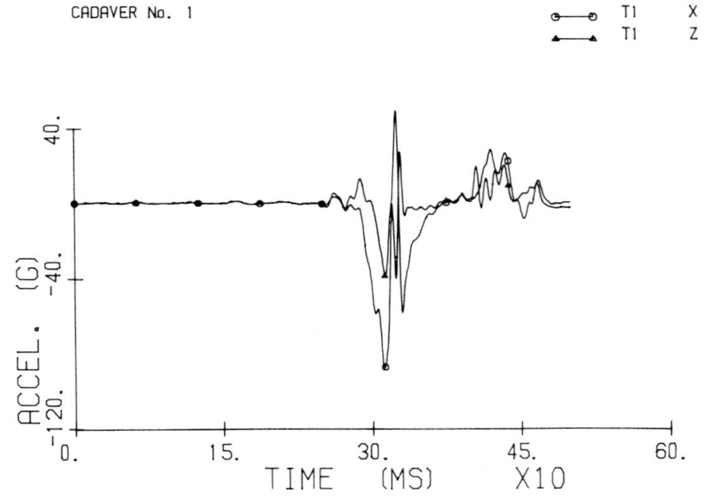

Figure 5.

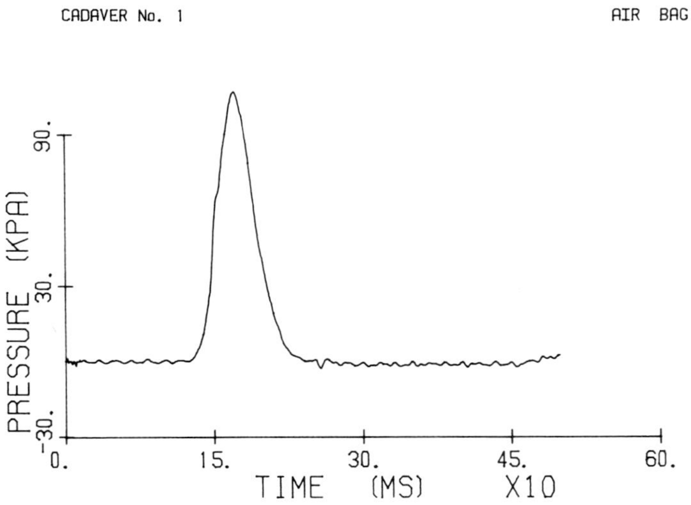

Figure 6.

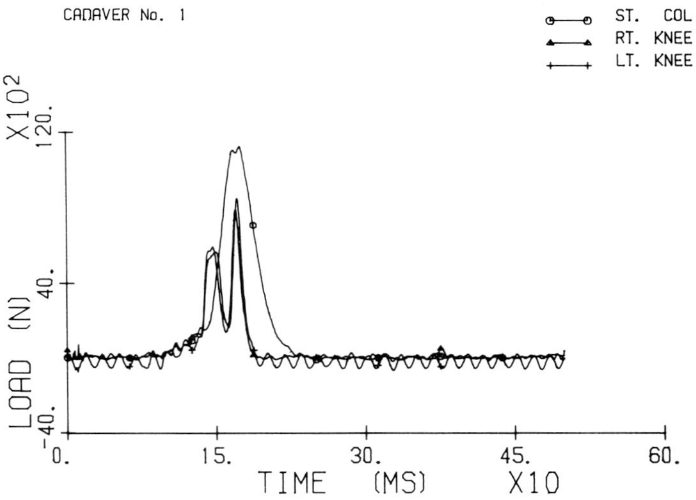

Figure 7.

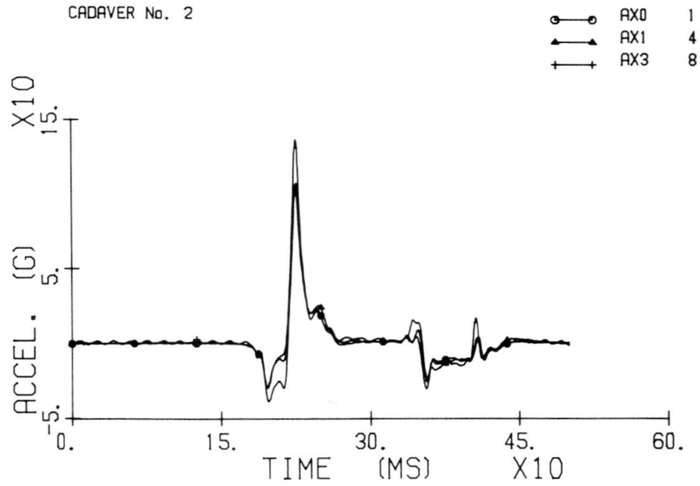

Figure 8.

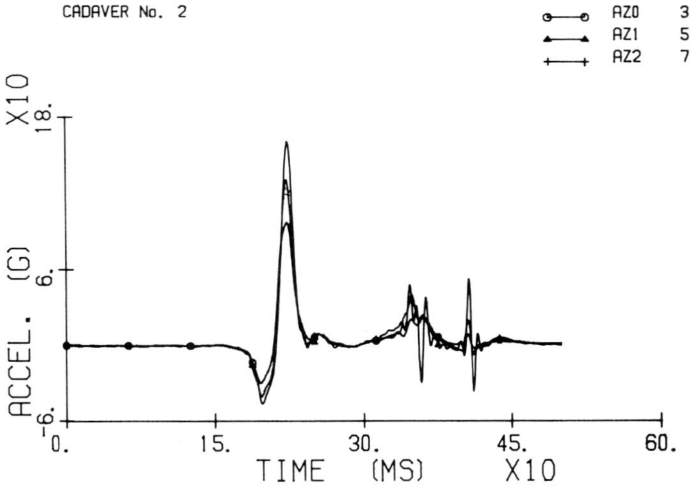

Figure 9.

The corresponding head T1 accelerations are shown in Figures 8 through 10. The bag pressure and column and knee loads are shown in Figures 11 and 12.

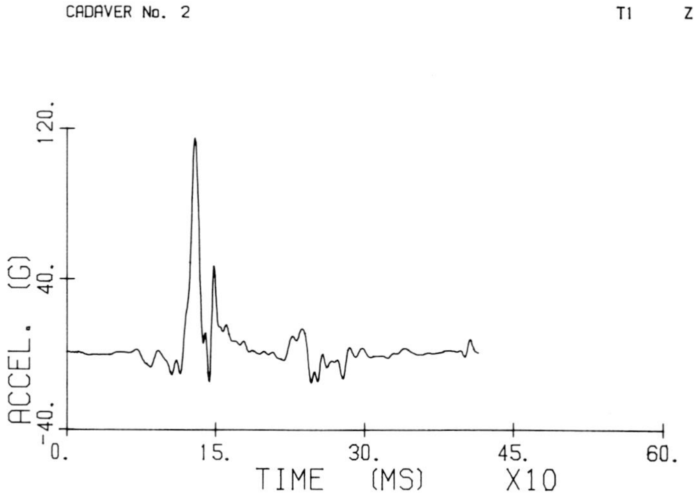

Figure 10.

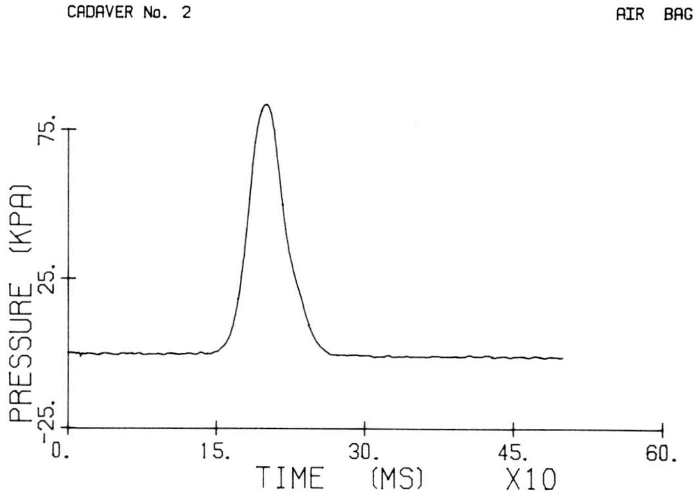

Figure 11.

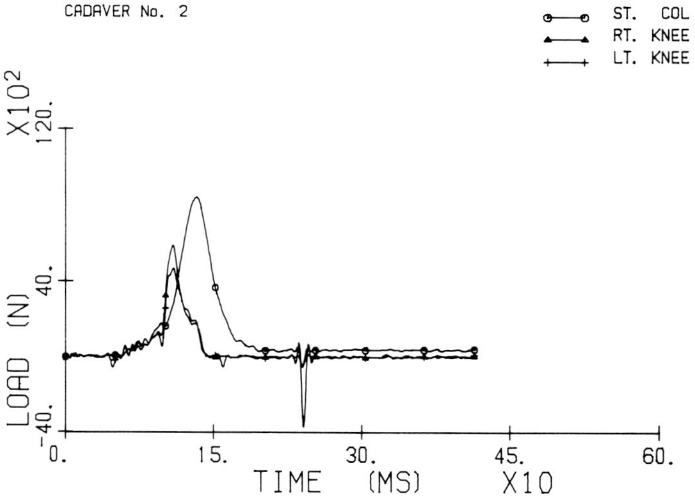

Figure 12.

3. Hybrid III ATD

The head (c.g.) and T1 (chest) accelerations for the Hybrid III ATD are shown in Figures 13 and 14, the neck loads and moments in Figures 15 and 16 and the bag pressure and column and knee loads in Figures 17 and 18.

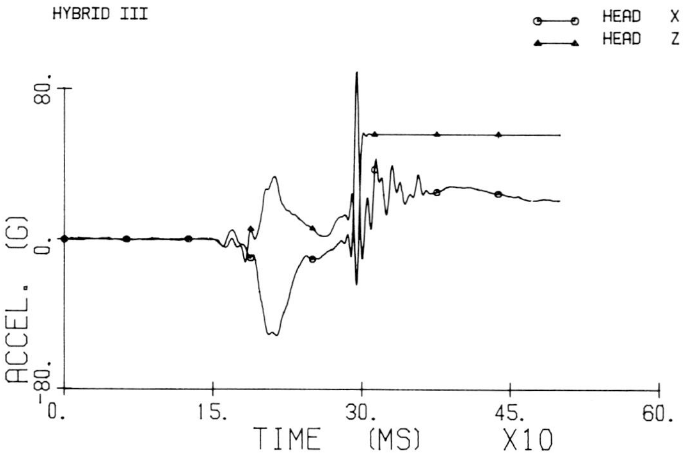

Figure 13.

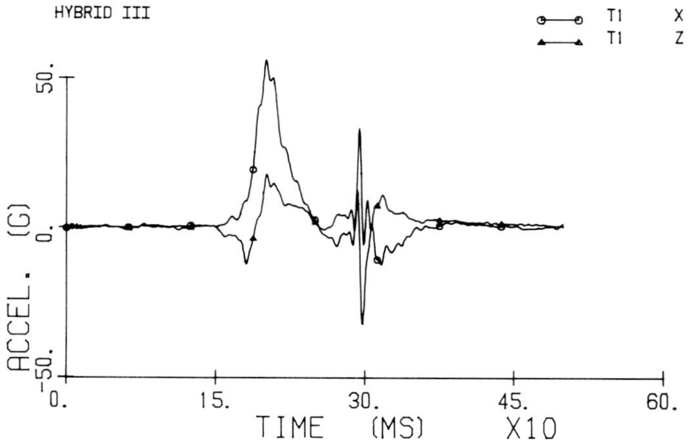

Figure 14.

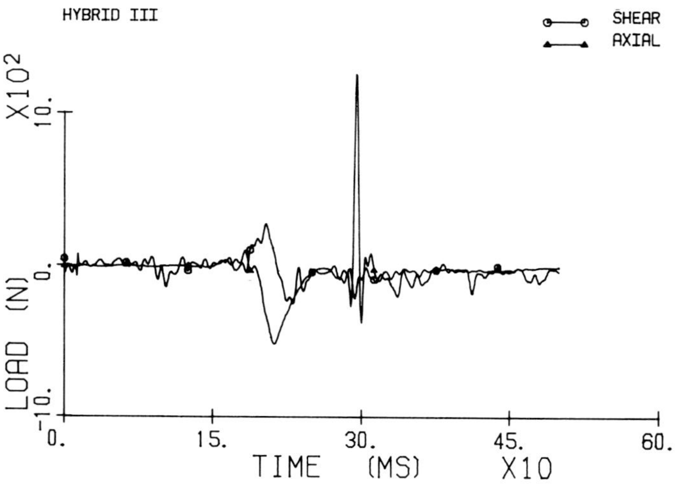

Figure 15.

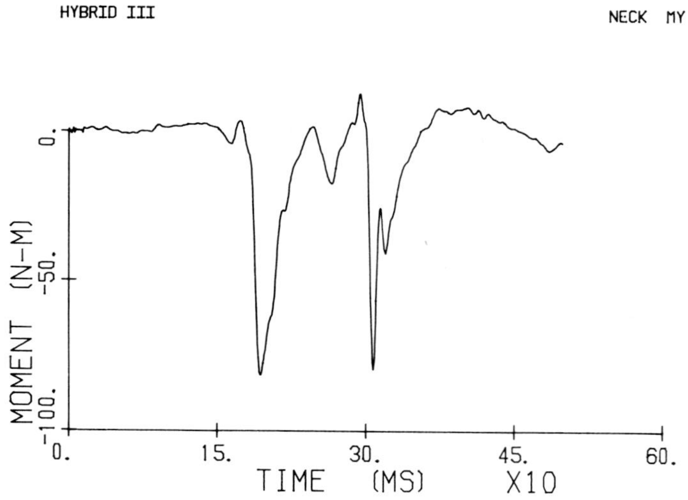

Figure 16.

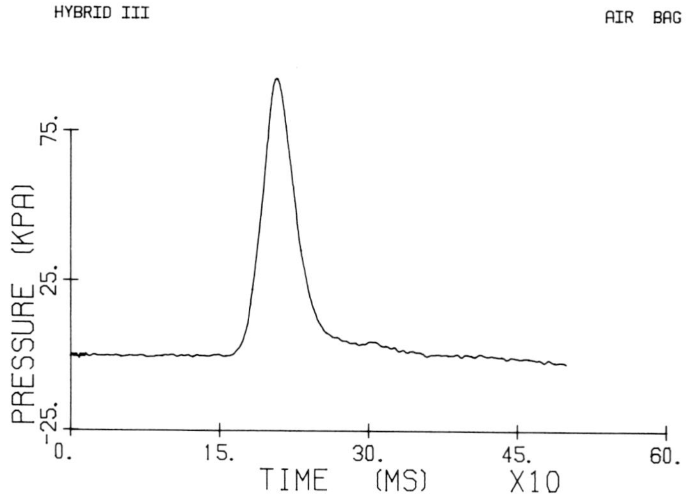

Figure 17.

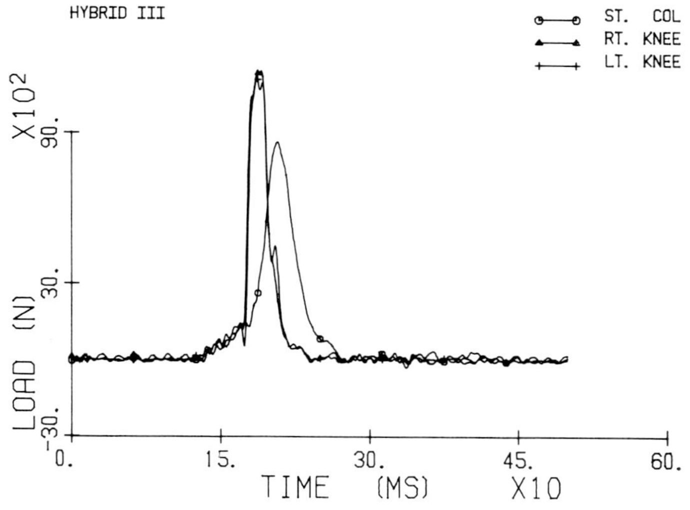

Figure 18.

4. Cadaver 3

This cadaver was almost 95th percentile in height and weight and did not sustain any severe neck injuries. There were several rib fractures, however.

Figures 19 through 21 show head and T1 accelerations while Figures 22 and 23 show air bag and steering column and knee loads.

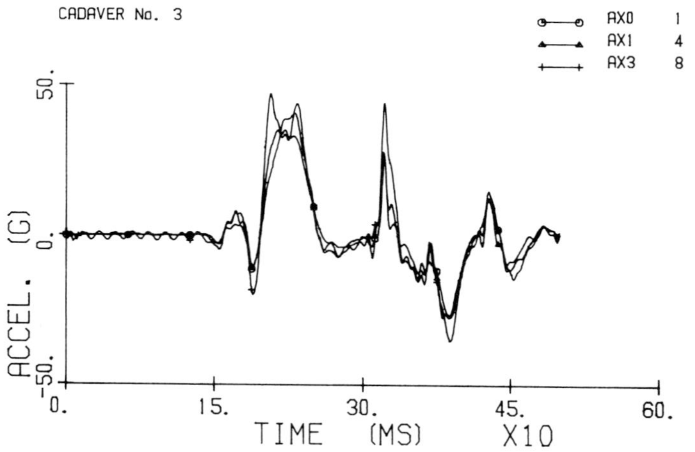

Figure 19.

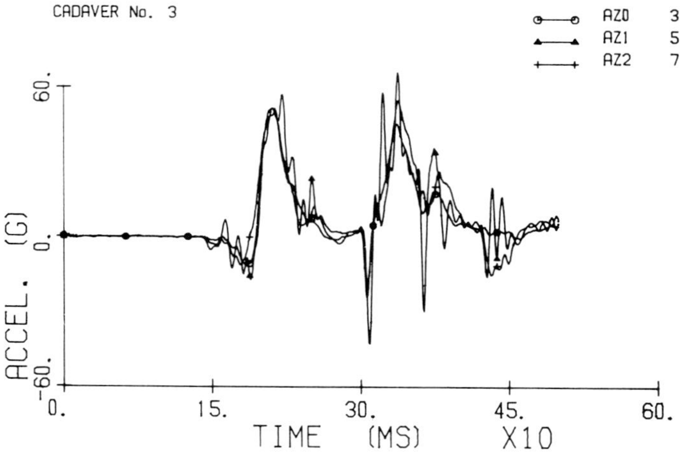

Figure 20.

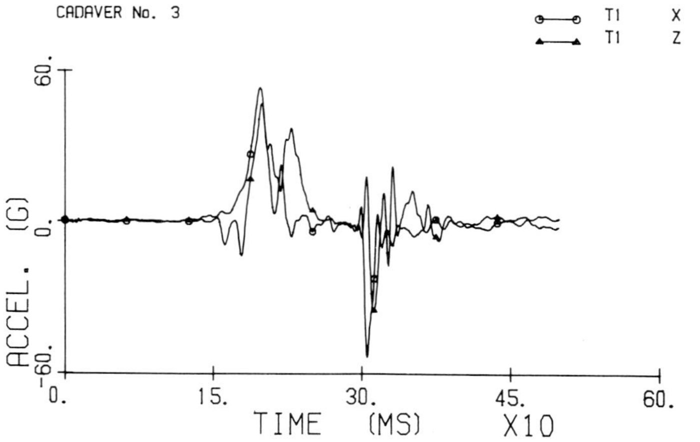

Figure 21.

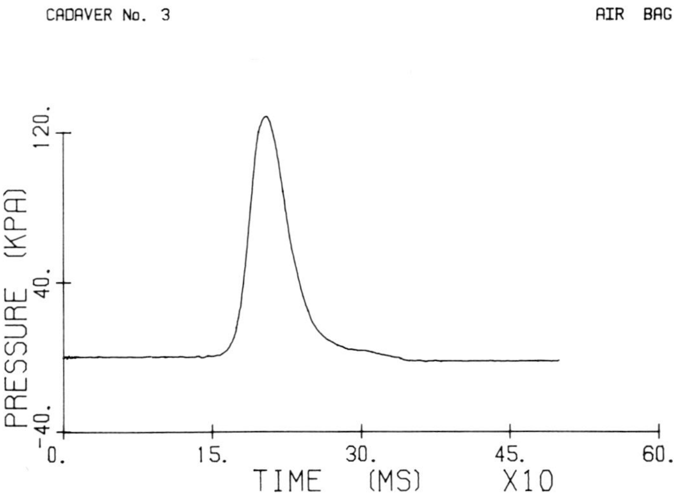

Figure 22.

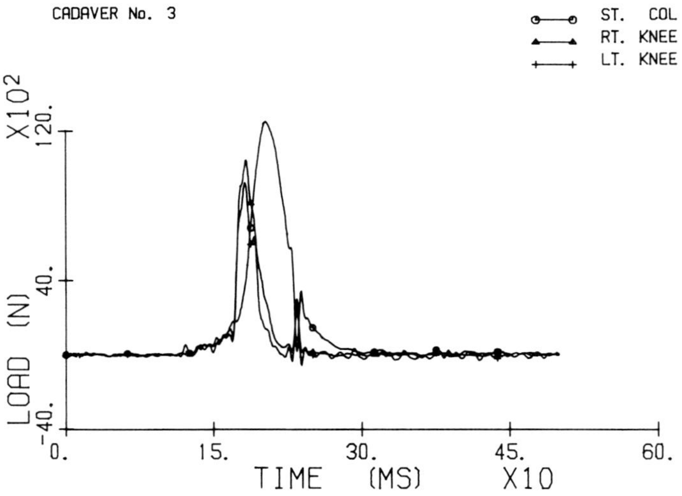

Figure 23.

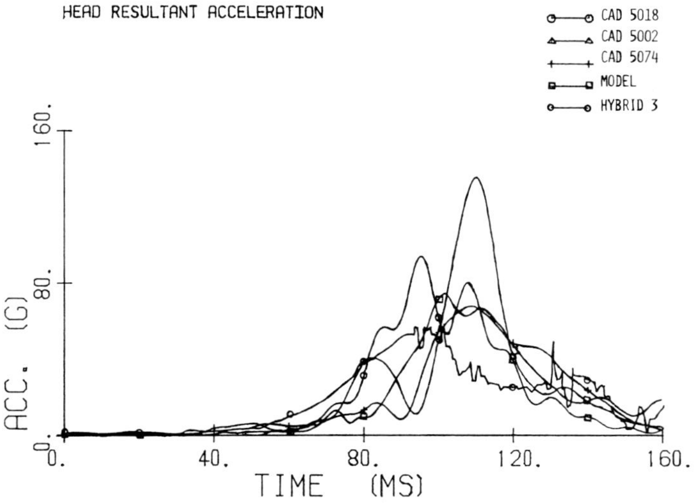

Figure 24.

Analysis of Model and Experimental Results

The resultant head accelerations of the three cadaver runs are compared with that of the Hybrid III ATD and the model in Figure 24. It is seen that the peak values for the two cadavers that sustained neck fractures were much higher than those of the dummy or of the cadaver which did not suffer a neck injury. The model results compared well with the latter case. The resultant acceleration for cadaver 2 reached a first peak of about 40 g, dipped to 10 g before it attained a second peak of 150 g. The ring fracture could have occurred at 40 g and the higher second peak was due to a lack of bony restraint of the head.

Neck loads are compared in Figures 25 through 27. The peak load is estimated to be about 7 kN in the cadaver. This may not be tolerable in weaker subjects.

The model was used to resolve the apparent paradox that severe neck injuries resulted in two of three cadavers that were run at the limits set by FMVSS 208. Had the subject been restrained by a belt system

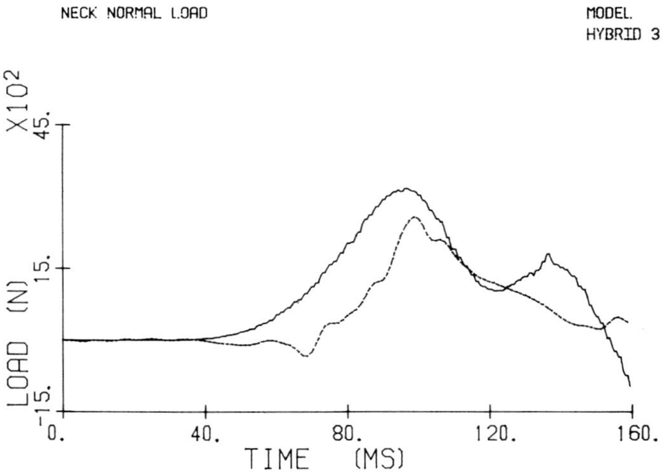

Figure 25.

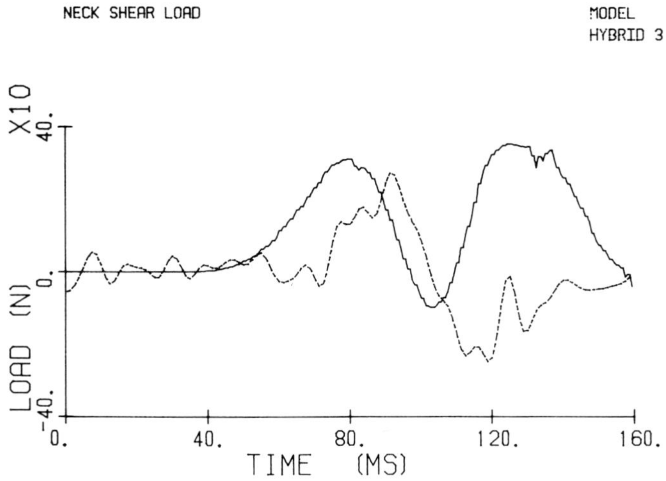

Figure 26.

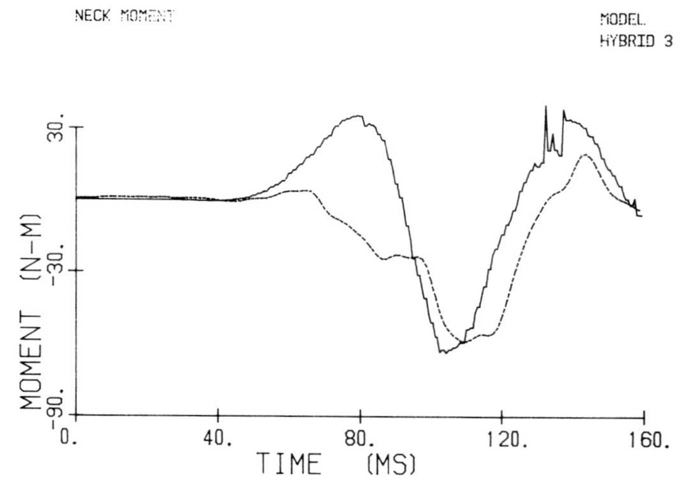

Figure 27.

which is approximately twice as stiff as the air bag, the neck loads were found to be higher than those encountered during an air bag run. If the shoulders were allowed to roll inside the shoulder restraint, there was no decrease in neck load. The air bag neck loads were found to be lower, as shown in Figures 28 through 30. A comparison of resultant head accelerations is shown in Figure 31. Those due to the belt, with or without rolling of the shoulders, were found to be higher than that of the air bag case.

The extent of neck stretch was about the same for the three cases shown in Figure 32. However the predicted motion of the odontoid process into the spinal canal was higher when the belt was used instead of the air bag, as shown in Figure 33.

Discussion and Conclusions

The air bag experiments described in this paper are not tests of the production air bag restraint system. They were part of a program to evolve a standardized test for the air bag and the results are not to be taken as representative of those of an air bag restraint. The tests were rather severe in view of the fact that all three limits of FMVSS 208 were reached simultaneously. Under these conditions, the neck may be the limiting element and a criterion of neck injury is definitely needed. However, this deceleration level of 38 g is not unattainable as vehicle downsizing continues.

The major conclusions are:

1. A neck injury criterion is needed.
2. Head impact does not affect the neck adversely.
3. Rolling of shoulders inside a belt restraint does not alternate head acceleration.

Acknowledgements

This work was sponsored in part by the National Highway Traffic Safety Administration under Contract No. DOT–HS–7–01792 and by the Office of Naval Research under Contract No. N000 14–75–C–1015.

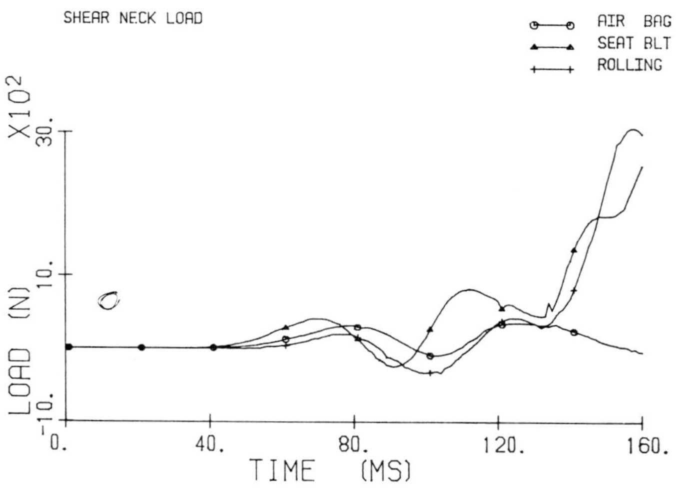

Figure 29.

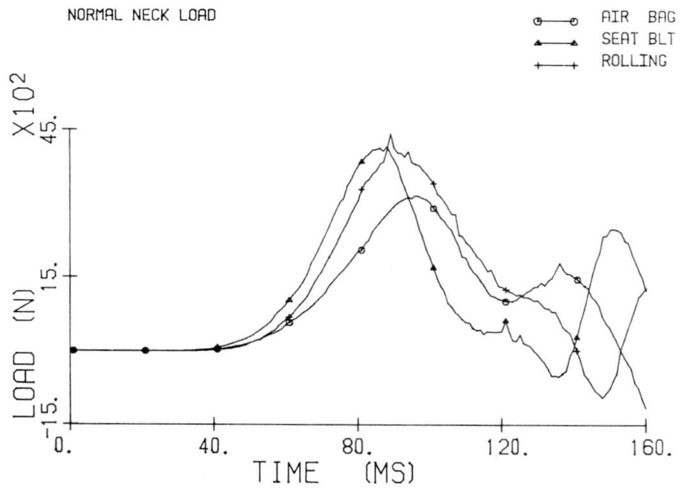

Figure 28.

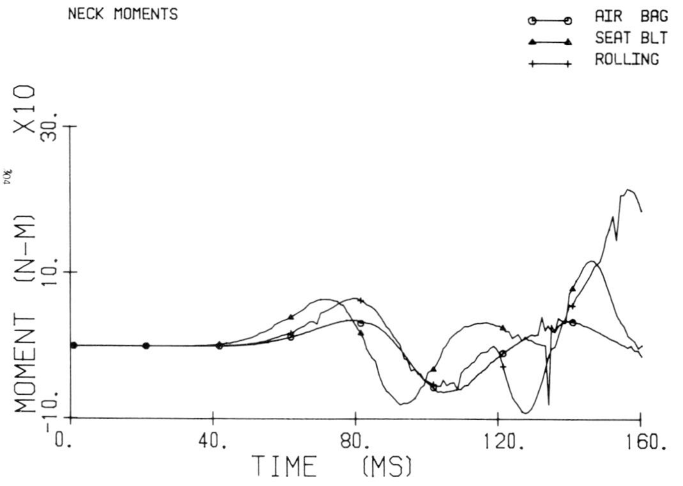

Figure 30.

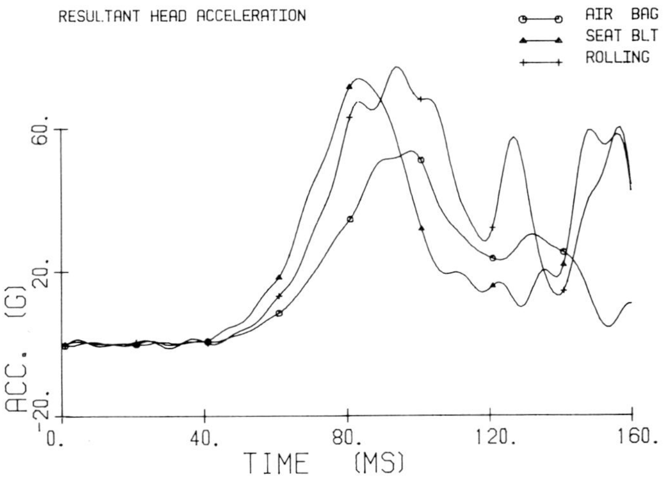

Figure 31.

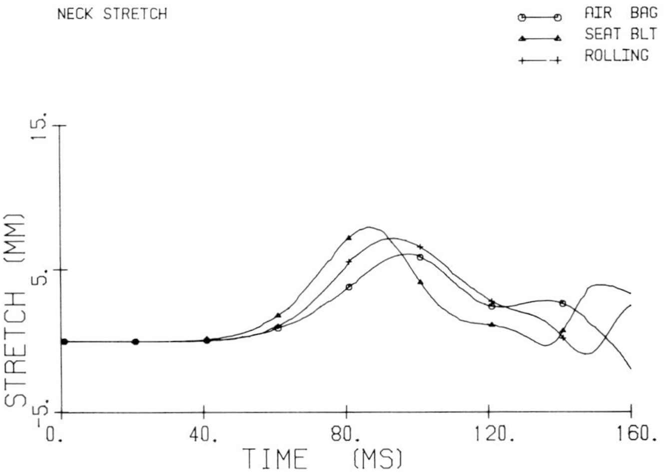

Figure 32.

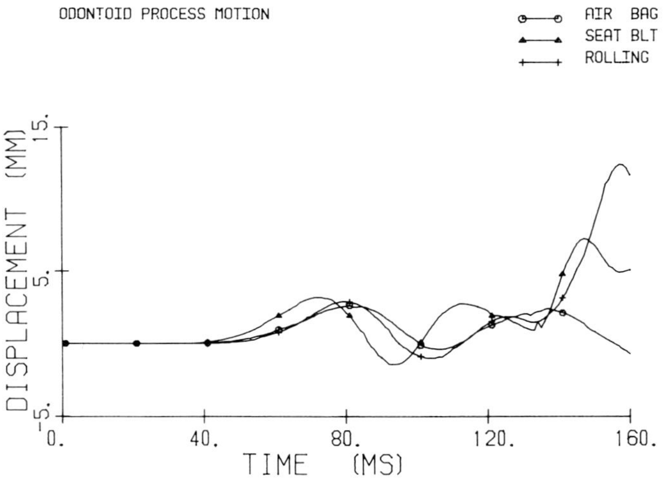

Figure 33.

References

1. Patrick LM, Bohlin N and Andersson A: Three point harness accident and laboratory data comparison. *Proc 18th STAPP Car Crash Conf:* SAE Paper No. 741181:201–282. 1974
2. Ewing CL: Human tolerance levels of injury. *Proc Workshop on Biomedical and Bioengineering Analysis of Injuries to the Head and Neck and Central Nervous System (Key Biscayne FL):* Dec 1980 (in press)
3. Huelke, DF, Mendelsohn RA, States JD and Melvin JW: Cervical fractures and fracture-dislocations sustained without head impact. *J Trauma 18 (7):*533–538. 1978
4. Prasad P and King AI: An experimentally validated dynamic model of the spine. *J Appl Mech 41:*546–550. 1974
5. Tennyson SA and King AI: A biodynamic model of human spinal column in *Mathematical Modeling Biodynamic Response to Impact.* SAE Publication SP-412 (SAE Paper No. 760771):31–44. 1976
6. Eppinger RH, Augustyn K and Robbins DH: Development of a promising universal thoracic trauma prediction methodology. *Proc 22nd STAPP Car Crash Conf* (SAE Paper 780891):209–268. 1978
7. Padgaonkar AJ, Krieger KW and King AI: Measurement of angular acceleration of a rigid body using linear accelerometers. *J. Appl Mech 42*:552–556. 1975

Status of Head Injury Modeling

Carley Ward

Introduction

The finite element method is the most widely used procedure for modeling irregular structures including the human head. Finite element brain models predict brain stresses, strains and tissue failure; finite element skull models determine the effects of skull deformation.

Using this method the structure to be analyzed is divided into small elements—blocks, tetrahedrons, plates, etc.—each having the continuum material properties of the host structure. The corners and elements are numbered and the coordinates measured. Once the model is developed, the data are input to a finite element computer program which calculates the dynamic response. Models are readily changed and modified, making parametric studies routine. Because the computer programs are widely used in civil and structural engineering, they are reliable, well-documented and easy to use.

The difficulties arise in the idealization of the structure and in model validation. Many assumptions are required when modeling biological systems. The material properties are difficult to define because they are nonlinear, nonelastic and strain rate dependent. The central nervous system is especially difficult to characterize because it is composed of soft tissue, vasculature and fluid. Furthermore, mass is not constant—there is flow through the arteries, veins and foramen magnum (the opening for the cervical cord). Material constants selected must be considered effective values.

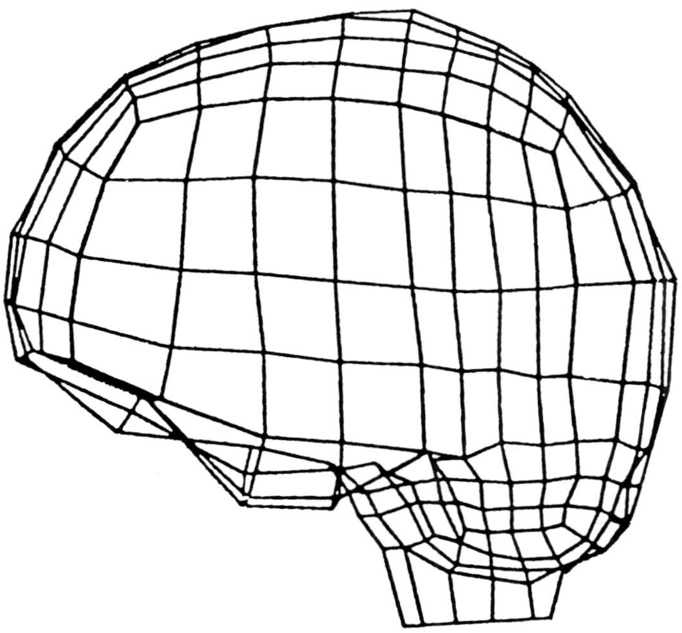

Figure 1.

For the head, the only check on the assumptions and idealizations is correlation with experimental data, such as measurements made in pressurized cadavers and live animal tests. These tests provide benchmarks for the models which must be met; good correlation is imperative.

Finite Element Skull and Brain Model Development and Design

The first model to approximate the irregular shape of the skull appeared in 1971 (1). It was a static model which employed triangular elements. Others soon followed (2) (3). In the most detailed model, three layers of eight node brick elements were used, representing two surface layers of dense bone and a center porous layer.

The first finite element model approximating the exact geometry of the brain was developed in the early seventies and was reported in 1974 (4). The model was refined and additional models of test animal brains were developed from 1975 to 1978 (5 through 8) (Figures 1 and 2). In these models, the brain tissue and contained fluids are modeled with eight node brick elements. The partitioning internal folds of dura are simulated with four node membrane elements and the opening for the cervical cord is represented. Later, a skull and cervical cord were added (9). In 1980, the brain model was integrated into a head and spine model (10).

Currently, the element grid in the brain stem and cerebellum are being modified. The number of elements is being increased to improve the accuracy of the shear strain calculations. A yielding capability is also being included to approximate the stress release which occurs when the brain or subarachnoid tissues fail.

Validation or Experimental Verification

To validate a biodynamic model, an experimental test is simulated on the computer and the measured and model-computed responses compared. If they do not agree, the model is modified and the simulation repeated. The procedure is continued until correlation

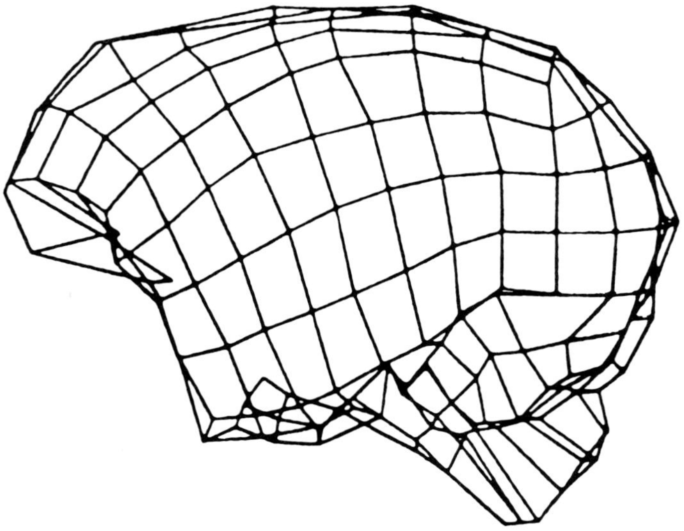

Figure 2.

is obtained. After successfully simulating many different tests with varying conditions, the model is considered valid.

Problems with skull model validation

Skull models have been checked statically on a few occasions (3), but they have not been dynamically validated. Before the models can simulate actual head impacts, some major modeling problems must be solved. First the boundary condition, the neck, is difficult to represent. The neck is very nonlinear and hard to characterize mathematically. Face and scalp effects must be included, and since impact force is the input to the model, the force direction, magnitude and location must be precisely defined.

Structural variations in the skull also create problems. Skull stresses, strains and displacements are exponential functions of skull thickness a thickness which varies from point to point and from skull to skull. Small inaccuracies in skull thickness, due to the straight element edges, produce errors in the computed response.

At present, the finite element skull models are restricted to head translation. Neglecting rotation also introduces errors.

Although the skull models cannot be used to predict dynamic skull stresses and strains, they can be used to study trends, such as the effect of skull deformation on brain response (11). They can also be useful in studying extreme conditions, like estimating the maximum possible skull stress in a given event.

Brain model validation

Finite element brain models, on the other hand, have been dynamically validated. They have accurately predicted measured brain responses in more than 50 different test simulations (12).

Brain models were easier to validate because fewer assumptions are required. Head acceleration measured in the test or obtained from a lumped parameter head-neck idealization are the input to the model. Mathematically, the brain is forced to move in space just as the head moves in the experiment. The neck, face, scalp and skull are not required. Only the internal shape of the skull is maintained to contain the brain. Thus, the number of variables is greatly reduced.

One of two finite element computer programs, EASE2 or modified SAPV, can be used. These programs have been especially modified to treat large head rotations and the nearly incompressible brain material. Any three-dimensional head rotation and translation can be simulated. A new element known as the split energy element, was developed to treat all values of compressibility.

Brain Model

Design requirements

For the model to compute the correct response in a test simulation, certain design requirements must be met. There are the obvious requirements that the model must have, approximately the same size and shape as the actual brain, but there are also less obvious requirements which were not satisfied in earlier head models. They are:

1. The opening in the base of the skull, the foramen magnum, must be simulated because tissue and fluids move through the opening. It acts as a pressure release mechanism for the brain (8).

2. The internal folds of dura, the falx and tentorium, partition the cranial cavity and influence the brain response. These membranes must be included in the model (5).

3. The brain must not be simulated as incompressible by using a brain specimen bulk modulus of approximately 300,000 psi. Flow into and out of the cranial cavity provides some compressibility or volume elastance. To model this effect, a lower bulk modulus or an effective Poisson's ratio must be used. The value selected is related to the acceleration pulse duration. Shorter pulses permit less flow and consequently are modeled with less effective compressibility (8).

Brain response

The inertia of the brain produces stresses and strains in the tissue as the brain tends to lag the motion of the skull. Brain tissue compresses against the skull near the impact site and is in tension opposite the impact. The result is a pressure or stress gradient through the brain. When the head rotates, the brain again lags behind, producing stresses and strains on the brain-skull interface. The falx and tentorium help to keep the brain in position, and instead of a single rotational displacement inside the brain as hypothesized by Holbourn (13), separate rotational motions develop in each compartment (Figure 3). These rotations in the cerebrum and cerebellum produce a complex interaction with the brain stem, the interconnecting brain structure.

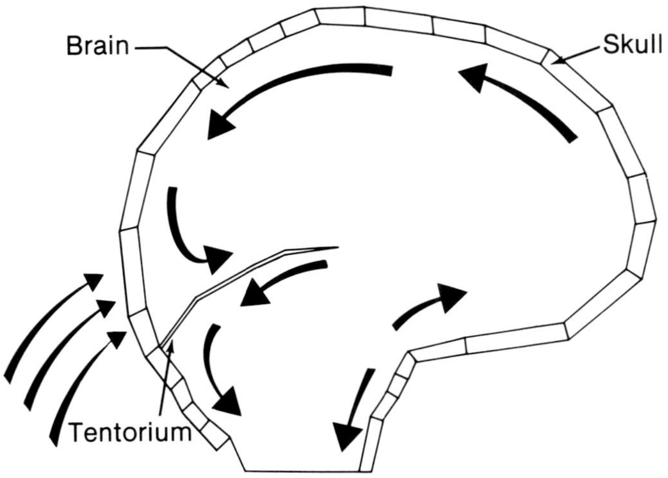

Figure 3.

The brain displacements are small, a few millimeters in most cases. Though the displacement pattern depends on the event, in general they are largest in the brain stem and cerebral cortex.

Displacements in the cervical cord are larger and influence the brain response when motion is in the superior-inferior or inferior-superior direction ($\pm$Z anatomical direction). A model with a cervical cord is necessary to simulate this motion (9).

Skull deformations have only a minimal effect on the brain. Comparisons of brain stresses from deformable and rigid skull simulations showed the maximum difference to be less than 15 percent (Figure 4) (11).

Displacements and stresses in an unpressurized dead test subject are different from those in the living or pressurized subject. The response is slower and more damped and, in some cases, the displacements are larger. Also, brain and cervical cord motions do not couple in the dead unpressurized animal. Because of these differences, dead unpressurized subjects should not be used in head injury research (9).

Correlation between response and injury

Once validated, the models become useful tools in the investigation of injury. Computed response is compared to the trauma produced in head injury tests. Because the results have been reported in many earlier publications (8) (12) (14) (15) (16) they are only summarized in the following paragraphs.

The high, nearly hydrostatic, normal stresses in the brain cause injury. Compression stresses of 34 psi can cause serious brain trauma near the impact site. Tension stresses of 27 psi can cause contrecoup contusions opposite the impact site (15). Combined tension and shear stresses produce subarachnoid hemorrhage. The tension and compression stresses producing these injuries are directly related to the head translational acceleration. Head rotation has only a minor effect on these stresses (17).

Shear strains are the largest strains in the brain. The high-strain regions are the brain stem and cerebellum, and along the brain external surface and cerebral cortex. Petechial hemorrhages, tear lesions and subdural hematomas develop in these regions. The actual shear magnitudes which fail the tissue are currently being researched. These shear strains are related to head rotational accelerations but do not disappear when rotation is eliminated (17).

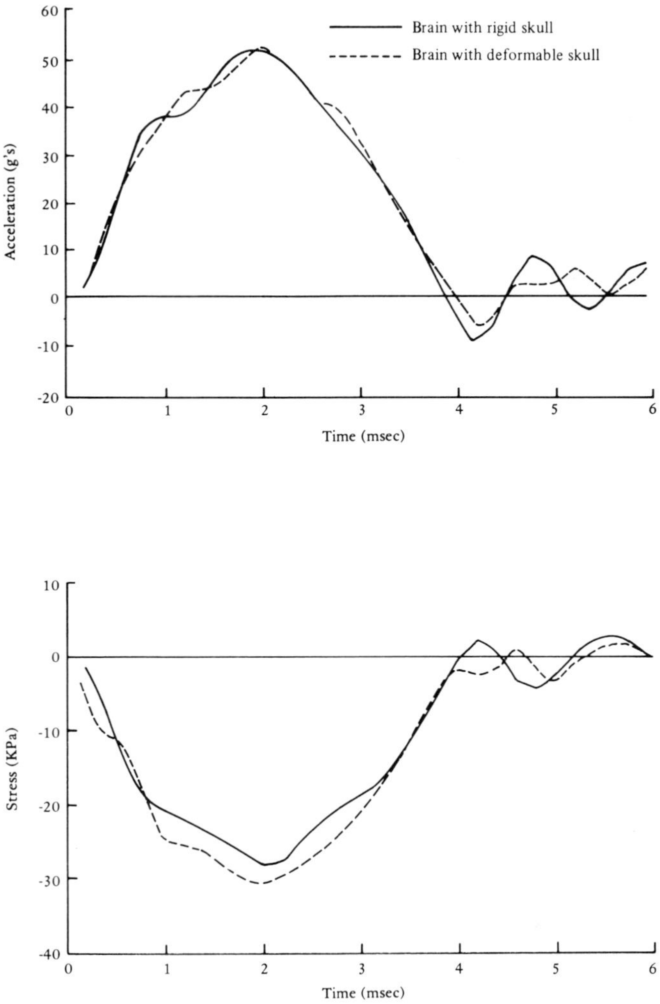

Figure 4.

Concussion is most likely related to shear strain, since the strains are high in the regions controlling consciousness and memory. The occurrence and duration of traumatic unconsciousness has been related to the magnitude of the brain response (15). Although maximum stress was the response measure used in the comparison, a similar relationship with maximum shear strain would be expected.

Brain tissue failure stresses are approximately the same in humans and animals (16). Because of differences in brain shape and response characteristics, the animal data cannot be directly related to the human through scaling, but it is possible to relate animal brain tissue failures to humans through the use of models.

Injury Criteria

Information obtained from the brain model simulations can be used to establish a head injury criterion (16). The minimum brain pressures for serious and moderate injury were determined from the relationship between peak brain pressure and overall brain injury severity shown in Figure 5. Pressures of 34 and 25 psi were selected and used to develop the severe and moderate injury curves shown in Figures 6 through 9. The curves define the translational acceleration pulses which will produce 34 and 35 psi pressure or stress in the brain.

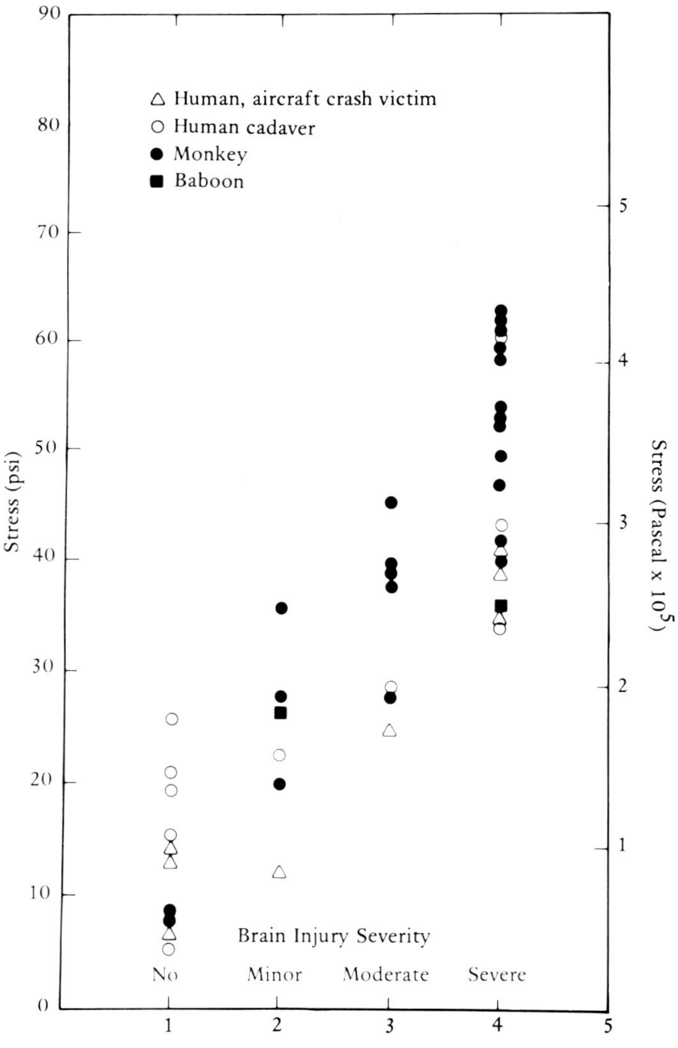

Figure 5.

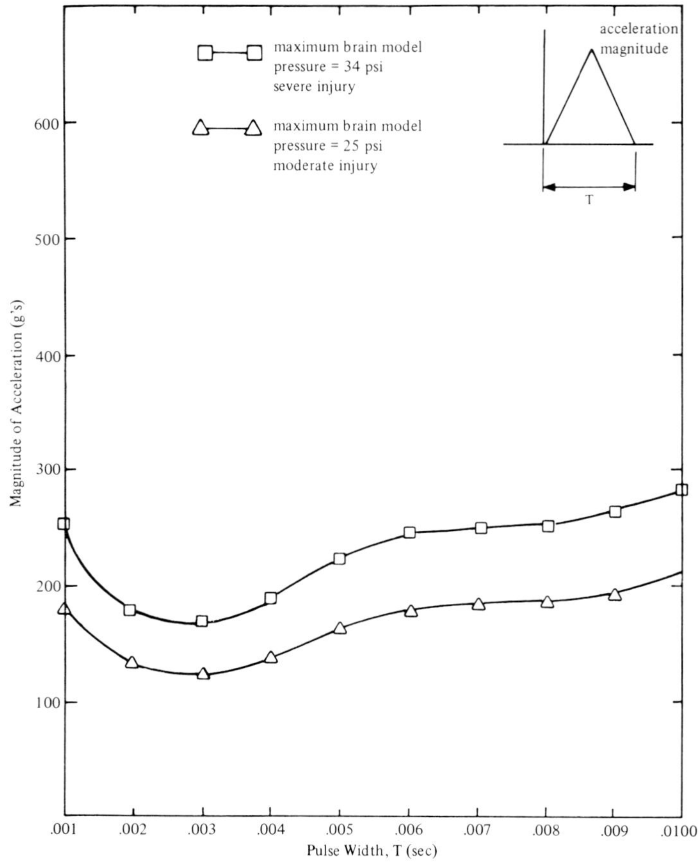

Figure 6.

If in a given event the head acceleration magnitude and pulse duration define a point above the severe injury curve, the brain could sustain serious or fatal injuries. If the point falls between the curves, moderate injuries could result. If the point lies below the curves, the injury would be minor at most. These curves represent the lower limits, and individuals having a high tolerance would sustain less injury.

The brain injury curves were compared to existing head injury criteria (16). As shown in Figures 8 and 9, the Wayne State Tolerance (WST) curve and the Department of Transportation Head Injury Criterion (HIC) curve differ from the brain pressure curves. The WST and HIC curves permit higher accelerations for short-duration impacts (less than 4 ms) and require lower accelerations for long impacts (greater than 8 ms).

Although the HIC and WST curves do not protect the brain in short-duration impacts, it is unlikely that

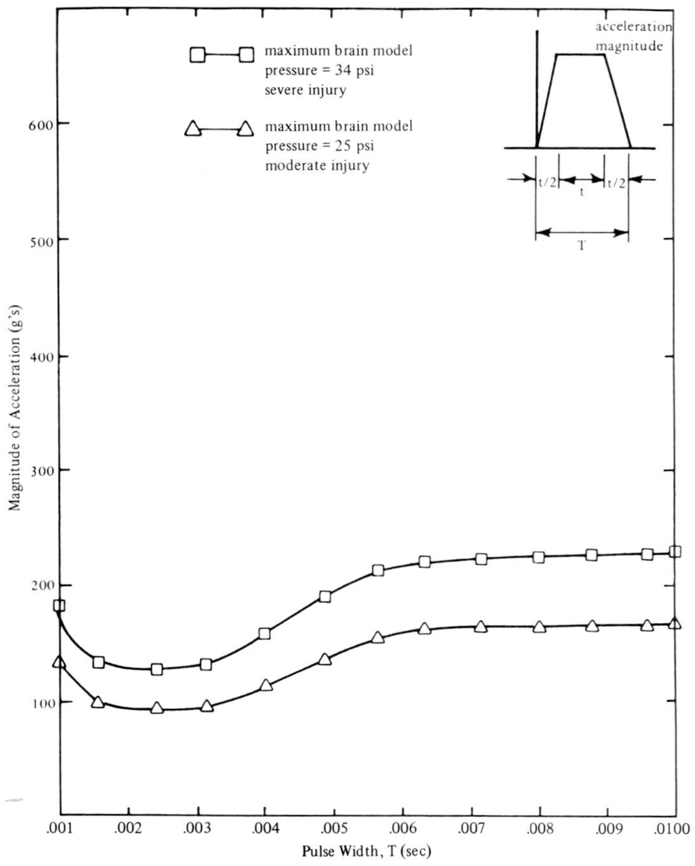

Figure 7.

such impacts would occur inside the vehicle. These are rigid-surface or ineffectually padded rigid-surface impacts.

Brain pressure is a function of the head acceleration pulse shape while the other indices are not. The HIC is an integration over the pulse, and the WST curve is based on average acceleration. To determine the maximum variation in pressure for a given pulse duration and HIC value, three triangular pulse shapes were considered. They had HIC values of 75, average accelerations equal to 50 g's, a pulse duration of 3 ms and acceleration onset rates of 1,000, 66.7 and 34.5 g's per ms. The computed peak pressures were 21.2, 20.1, 16.5 psi; the faster rise time produced higher pressures. For this extreme case, the maximum variation in peak pressure was 24 percent. In the lower stress regions, the variations were as high as 35 percent. This is the maximum pressure variation which could be expected for a given pulse duration and HIC value. It is interesting to note that the HIC value is low, but the brain pressures are approaching the moderate injury level.

For long pulses, the HIC and brain pressure curves diverge. For a HIC value of 1,000, a 15-ms pulse would produce brain pressure and stresses in the 14 psi range. For a 50-ms pulse, the pressures would not exceed 6 psi. Clearly, the HIC is overly conservative for long acceleration pulses.

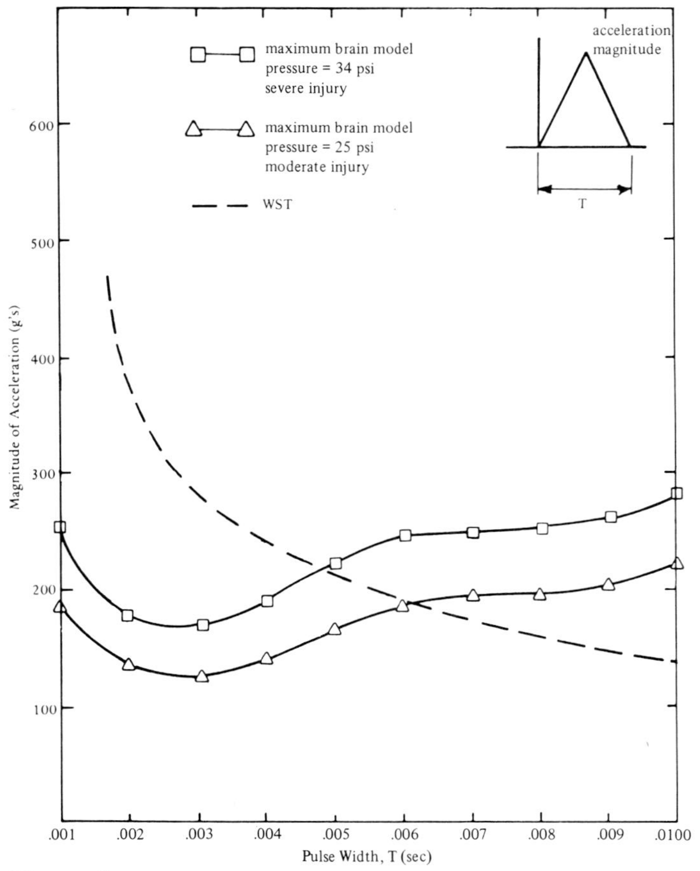

Figure 8.

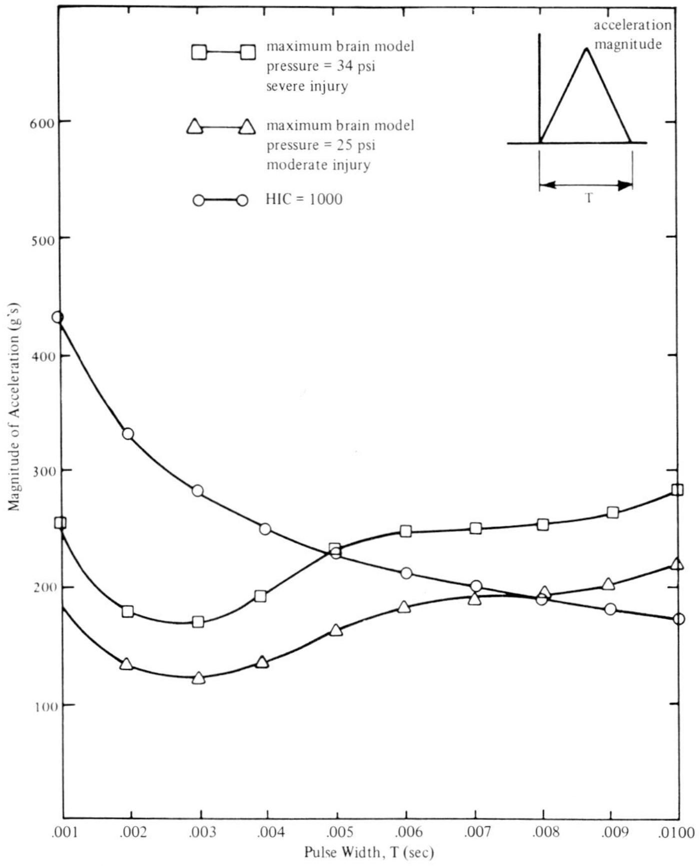

Figure 9.

High brain pressures are not the only injury mechanisms. Shear strains also produce injury and are related to head angular acceleration. Since none of the existing criteria consider rotational acceleration, they may not be providing adequate protection. The magnitudes of the injury producing strains, and the head rotations which produce these strains, need to be determined.

Conclusions

Finite element skull models have been developed, but have not been experimentally verified. Although these models cannot be used to predict skull stresses and strains versus time, they are useful in investigating trends.

Finite element brain models have been developed and verified. In more than 50 simulations, they have accurately predicted brain stresses or displacements. To obtain good correlation with experimental results, brain models must include the partitioning folds of dura, the foramen magnum and effective compressibility.

The verified brain models are revealing new information about brain response and injury. Stresses and strains develop in the brain as it lags the motion of the skull. Coup and contracoup injuries are caused by high compression and tension stresses, 34 and 27 psi respectively. The stresses are produced by translational head acceleration.

Petechial hemorrhages and tear lesions in the brain stem and cerebellum and subdural hematomas along the brain-skull interface are caused by high shear strains. The strain magnitudes and head rotations which produce these injuries have yet to be determined.

Injury severity has been related to peak stress in the brain. Brain injury curves have been developed and compared to the WST and HIC equal 1,000 curves. The comparison shows that for 5- to 10-ms pulses, the HIC and WST provide adequate protection for the brain. For longer pulses, the HIC becomes overly conservative.

None of the current injury criteria consider rotation acceleration. Brain tolerance to rotational motion needs to be determined.

References

1. Hardy CH and Marcal PV: Elastic analysis of a skull. Tech Rpt 8 Office of Naval Res.; Contract N00014-67-A-0191-0007, Div. of Engr. Brown Univ. 1971
2. Khalil TB and Hubbard RP: Parametric study of head response by finite element modeling. *J Biomech 10*:119–132. 1977
3. Shugar TA: A finite element head injury model vol 1 theory development and results. Civil Eng Lab Tech Report R-854-1; Naval Constr. Battal Ctr (Port Hueneme CA) 93043. 1977
4. Ward CC: A dynamic finite element model of the human brain. PhD Dissert. UCLA. 1974
5. Ward CC and Thompson RB: The development of a detailed finite element brain model. *Proc. 19th STAPP Car Crash Conf*:641–674. 1975
6. Ward CC: Analytical brain models for head impact. *Proc Int'l Conf on Impact Trauma IRCOBI (Berlin)*. 1977
7. Ward CC, Nikravesch PE and Thompson RB: Biodynamic finite element models used in brain surgery research. *J Aviation Space and Environ Med 49*:136–142. 1978
8. Ward CC: A head injury model. *NATO Adv Grp for Aerospace R&D Conf Proc 253*. Models and analogues for the evaluation of human biodynamic response, performance and protections. 1978
9. Nusholtz GS, Axelrod J, Melvin J and Ward C: Comparison of epidural pressure in live anesthetized and post-mortem primates. Highway Safety Res Inst Rpt UM-HSRI-79-90. 1979
10. Hosey R and Liu YK: A homeomorphic finite-element model of impact head and neck injury. *Proc Int'l Conf on Finite Elements in Biomechanics (Tucson AZ)*:829–850. 1980
11. Chan C, Ward C, Schneider D and Adams S: Relative importance of skull deformation. ASME Biomechanics Symp (CO) 1981
12. Ward C and Chan M: Finite element modeling of the head and neck. Chapt in *Impact Injury to the Head and Spine* (to be pub. by CC Thomas Co, Springfield IL)
13. Holbourn AH: Mechanics of head injuries. *Lancet*:Oct 9, 1943
14. Ward CC, Chan H and Chan M: Simulation of brain injury tests using a finite element brain model. *Proc of Internat'l Conf on Finite Elements in Biomechanics (Tucson AZ)* 2:829–849. 1980
15. Ward CC: Correlation between brain response and cerebral concussion. To be pub. in *J of Aviation, Space & Env Med*
16. Ward C, Chan M and Nahum A: Intracranial pressure—a brain injury criterion. *Proc 23d STAPP Car Crash Conf (Troy MI)*. 1980
17. Ward C and Chan C: Rotational generated shear strains in the brain. Human Subj. Symp. 1980

Patterns of Deformation in Brain Models Under Rotational Motion

Bertil Aldman
Lennert Thorngren
Christer Ljung

Abstract

A physical model of the human brain is developed using a transparent silicone gel in simplified head forms of acrylic plastic. Photographic targets are placed in the gel during the curing period. The displacement of these targets during rotational motion of the model is recorded by high-speed cinematography. The methods for assessment and comparison of the material properties of human brain material and that of the gel are described. The changing patterns of deformation of the brain model under rotational motion during stepwise development of the model into anatomically more realistic shape are described.

Background

Over the years a great number of investigations in the field of brain injury have demonstrated the importance of translational and rotational head motions. Studies by Ommaya et al. in 1967 (1) and in 1971 (2) as well as by Lowenhielm 1975 (3) indicate that angular accelerations can produce cerebral concussion and brain injuries if the angular velocity change exceeds a certain level. In human volunteer tests performed by Ewing et al. 1975 (4) no obvious damage occurred at angular accelerations up to 1700 rad/s^2 resulting in angular velocities of 32 rad/s. However, Ommaya claims that angular acceleration greater than 1800 rad/s^2 and change in angular velocity above 60–70 rad/s will result in cerebral concussion and Lowenhielm suggests tolerance levels of 4500 rad/s^2 for bridging vein rupture. Hypotheses put forth to explain the mechanical reactions of various parts of the brain have been examined in physical and mathematical models. In these studies it has often been difficult to separate fully the effects of translational and rotational motions. The aims of the project, of which the initial steps are reported here, are to develop a physical brain model and experimental devices in which this model can be studied under rotational and translational motions separately as well as combined.

In this early phase the model consists of a number of mainly two-dimensional projections of the brain in the sagittal (x-z) and transversal (y-z) planes. In order to study the influence of various anatomical structures on the deformation of the brain under rotational motions the shape of these two-dimensional projections are made increasingly more anatomically realistic.

Methods

Assessment of material properties

To enable studies of the influence of anatomical structures during linear and angular motions it appeared advantageous to have a model material which was transparent and in which the material properties could easily be changed within certain limits. After a series of tests it was found that a silicone gel (Dow Corning dielectric gel Q3 6527) best fitted the requirements. The gel is produced by mixing two components and cures in about 24 hours at room temperature. By varying the proportions of the two components the material properties changed within certain limits.

A series of cylindrical vessels with tight-fitting lids were made of acrylic plastic in such a way that they could easily be fastened on a rotor. The radius of the vessel, 95 mm, was chosen to be not too far from that of the skull in different planes. The height of the vessels were 80 or 120 mm (Figure 1).

For the assessment of the material properties the two components of the gel were mixed and poured into the vessel to cure at room temperature. A few hours before the curing was completed photographic targets—consisting of confetti-like pieces of black paper—were carefully placed in a straight line on the surface of the gel (Figure 2).

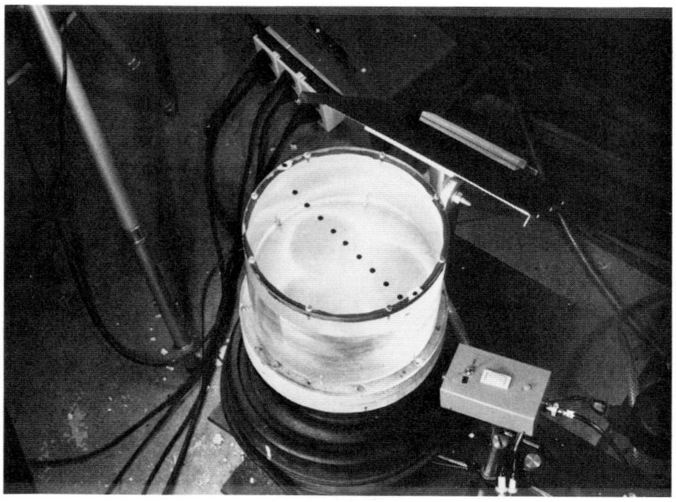

Figure 1. The Cylindrical Vessel Containing Silicone Gel and Water Fitted on the Rotor for the Assessment of the Materical Properties of the Gel.

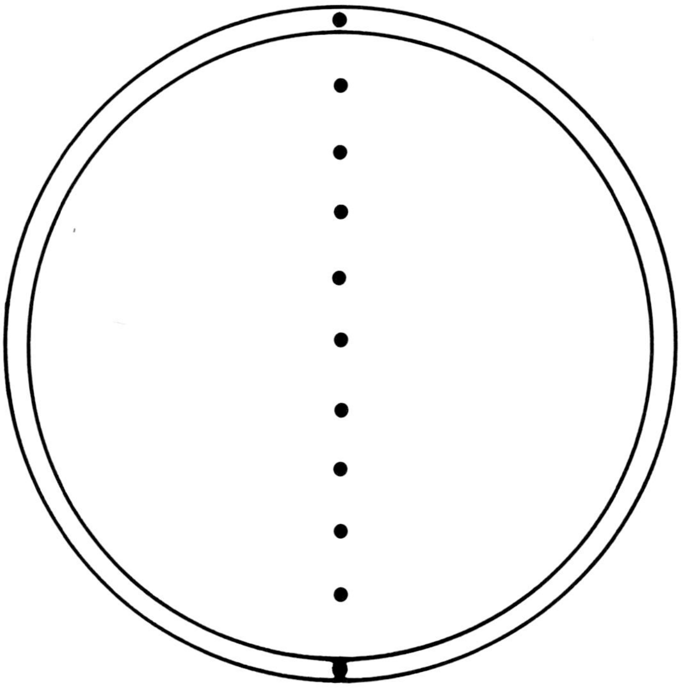

Figure 2. Black Photographic Targets Placed in a Straight Line on the Gel.

When cured, the gel sticks to the sides and the bottom of the vessel. The distance from the surface to the bottom—90 mm—was chosen big enough to ensure that the influence from the bottom on the displacement of the targets under angular acceleration of the vessel was negligible. In order to prevent the gel from getting in contact with the lid during rotation the

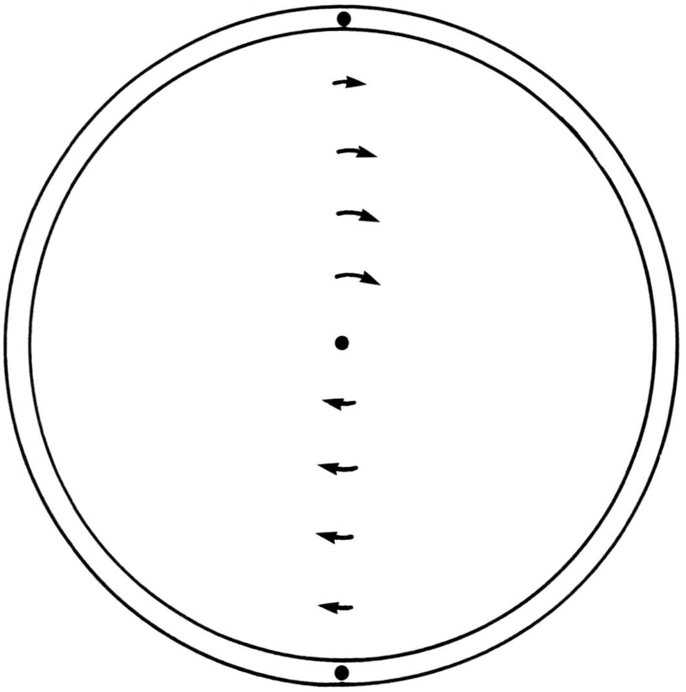

Figure 3. The Arrows Indicate the Deformation of the Gel During Deceleration as Revealed by the Displacement of the Targets.

vessel was filled with water and closed in a careful way so as to avoid having air bubbles trapped under the lid (Figure 3).

The rotor used in these experiments consisted of a circular wooden table fixed to a hub and brake drum taken from the front wheel of a motor car. The brake drum was connected with an electric motor by a belt, and the brake could be actuated by a pneumatic cylinder. Accelerometers were fitted under the wooden table and via a slip-ring device and cables connected to amplifiers, the signals were recorded on tape. The vessel could be rotated at a pre-chosen velocity and stopped by applying the brake. The deceleration pulse used was a ramp function which from the peak rapidly dropped to zero. The film from a high-speed camera operating at 500 fps and placed vertically above the center of the vessel was analyzed with respect to the tangential displacement of the targets relative to the surrounding vessel.

In a previous study by Ljung 1975 (5) mathematical models were developed for a Kelvin-Voigt viscoelastic material contained in cylindrical and spherical rigid shells subjected to sudden rotational motion. The two material parameters of a Kelvin-Voigt material are in such cases shear modulus and kinematic viscosity. In order to determine those parameters for brain tissue, experiments were performed using brain matter from human cadavers. The temporal lobe was inserted in a cylinder which was then subjected to an angular acceleration of a magnitude which ascertained that the experiment was realistically simulating an injurious situation. The two material parameters of the mathematical model were then chosen so as to minimize the model and experiment displacement response differences in a least-squares sense.

In the present investigation the above procedure has been repeated in the opposite direction. Given the material properties of brain matter (as expressed by shear modulus and kinematic viscosity), the correctly mixed silicone gel is sought by comparison of experiment and model displacement responses.

It is true that in this way care is only taken to ensure that material properties of brain matter and silicone gel match in problems of rotational symmetry where shear modulus and kinematic viscosity suffice in describing the material. It is, however, maintained that the comparison of material properties made will give a reasonable result for the present study.

A cylindrical vessel like the one used for the assessment of material properties was divided into two halves by rigidly fitting a plate of acrylic plastic across the center. Each half cylinder would then roughly resemble a lateral projection of a middle portion of the skull where the flat plate represented a straight approximation of the skull base and the tentorium (Figures 4 and 5).

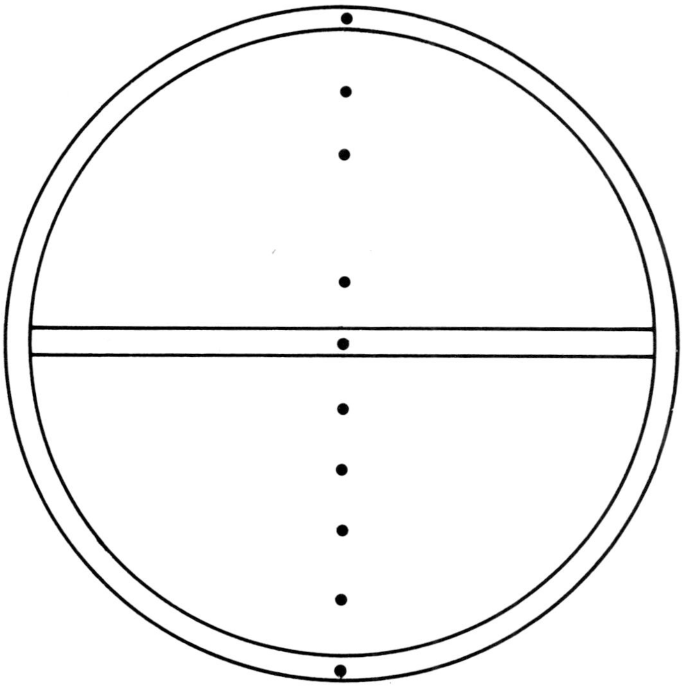

Figure 4. The Cylindrical Vessel Divided into Two Halves by a Rigid Plate.

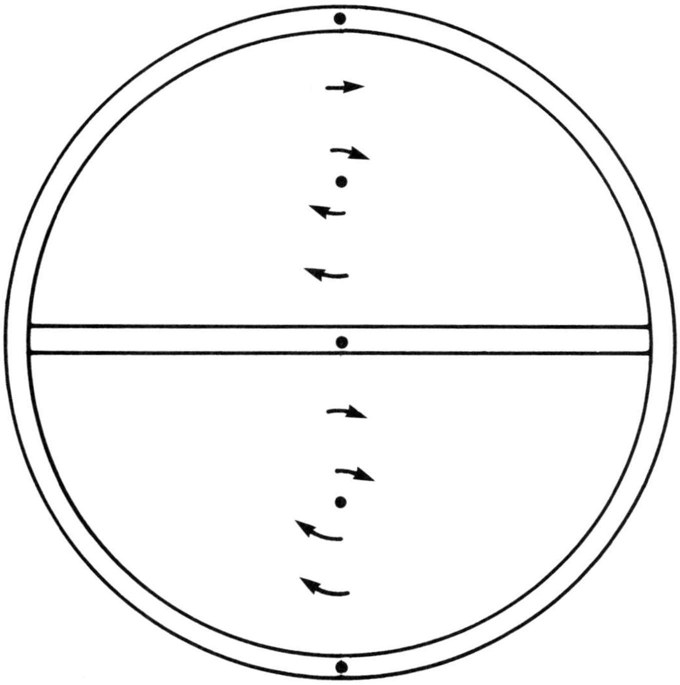

Figure 5. In Each Half Cylinder the Deformation Takes Place About a Center.

In one of the two half cylinders a shorter plate was fitted to the concave wall at approximately right angles with the longer plate. This new plate was intended as a simulation of the falx cerebri in a frontal projection of the skull. The two quadrants joined in their central parts could then approximately represent cross sections of the two cerebral hemispheres and the mid brain (Figures 6 and 7).

In the next step a more elaborate system of plates was fitted in a cylindrical vessel in order to simulate a mid-sagittal section of the whole brain and upper spinal cord. The skull base and the tentorium are still

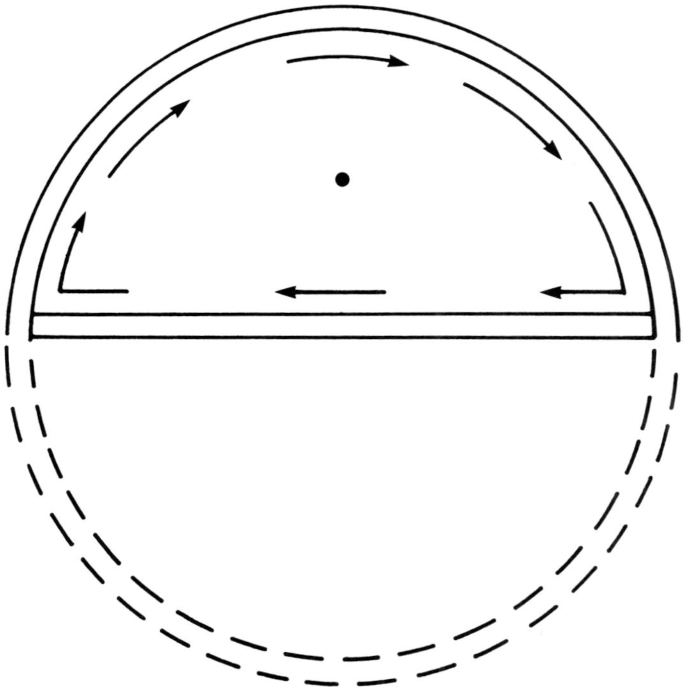

Figure 6. The Arrows Indicate the Main Pattern of Deformation in a Half Cyclinder.

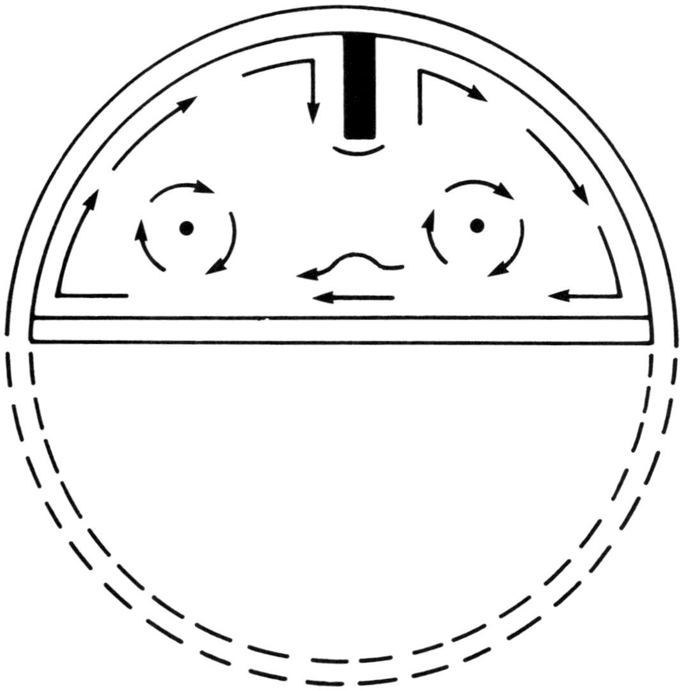

Figure 7. The Pattern of Deformation Changes Upon the Introduction of a Short Plate Simulating the Falx Cerebri.

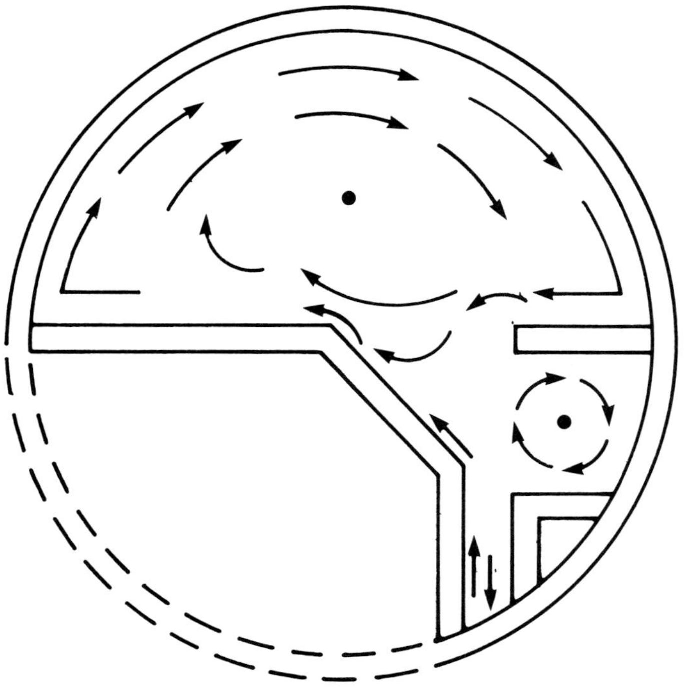

Figure 8. The Pattern of Deformation in a More Realistic Container Where the Gel Sticks to the Walls.

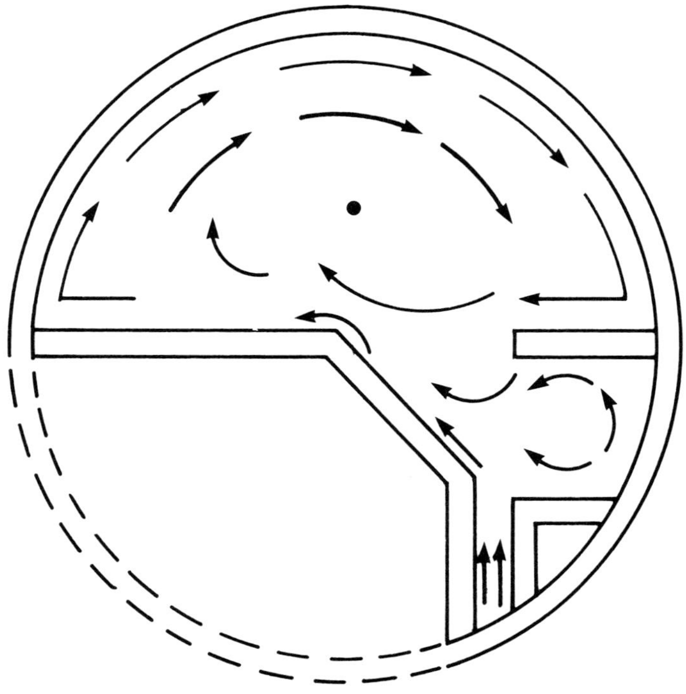

Figure 9. If the Gel is Cured in a Soft Bag and Separated from the Walls by Water the Pattern of Deformation Below the Tentorium Changes.

represented by an approximately straight plane but with an opening simulating the tentorial opening (Figures 8 and 9).

During all the steps of development so far the gel simulating the brain matter had been left to cure in the different acrylic vessels. This implies that the gel will stick to the side walls of the container and all the displacement takes place in the gel itself. In the next step of development measures were taken to separate the gel from all the walls of the container simulating the skull. For this purpose bags of thin transparent vinyl plastic were produced. The bags were made a few millimetres smaller than the container but of the same shape. The mixed gel was left to cure in the plastic bags and the photographic targets placed at halfway between the bottom and the vinyl lid of the bag. The acrylic vessel was then filled with water before the plastic bags with the gel were transferred to the vessel. Great care was taken to avoid air bubbles to be trapped in the vessel when the lid was finally fitted.

It would also be of interest to simulate displacements in the brain matter in a horizontal plane (x-y). In order to do so a rigid plastic mould and three soft and transparent vinyl bags were made to fit the base of the skull. The rigid mould was secured inside a cylindrical acrylic vessel by means of a rigid polyurethane foam. The three soft vinyl bags were placed inside the rigid mould. In the inner bag a transparent tentorium and parts of the falx cerebri were welded in position. It was then filled with silicone gel which was left to cure when photographic targets had been placed in the cerebellar as well as in the cerebral parts. These were, in both of these structures, placed in a middle plane, which means at two different levels. The spaces between the rigid mould and the vinyl bags were then filled with water, air bubbles removed and the acrylic lid fitted on top of the cylindrical vessel (Figures 10 and 11).

Procedure

The deformation of the gel at angular deceleration was studied by recording the displacement of strategically arranged photographic targets by high-speed cinematography. The targets were not placed on top of the gel but in the substance itself at approximately the same distance from both horizontal surfaces. They were placed in a pattern which was thought to give the best information about the deformation of the simulated brain substance in each test.

For practical purposes it seemed better to decelerate the model from a pre-set angular velocity by actuating the brake rather than to accelerate it to the desired velocity. The rotation about the center of the cylindrical vessel in these tests would roughly represent rotation about the center of gravity of the head in the projections chosen. Two different velocities were chosen for these experiments: 30 rad/s and 60 rad/s. Two pressure levels, 3 and 5 bar, in the pneumatic cyl-

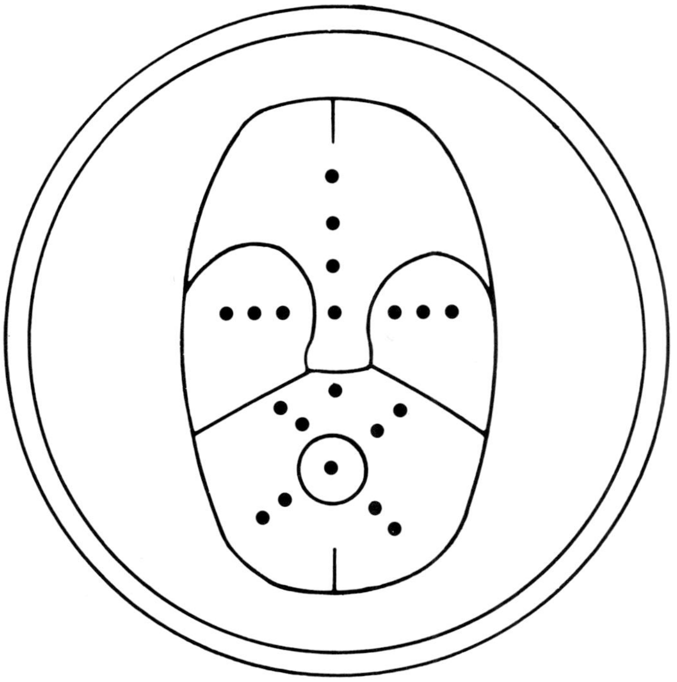

Figure 10. A Mould of the Base of the Skull with the Gel in a Soft Bag and Targets at Two Different Levels.

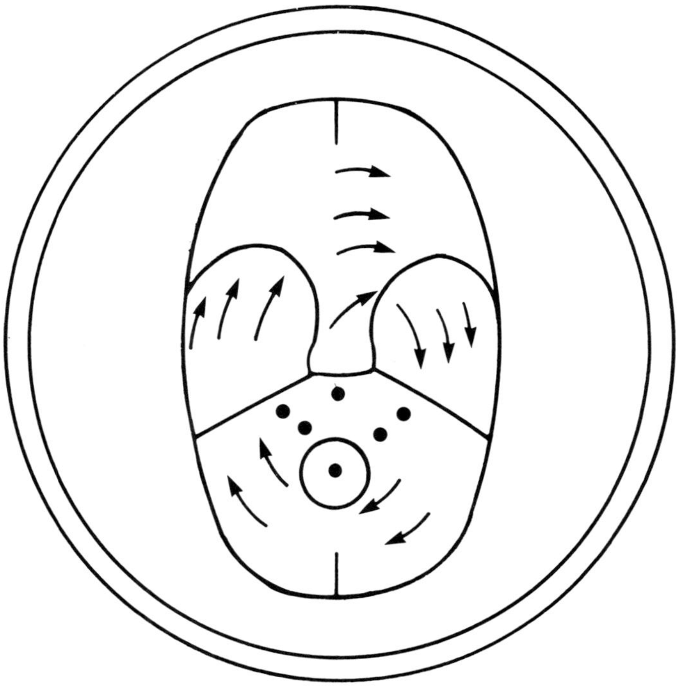

Figure 11. Deformation at Both Levels Seem to Take Place About a Center in the Brain Stem Area.

inder resulted in approximately the following peak values of deceleration at 30 rad/s: 1500 rad/s^2 and 2600 rad/s^2 and at 60 rad/s: 2000 rad/s^2 and 4700 rad/s^2. These values were used throughout these tests since they range from well below and up to what has been suggested as injury producing levels.

In previous investigations of oblique impacts of a dummy head wearing different types of approved crash helmets (6) peak angular accelerations ranging from 4500 to 14,500 rad/s^2 and peak angular velocities from 20 to 55 rad/s were recorded during the impact sequence in drop tests. The vertical velocity component 8.33 m/s (30 km/h) and the helmeted dummy head impacted different types of simulated road surfaces. In these tests the peak linear accelerations ranged from 90 to 135 g's and peak angular and linear accelerations occurred simultaneously.

It would seem therefore that the angular accelerations used in these experiments are not unrealistically high but could occur in many accident situations.

Results and Discussion

The patterns of displacement of the photographic targets as a result of the applied decelerations are illustrated by arrows in Figures 3 through 11. The introduction of a plate dividing the original cylinder into two halves results in displacements around two new centers situated at a distance of approximately one half of the radius from the center of the cylinder (Figure 5). If the dividing plate can be considered as a straight line approximation of the skull base and the tentorium, the direction of the motion would of course be expected to be in opposite directions above and below that plane (Figure 6).

In the next step the introduction of the shorter plate to simulate the falx in a frontal projection of the brain again results in a similar change in the pattern of displacement of the targets in the two quadrants (Figure 7).

In the more complete simulation of a lateral projection of the brain, brain stem, cerebellum and the upper spinal cord, considerable strain could be demonstrated already in the first simulation where the gel stuck to all the side walls of the container. Rotation in the same direction occurred in the cerebrum and in the cerebellum which implies that the direction of displacement of the targets were in opposite directions above and below the tentorium. This means that one can expect high values of shear strain in the vicinity of the tentorial opening.

When the gel was kept in a vinyl bag and water was introduced between this bag and the acrylic container, the displacement of the targets in the cerebellum and the upper cord changed. Obviously the shear strain in the vicinity of the container walls is reduced, while it appears that the more relaxed conditions for motion cause greater displacement and strain in the more central parts of the brain.

In the horizontal projection of the brain, deformation of the model brain material occurred in a similar pattern at both levels. Thus, large displacements of the targets were seen in the forward half and the rearmost part of the mould, while little or no displacement was recorded in the brain stem area. It should be pointed out, however, that the simulated parts of the falx in this experiment were not fixed to the mould at their upper ends but could move a little with the vinyl bag containing the gel.

At this stage of development no attempt has been made to assess the degree of deformation of the simulated brain material for different inputs of angular acceleration. The aim of this presentation is only to demonstrate the general patterns of deformation which will occur in a homogeneous model material under two separate conditions:

—the material sticks completely to the walls of the container
—the material is separated from the walls by vinyl bags and water.

In reality the brain is of course not a homogeneous structure and is probably connected to the skull with a certain slack. For this demonstration input pulses were chosen which were considered to be realistic and possibly injurious. The dimensions of the models were supposed to be reasonably realistic compared with the human skull and brain.

References

1. Ommaya, A. K., Yarnell, P., Hirsch, A. E., and E. H. Harris. 1967: "Scaling of Experimental Data on Cerebral Concussions in Sub-Human Primates to Concussion Threshold for Man." Proceedings of 11th Stapp Car Crash Conference Oct. 10–11, 1967. SAE, NY, USA.
2. Ommaya, A. K., and A. E. Hirsch, "Tolerances for Cerebral Concussion from Head Impact and Whiplash in Primates," *Journal of Biomechanics,* 4, 13, 1971.
3. Lowenhielm, P., "Brain Susceptibility to Velocity Changes. Relative and Absolute Limits for Brain Tissue Tolerance to Trauma and Their Relation to Actual Traumatic Situations," Proceedings of the International Interdisciplinary Symposium on Traffic Speed and Casualties held at Gl Averness, Funen, April 22–24, 1975. Denmark.
4. Ewing, C. L., Thomas, D. J., Lustick, L., Becker, E., Willems, G., and W. H. Muzzy. "The Effect of the Initial Position of the Head and Neck on the Dynamic Response of the Human Head and Neck to $-G_X$ Impact Acceleration," Proceedings of the 19th Stapp Car Crash Conference, November 17–19, 1975, SAE, Warrendale, USA.
5. Ljung, C., "A Model for Brain Deformation Due to Rotation of the Skull," *J. Biomechanics,* 1975, Vol. 8, pp. 263–274.
6. Aldman, B., Lundell, B., and L. Thorngren, "Oblique Impacts—A Parametric Study in Crash Helmets." Proceedings of the 3rd International IRCOBI Meeting, 1978, Lyon, France.

SESSION 2, PART 4:

Status of Current Criteria of Head Injury

Session 2, Part 4

Status of Current Criteria—Head Injury

Further Considerations of the HIC

James A. Newman

Introduction

A compilation of recent attempts to correlate HIC to head injury AIS is given in Figure 1 (1). These data have been used to demonstrate that there is little, if any, true correlation between the two. The reasons for the lack of correlation might include:

1. The surrogates, be they mathematical models, cadavers or anthropometric test devices, do not adequately model the living human system.
2. Documentation of the events simulated, e.g., free-fall, automobile crash, is incomplete.
3. The AIS, a discrete number assigned to an observed injury is too coarse a measure to provide a good correlation.
4. AIS is not correlated to HIC, i.e., head injury depends on factors other than the parameters that comprise HIC: A position first advanced by the author in 1975 (2).

Discussion

The HIC, and its predecessors, has withstood considerable criticism. The purpose of this brief discussion is not to reiterate all of those concerns but rather to concentrate on one aspect of the FMVSS 208 interpretation of the HIC.

The HIC is formulated specifically in terms of the function a(t); the acceleration-time response of the center of gravity of the surrogate head during impact. Different a(t)'s produce different HICs. Different HICs allegedly represent different levels of head injury severity or likelihood; the higher the HIC, the worse.

The utility, if not the validity, of the HIC has often been supported on the grounds that, when set to some chosen value (usually 1000) the variation of the average head acceleration $\bar{a}$ and the pulse duration T, is in general accord with experimentally observed trends such as the Wayne State Tolerance Curve (3) and the JARI tolerance curve (4). Attempts to support the model have even been made (5) on the basis of the predictions of Ward et al. (6) finite element brain model.

Notwithstanding its discouraging performance (Figure 1), attempts to shore up this unsound criterion will no doubt continue. Perhaps however it is not necessary to do so. Perhaps a simpler, more legitimate approach providing even greater assurance of limiting head impact injury is already available.

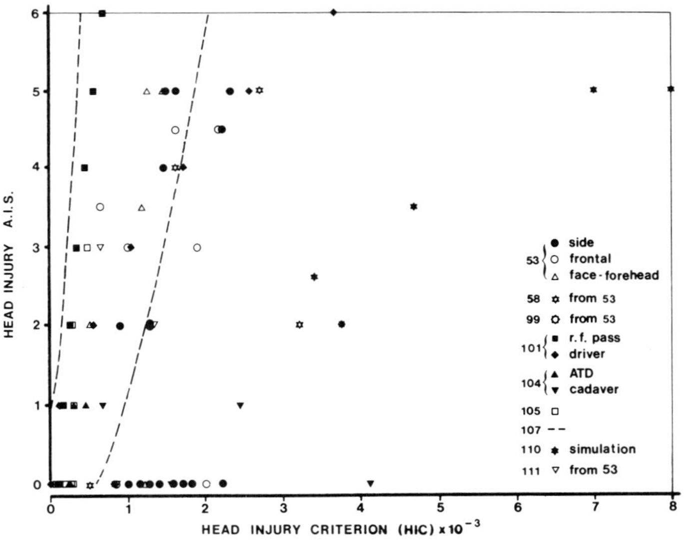

Figure 1. Head Injury Severity as a Function of HIC. Data from Various Sources. References Noted are from Reference 1.

Consider the following:

In general

$$a(t) = a_m g(t)$$

where a_m is the maximum acceleration

The average acceleration, for any a(t), is given by

$$\bar{a} = \frac{1}{T} \int_T a(t)dt$$

$$a(t) = \bar{a}g(t) \frac{T}{\int_T g(t)dt}$$

$$= \bar{a}g(t)f(T)$$

As a consequence, HIC, which is a function only of a(t), can be generally expressed as

$$HIC = HIC\,(\bar{a}, g(t), f(T))$$

That is, HIC will have a functional dependence on average acceleration, pulse duration and time.

If HIC is related to head injury, then head injury also depends on g(t) as well as ā and T. The basis of the HIC is the analysis of Gadd (7) and Versace (8) and the experimental data of Gurdjian et al. (3), Eiband (10) and Hodgson and co-workers (11). Their data, as well as the more recent data of Ono, et al. (4), provides a relationship between ā and T only. If these relationships are valid, then HIC cannot depend on g(t), i.e.,

$$HIC(a, g(t), f(T)) = HIC(\bar{a}, f(T))$$

The only way the time dependence can disappear from the formulation is if

$$g(t) = \text{Constant}$$

i.e., $a = a_m$, a square wave

Since square acceleration pulses are never produced in practice, the existing data cannot relate to the HIC. If in fact HIC does somehow relate to head injury, the Wayne State Tolerance curve (and other ā, T relations) therefore generally does not. Conversely, if the WST curve does not relate to head injury then the HIC cannot.

In consideration of tolerance limits such as the WST and the JARI curves, a reasonable question is: Can head injury be generally related (as implied by those curves) to ā and T only? The answer is: except for the specific conditions under which those tests and analyses were conducted, no! Both Gurdjian et al. and Ono et al. have acknowledged this.

The attractiveness of the concept that a biological system, such as a head, can tolerate higher average accelerations the shorter the time duration is embodied in fairly classical concepts concerning the exposure of systems to various hazard levels. Its relevance to mechanical inputs, such as head impacts, may be considered with the following simple model.

Figure 2 shows a rigid carriage that can be caused to accelerate. Placed upon the carriage is a block that will move with the carriage so long as the carriage does not accelerate more than some critical value a_c. If at any time t the carriage acceleration exceeds a_c, the block will move relative to the carriage. The concept is the same as that of static friction whereby a critical force is required before relative movement can occur. It can be assumed that inertial forces on the block exceed this limiting value if its acceleration exceeds a_c.

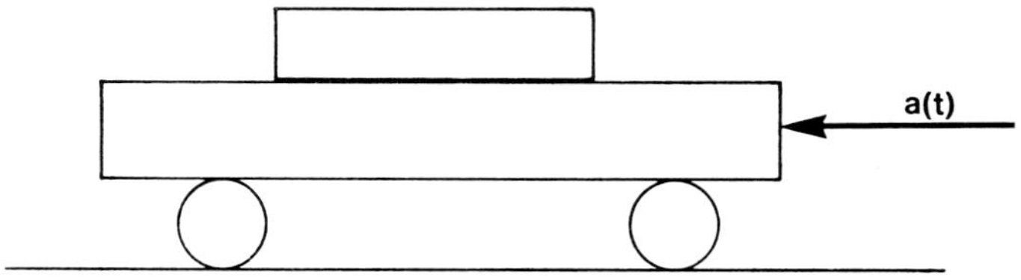

Figure 2. A Simple Mechanical Analogy. Rigid Block Will Move Relative to Rigid Carriage if the Maximum Value of a(t) Exceeds Some Critical Value a_c.

Assume that the carriage is caused to accelerate in accordance with

$$a(t) = \frac{am}{2}\left(1 - \cos\frac{2\pi t}{T}\right)$$

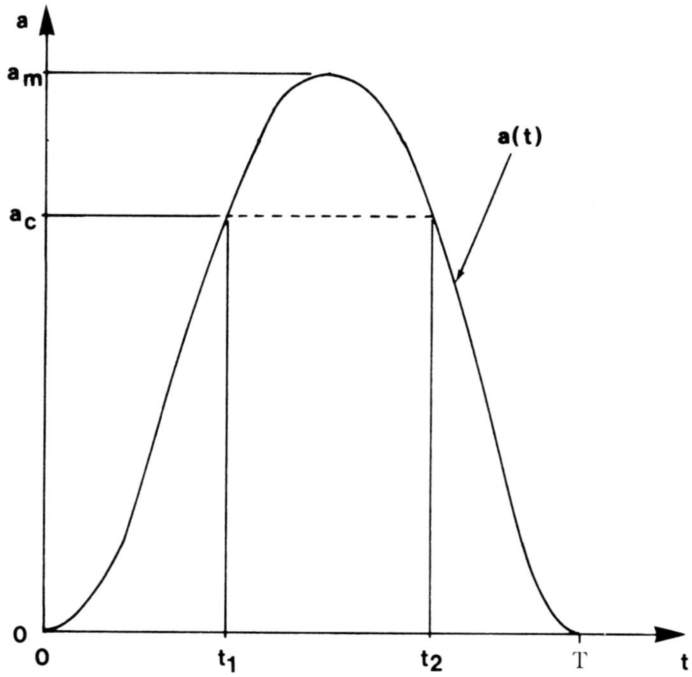

Figure 3. Haversine Acceleration Pulse: Maximum Acceleration Exceeds Critical Value During Time Interval t_1 - t_2.

During the time that the carriage acceleration is greater than a_c, the relative displacement s between the carriage and the block can be calculated by computing the difference in the absolute displacements of the two bodies.

Assume now that this simple mechanical analogy is representative of a biological system for which relative displacement, i.e., physical disruption of the system, is related to injury. Assume further that the greater this displacement, the more serious the injury.

Given the particular a(t) above, for a particular a_C and s, one can generate corresponding values of $\bar{a}$ and T. Figure 4 shows the results for a_C=200 g's for a series of values of s. Every point on a line of s=constant has an associated $\bar{a}$ and T. When $\bar{a}$ is high, T must be low to produce the same s in the same general way that the WST and JARI curves predict head injury dependence on $\bar{a}$ and T. For larger values of s (more serious injury?), the curves move upward in the expected manner. Note however that the curve for no relative displacement (no permanent disruption or injury) is in fact a straight line. This of course simply reflects the fact that if the maximum acceleration does not exceed the critical value, insufficient inertial forces are developed to produce permanent disruption. It does not matter therefore how long the acceleration persists; no permanent disruption of the system can occur.

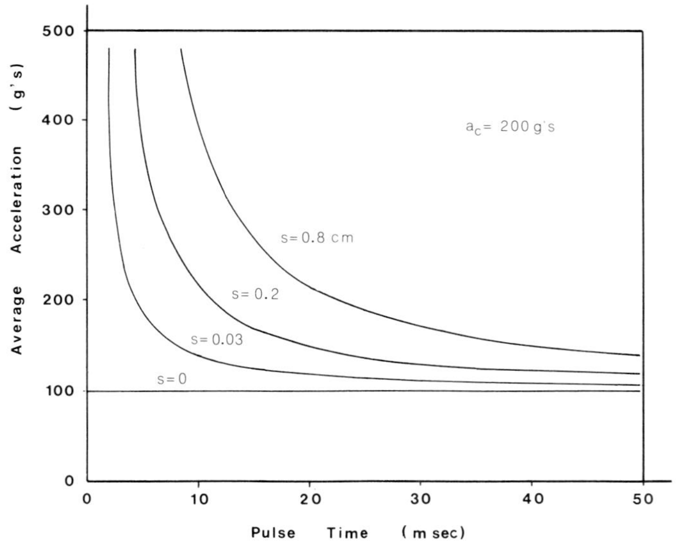

Figure 4. Lines of Constant Relative Displacement

As a matter of interest, this simple linear model can be used to represent the a, T relationship of the WST curve. By matching the a for long duration, one can seek the value of s which closely matches the WST curve. This is shown in Figure 5. Since indeed the WST (and the JARI) curve denote and a and T condition for some level of brain injury, the straight line a = constant might well denote the condition of no injury.

It is important to recall in this discussion that all the s = constant curves are based upon a particular arbitrary a(t). Clearly the amount of physical disruption to the similar linear model would depend upon the shape of the a(t) curve (above a_c). Hence these curves (like the WST and JARI) do

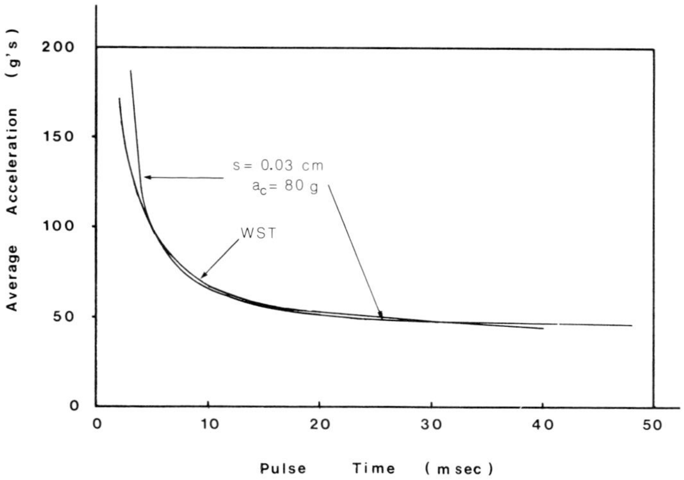

Figure 5. Predictions of Simple Mechanical Model Fitted to the Wayne State Tolerance Curve.

not, by themselves, provide any information regarding injury and the time dependence of the acceleration pulse; unless a_m is always less than a_c.

The next question then is; has head injury been shown to be specifically related to the functional form of the acceleration response g(t)? The answer may lie in the work of Ward et al, (6).

For a given a and T, different g(t)'s are associated with different normal stresses in the brain». Since intercranial pressure does relate to brain injury (based upon data other than that used to construct the HIC) then yes brain injury does relate to some g(t) as well as to a and T.

However, it is clearly evident, as shown in Figure 6, that the a vs T tolerance curves generated by HIC = constant, and those generated by P = constant are very different. Therefore the functional dependence on t is quite different for the two formulations; except when T is large. Then, for both cases, the tolerance boundaries appears to become essentially independant of t and of T. In the limit of long pulse duration, both models seem to predict that the limit for brain injury approaches some constant value of a.

On the basis of the simple linear model described earlier, it would appear that the above generalization would be even truer the lower the injury level one chose to adopt as the acceptable limit. Indeed, on the basis of available evidence, an acceptable translational acceleration-based index for head injury might simply be that, regardless of pulse shape, if T is greater than, say 7-8 msec (and it usually will be in automotive crash testing), the average acceleration may not exceed some prescribed level (80-100 g's would appear to be a reasonable number). Notice that if T is much less than 10 msec, such a criterion is still, according to the HIC, very conservative.

As a final note, it is of interest to observe that the extrapolated concussion data for humans derived by Ono et al (4) is in direct accord with the concept of limited average acceleration irrespective of pulse duration. With one exception, for both occipital and frontal impacts, a tolerance boundary of a = 100 g's appers valid even down to 2 msec.

»A traingular pulse with a = 100 g's and T = 5 msec is associated with much higher pressures than a trapezoidal pulse of the same a and T.

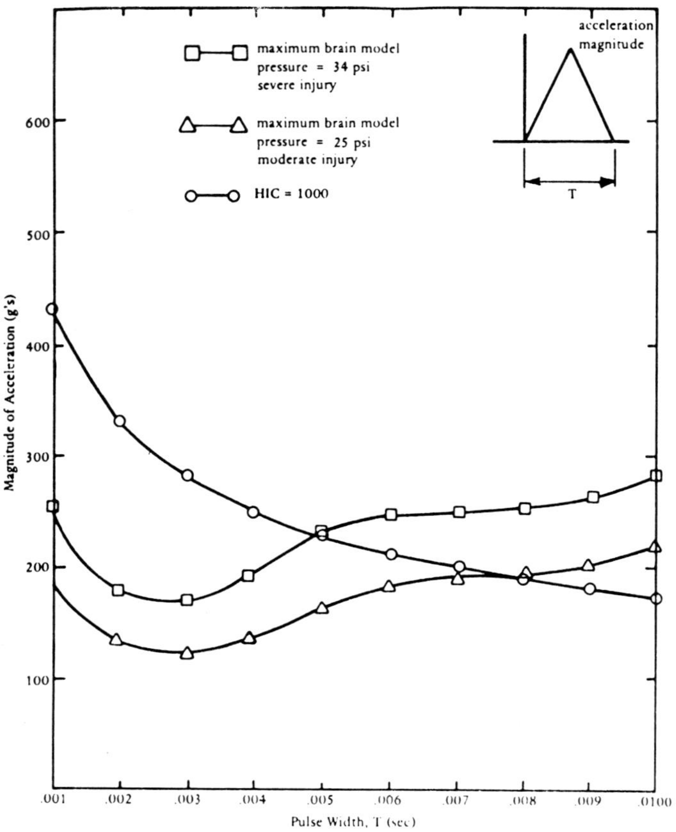

Figure 6. Comparison of NHTSA Head Injury Criterion and Brain Pressure Tolerance Curves for Moderate and Severe Injury. From Reference 6.

Summary

- Head injury tolerance boundaries showing the variation of average head acceleration with pulse duration do not accurately depict the conditions for head injury except possibly for very unique and special circumstances.
- Such tolerance boundaries do not by themselves provide data concerning the influence of associated a(t) functions.
- Head injury does appear to be related to the shape of the corresponding acceleration pulse.
- HIC invokes a(t) variations in a way that is not supported by data.
- Average translational acceleration set to some limiting value is in accord with experimental data and can be a more conservative measure of head injury tolerance than the HIC.

References

1. J. A. Newman, "Head Injury Criteria in Automotive Crash Testing," SAE Paper No. 801317, Proceedings of the 24th Stapp Car Crash Conference, October 15-17, 1980.
2. J. A. Newman, "On the Use of the Head Injury Criterion (HIC) in Protective Headgear Evaluation," SAE Paper No. 751162, Proceedings of the 19th Stapp Car Crash Conference, November 17-19, 1975.
3. E. S. Gurdjian, V. L. Roberts, and L. M. Thomas, "Tolerance Curves of Acceleration and Intercranial Pressure and Protective Index in Experimental Head Injury," *Journal of Trauma,* p. 600, 1964.
4. Koshiro Ono, Astumi Kikuchi, Marumi Nakamura, Hajime Kobayashi, and Norio Nakamura, "Human Head to Tolerance to Sagittal Impact Reliable Estimation Deduced from Experimental Head Injury Using Subhuman Primates and Human Cadaver Skulls," SAE Paper No. 801303, Proceedings of the 24th Stapp Car Crash Conference, October 15-17, 1980.
5. R. R. Stephenson, Written communication to Road and Motor Vehicle Traffic Safety, Transport Canada, October 17, 1980.
6. Carley Ward, Marian Chan and Alan Nahum, "Intracranial Pressure—A Brain Injury Criterion," SAE Paper No. 801304, Proceedings of the 24th Stapp Car Crash Conference, October 15-17, 1980.
7. C. W. Gadd, "Use of a Weighted-Impulse Criterion for Estimating Injury Hazard," SAE Paper No. 660793, Proceedings of the 10th Stapp Car Crash Conference, November, 1966.
8. J. Versace, "A Review of the Severity Index," SAE Paper No. 710881, Proceedings of the 15th Stapp Car Crash Conference, November, 1971.
9. A. Eiband, "Human Tolerance to Rapidly Applied Accelerations: A Summary of the Literature," NASA Memorandum 5-19-59E, June, 1959.
10. V. R. Hodgson, L. M. Thomas, and P. Prasad, "Testing the Validity and Limitations of the Severity Index," SAE Paper No. 700901, Proceedings of the 14th Stapp Car Crash Conference, November, 1970.

The Head Injury Criterion

S. H. Backaitis

During the last several years the Head Injury Criterion (HIC) has been examined, compared, criticized and sometimes praised for its suitability as a measuring norm to evaluate the occupant protection capability of passenger car compartments in the event of a crash. In some instances the HIC was found to be a good discriminator, in others it was thought to be inappropriate, fundamentally wrong, etc. Perhaps there is some truth in all of these statements, for they are relative, and anyone's relative assessment of its quality will depend on whether the person is a researcher or a regulator, whether the application requires fine gradations or just merely being on one or the other side of the limit in a particular impact mode.

Looking at the head injury problem from the point of view of a researcher, one cannot do anything but to observe that we have made great strides in the effort to comprehend a very complex set of problems. However, we are certainly still far away from fully understanding the details which make up the injury spectrum in the crash environment. It is certainly necessary to understand the injury mechanisms at the fundamental level, but, it would be naive to believe that only one injury mechanism may be involved. Current studies of the accident environment (1) shows (Table 1) that severe, critical and fatal head injuries are induced nearly always by hard contacts, which undoubtedly include localized skull deformations and various load transmissions mechanisms, as noted by Dr. Goldsmith. Different types and areas of brain tissue damage as well as different physiological consequences certainly indicate the presence of more than just one injury mechanism as Drs. Gennarelli and Graham indicated this morning.

Table 1. Head Injury Data in NCSS

Contact Area/Injury	AIS-3	AIS-4	AIS-5	AIS-6
1. Instrument Panel	14	3	5	1
2. Steering Assembly	38	9	8	1
3. Windshield	36	19	9	1
4. Glove Compartment	7	2	1	0
5. Front Hardware	0	0	2	0
6. Mirror, Roof, Hood	27	37	25	6
7. Other Occupant	0	0	1	0
8. Loose Object	0	1	0	0
9. Window	9	5	6	1
10. Front Seat Back	6	4	1	0
11. Restraint Hardware	3	1	2	0
12. Exterior Object	19	11	27	17
13. Side Interior	10	3	2	0
14. A-Pillar	15	16	25	4
15. B-Pillar	0	1	2	1
16. C-Pillar	0	0	2	0
17. Rear Window	0	1	0	0
18. Contact Areas Unknown	133	85	67	29
19. Non-Contact	0	0	1	0
Total	310	198	186	61

The resolution of head injury at the fundamental level would provide maximum latitude in predicting the injury consequences to a variety of loading inputs. That is a highly desirable goal, as long as it is remembered that it must be practical and objective and be significantly more effective than the criteria it intends to replace. From the point of view of the regulator, it would be adequate to quantify the force, moment or energy dosage to the head if serious injury or death is to be prevented. This approach, while appearing simple on the surface, in reality is almost as difficult to attain as the understanding of brain injury at the fundamental level. For one, the dosage may not be uniform for various areas of the head, and its magnitude may also be rate, direction and time dependent as noted by Dr. Tarriere. Of even more significance is the question as to how the determination of dangerous loading could be established in view of the fact that testing of humans at an injury level is out of the question, and tests with cadavers and animals do not necessarily produce the needed answers. Nevertheless, work is being pursued along both of these paths even though the progress is painstaking and slow.

In the meantime, the HIC is being used nearly universally to judge the adequacy of vehicle occupant protection systems. It is a reasonably good measure, especially, when one considers allegations that the Wayne State Tolerance (WST) (2, 3) Curve might be in error. To begin with, I am not sure that the critique of the WST is fully justified. Extensive studies by Japanese researchers (4), based on live monkey and human cadaver tests, have established a tolerance curve which exhibits similar exponential power relationship and magnitudes (Figure 1) of impact acceleration as that shown in the WST curve. This finding thus reaf-

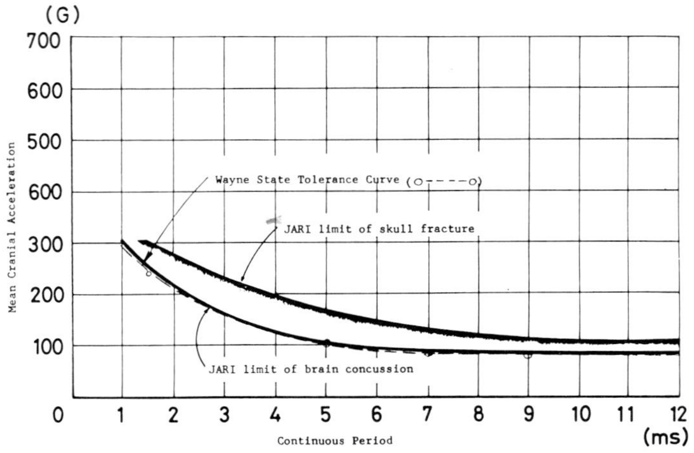

Figure 1. Human Tolerance Limits in Sagital (Frontal) Impacts

firms the credence in the WST formulation and at the same time supports the Gadd Severity Index (5) concept in spite of its certain limitations. The HIC (6), which was initially synthesized from the Gadd Severity Index by Versace (7), provided a practical and an objective means to focalize on the portion of the response curve having the highest power content (Figure 2). The argument, that there is no general relationship between head kinematics as determined by the HIC and the head injury, appears to ignore voluminous experimental and statistical test evidence at least in the frontal impact mode with either belt or air cushion restrained occupants. In these impact configurations the HIC appears to work well as a practical and effective discriminator in crash tests between those systems which allow head impacts of hard vehicle surfaces and those that do not. Experimental tests of restrained cadavers also support the ability of the HIC to act as a discriminator between those restraint systems which do not allow hard impacts to occur and those that do. Those experiments that do not permit hard impacts, usually produce no injury to the head and its content, while those that do, usually result in a variety of injuries. Also, statistical accident data overwhelmingly support the conclusion that serious head injury will occur only with evidence of hard surface impact. As shown in Table 1, of some 755 occupants injured to AIS=3+ level injuries in the NSS data file, only one noncontact injury at AIS=4 level is found. Although the HIC=1000 as originally conceived was meant to represent the threshold of serious injury, further extrapolation of it to measure the degrees of injury severity resulted in Langwieder's conclusion (8) that AIS=3 head injuries have a mean HIC value of 1000, while Ward (9) in her modeling work concluded that HIC provides as good a correlationship with intracranial pressure as any other indicator developed to date.

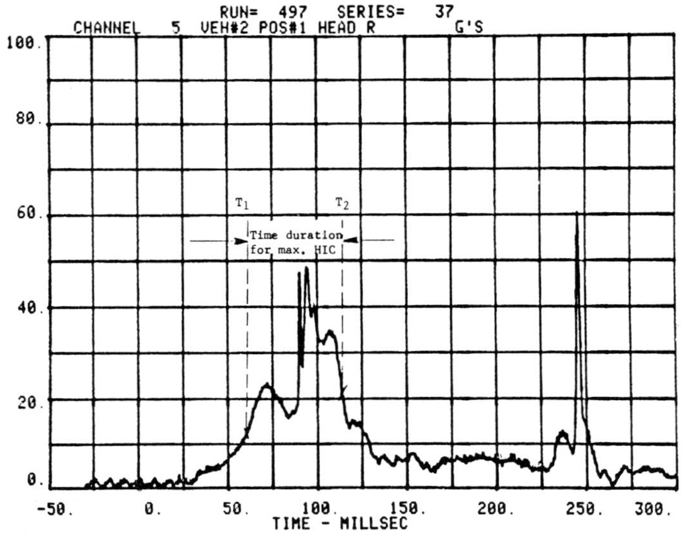

Figure 2.

Those critics, who make the allegation that the HIC has no theoretical basis, should realize that the HIC formulation contains the peak power term or the rate of change of the energy level as seen by the head during the impact process. It is reflected in the equation:

$$HIC = \left(\frac{1}{t_2 - t_1}\int_{t_1}^{t_2} a\,dt\right)^{2.5}(t_2 - t_1) = (a^{-2.5}\,\Delta t)_{max} =$$

$$((a^{-2}\,\Delta t)\sqrt{a})_{max} = \left(\left(\frac{V^{-2}}{\Delta t}\right)\bar{a}\right)_{max}$$

The V2/Δt term represents the peak power or the energy level over a searched out time duration $(t_2 - t_1)$ until the maximum value is found. The power to injury correlation was discussed by DiLorenzo (10) in an SAE technical paper in 1976.

Is the HIC applicable to response measurements of other than those occupants not experiencing a direct head impact contact? This is an area that needs to be investigated further both at the experimental laboratory level and in terms of accident statistics. Some scattered data indicate that the HIC measurement might appropriately discriminate between any hard and soft surface impacts. These judgments, however, must be based on an extremely careful review of the evidence on hand, such as direction, rate and magnitude of loading, its time duration and location with respect to crash initiation, etc. Cadaver testing and accident reconstruction programs should be conducted to yield information on the above parameters and also to establish whether the present HIC formulation correlates with the observed injuries and whether its levels and durations need to be adjusted and/or other injury producing parameters considered for indication of life threatening exposure.

In conclusion, it should be said that while the HIC was developed empirically, its general concept is in agreement with the basic laws of mechanics. It has been found to be a reasonably good discriminator between occupant contact and noncontact type impact conditions corresponding with differences between serious and nonserious injuries in real-world accidents. The variety of head injuries occurring in the accident environment calls for research to understand the injury mechanisms and trauma, so that more effective countermeasures could be developed or the one in existence would be supplemented with additional injury control parameters. HIC, for the time being, is a good objective threshold indicator of the effectiveness of occupant protection systems. Replacement of HIC should be considered only if a practical and significantly more effective tolerance criteria is found.

References

1. L. L. Ricci. *NCSS Statistics: Passenger Cars—* Technical Report UM-HSRI-80-36, The Highway Safety Research Institute, Ann Arbor, MI, 1980.
2. L. M. Patrick. *"Human Tolerance to Impact—Basis for Safety Design,"* SAE, Paper 650171, 1965.
3. L. M. Patrick, H. R. Lissner, E. S. Gurdjian. *"Survival by Design—Head Protection,"* Proceedings, Seventh Stapp Car Crash Conference, 1965.
4. K. Ono, A. Kinkuchi, M. Nakamura, H. Kobayashi, N. Nakamura. *"Human Head Tolerance to Sagittal Impact-Reliable Estimation Deduced From Experimental Head Injury Using Subhuman Primates and Human Cadaver Skulls,* Proceedings, Twenty-Fourth Stapp Car Crash Conference, SAE 801303, 1980.
5. C. W. Gadd. *"Use of a Weighted-Impulse Criterion for Estimating Injury Hazard,"* Proceedings, Tenth Stapp Car Crash Conference, SAE 660793, 1966.
6. 37 FR 12393, June 1972. *FMVSS No. 208,* Rule Docket 69-7, Notice 19, Occupant Crash Protection.
7. J. Versace. *"A Review of the Severity Index,"* Proceedings, Fifteenth Stapp Car Crash Conference, SAE 710881, 1971.
8. K. Langwieder, M. Damner, W. Schmelzing, H. Appel, F. Kramer, J. Hoffman. *"Comparison of Passenger Injuries in Frontal Car Collisions With Dummy Loadings in Equivalent Simulations,"* Proceedings, Twenty-Third Stapp Car Crash Conference, SAE 751165, 1975.
9. A. Nahum, C. Ward, E. Raasch, S. Adams, D. Schneider. *"Experimental Studies of Side Impact to the Human Head,"* Proceedings, Twenty-Fourth Stapp Car Crash Conference, SAE 801301, 1980.
10. F. DiLorenzo. *Power and Bodily Injury,* SAE Paper 760014, 1976.

Head Injury Discussion Paper

Charles W. Gadd

It has been requested that the first portion of this paper consists of commentary on the paper of James Newman, the previous speaker. Since his manuscript was not available in advance, this commentary will be based on other papers written by him during the past year (8, 9). In these papers, various statements and implications regarding the foundation for the exponentially weighted impulse head injury criterion (Severity Index of HIC) are in need of correction to set the record straight.

Firstly, it was clearly shown in reference 1 that the criterion was not based solely upon the Wayne State data or curve, but upon three principal sources of data, which included the 1959 NASA summary of tolerance information by Eiband and the accident simulation data by Swearingen of the FAA. Eiband summarized data from living people and animals, while Swearingen reconstructed in the laboratory a large number of actual car accidents. Because he knew in each instance the degree of injury and whether death had occurred, he could correlate injury severity with "g" profiles obtained in the laboratory with cadaver subjects. He restricted himself to cases in which it was known that the head had struck frontally against instrument panels having differing configurations.

It was shown in reference 1 that the 2.5 power weighting exponent was really a very close approximation of the previously published NASA tolerance curve, and that it also fell within the (rather broad) scatter band of dog pressure-induced brain tolerance data of Wayne State.

Regarding the choice of a Severity Index of 1000, it was also stated in reference 1 that this value stemmed firstly from the NASA curve for forward-facing deceleration, which it matched almost exactly. Also it was stated that 1000 was in reasonable agreement with the Wayne Curve, but there was some uncertainty here because of Wayne's use of an "effective" g. It was then stated that to clear this up we went to the original Wayne acceleration oscillograms and integrated these to the 2.5 power. Although there was of course scatter (unavoidable with biological materials) agreement was reasonable with a value of 1000. Finally, it was also stated that the value of 1000 rested in addition upon our analysis of the FAA study, whose oscillograms were also integrated.

Reference 1, further discussed reasons for believing that a value of 1000 was conservative; that this severity entailed danger to life but not death. However, since this paper's publication it has been customary to take accelerations triaxially rather than uniaxially. For this and other reasons a value of 1500 was suggested for design purposes. Substituting the HIC modification for the original SI generally in practice gives somewhat lower numerical values as well. The football helmet manufacturers, under the guidance of Dr. V. Hodgson, elected to stay with the simpler SI, but raised the design guide to 1500. They have incidentally reduced the death rate on football fields about in half over the past seven years through their test program which qualifies helmets for use providing they do not exceed an SI of 1500.

Thus Newman misleads the reader when he implies that the SI or HIC rest solely upon some narrow or questionable interpretation of the Wayne Tolerance Curve, and that they should therefore not be taken seriously.

Still other studies which serve as a further basis for continued use of the experimental weighting criterion were cited in Discussion Papers by the writer, published in the proceedings of the 14th and 15th Stapp Conferences of 1970 and 1971. Some of this work is summarized in Figure 1. For example, Sonntag (3) stopped chimpanzees from 90 mph in only 28 inches without appreciable injury. Even with scaling the tolerance down to human size as discussed in the 14th Stapp Conference proceedings, one arrives at SI values of about 2000 for this test series. The extensive later NASA summary compiled by Fraser (2) is pertinent, in particular the forward-facing decelerations of humans extending out to very long time durations of 10 seconds. Here there is a departure from the 2.5 power exponent toward a horizontal asymptote. This will be touched upon further below.

The pioneering work of Col. Stapp is also pertinent. Considerable study of this work, including examination of high speed movies, was made by the writer and summarized in the 15th Stapp Conference Discussion paper. It was concluded that in sled runs 133 and 135, the subjects sustained SI's of at least 1500. Still

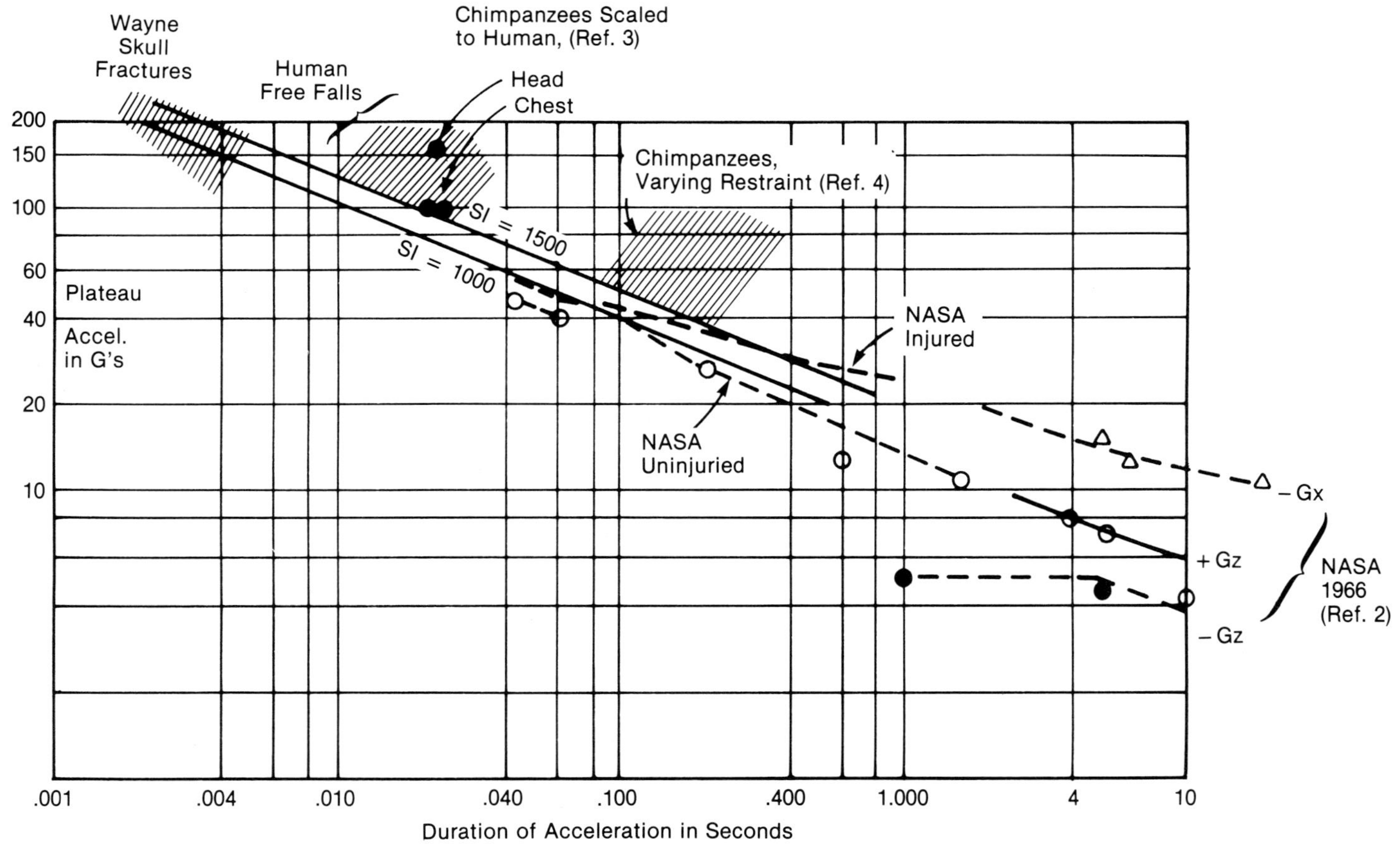

Figure 1. NASA 1959 and 1966 Literature Summaries for Tolerable Plateau Accelerations, Harnessed; with Other Data Superimposed.

other volunteer runs on the Daisy Track under Eli Beeding in 1960, stopping from 46 ft/sin 60 to 70 ms, undoubtedly produced similar exposures.

The free-fall survivals are rather controversial, but various biomechanics specialists do feel these represent maximum survivability providing the victim is fortunate enough not to sustain severe localized loading (stress concentration) or severe distortional loading. In one case that we investigated, a person fell horizontally onto the roof of a Chevrolet sedan from a height of 12 stories. He reported the next day for his window washing job. The countless instances of such survivals against both hard and soft surfaces, while they should not be taken as tolerance limits generally, do reinforce the belief that the body is designed to minimize resonances or "dynamic overshoot" which, if present, would certainly aggravate injury under suddenly applied loading. This appears especially true of the brain, where partitions, bony ridges and a multitude of attachments to the skull appear to be designed at least in part to minimize dynamic reactions. The high-speed x-ray movies of Schatsky also showed little evidence of transient resonance.

Carefully conducted air bag tests on volunteers have more recently confirmed the tolerances estimated above from the Air Force studies. While this discussion will not take up the question of overall adequacy of this device under various kinds of accidents, the frontal loadings imposed upon the volunteers in the 30 to 31 mph Daisy Track runs yielded perhaps the most accurate data available in support of any head injury criterion for the time domain of 50–60 ms. Contrary to Newman's assertion that head cg acceleration readings cannot be valid because the accelerometer cannot be placed at the cg in the living head, this problem was essentially overcome in this test series, by first conducting a number of dummy runs with accelerometers both inside and at the sides of the head to verify that similar readings were obtained. Figure 2 illustrates typical results. Impacts were approximately 50 ms in duration, rather abrupt, in that the head was arrested not only by the bag but in addition by subsequent denting of an aluminum cowl against which the

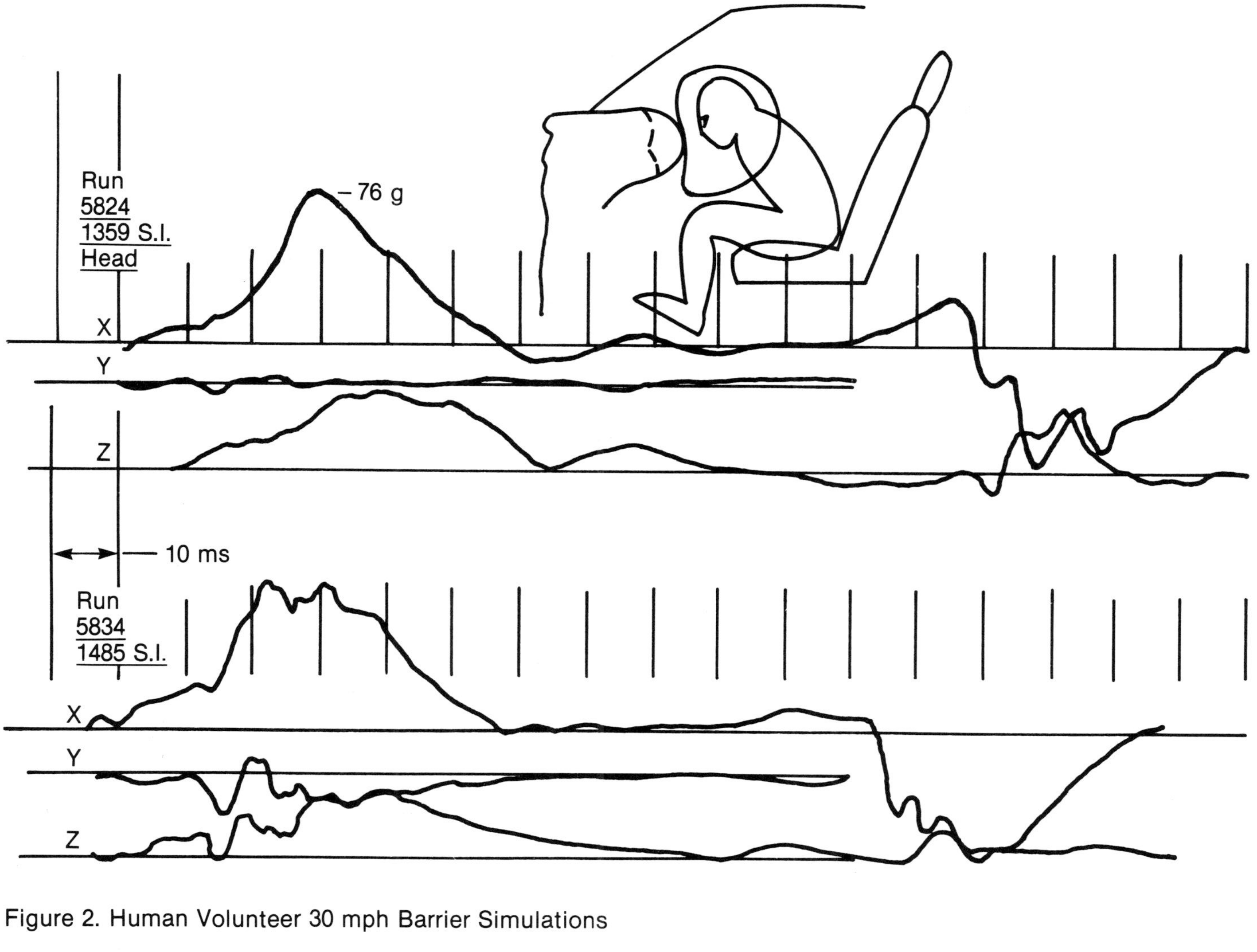

Figure 2. Human Volunteer 30 mph Barrier Simulations

bag pressed. The most interesting aspect of the work in the writer's opinion was the fact the SI approached 1000 on the forward onset and another 500 on rebound against the head rest for a total of as much as 1500 without appreciable injury to the subjects.

The foundation for use of a 2.5 power exponential weighting for head injury hazard is, thus, far more broadly based than Newman's articles would lead one to believe.

Accuracy of Biomechanics Data in General

Criticism of head injury data is that it is not accurate enough. It would of course be naive to believe that any particular study can give the whole answer, in view of the many modes of possible injury to the head, but it is equally wrong, as implied by Newman, to wait for some fancied breakthrough in our knowledge before using what we have for design guidance. Using what we have can help fulfill a moral obligation to build the safest products consistent with practical considerations. Strangely, Newman does not apply any requirement of accuracy or consistency in support of his own alternative recommendations, and one can only conclude that he in fact recommends no design guides for some time to come. His several recommendations, namely eliminating head impact, measuring velocity change (ΔV), limiting head impact force, measuring external head pressure distribution and monitoring an array of pressure transducers in an artificial brain, are in various ways mutually contradictory. Certain of them have merit, but require further research before their range of utility can be established and whether problems of instrumentation and practical test procedures can be solved.

We all realize that head can be injured as a result of a multitude of different mechanisms as well as in differing degrees from impulses from differing direc-

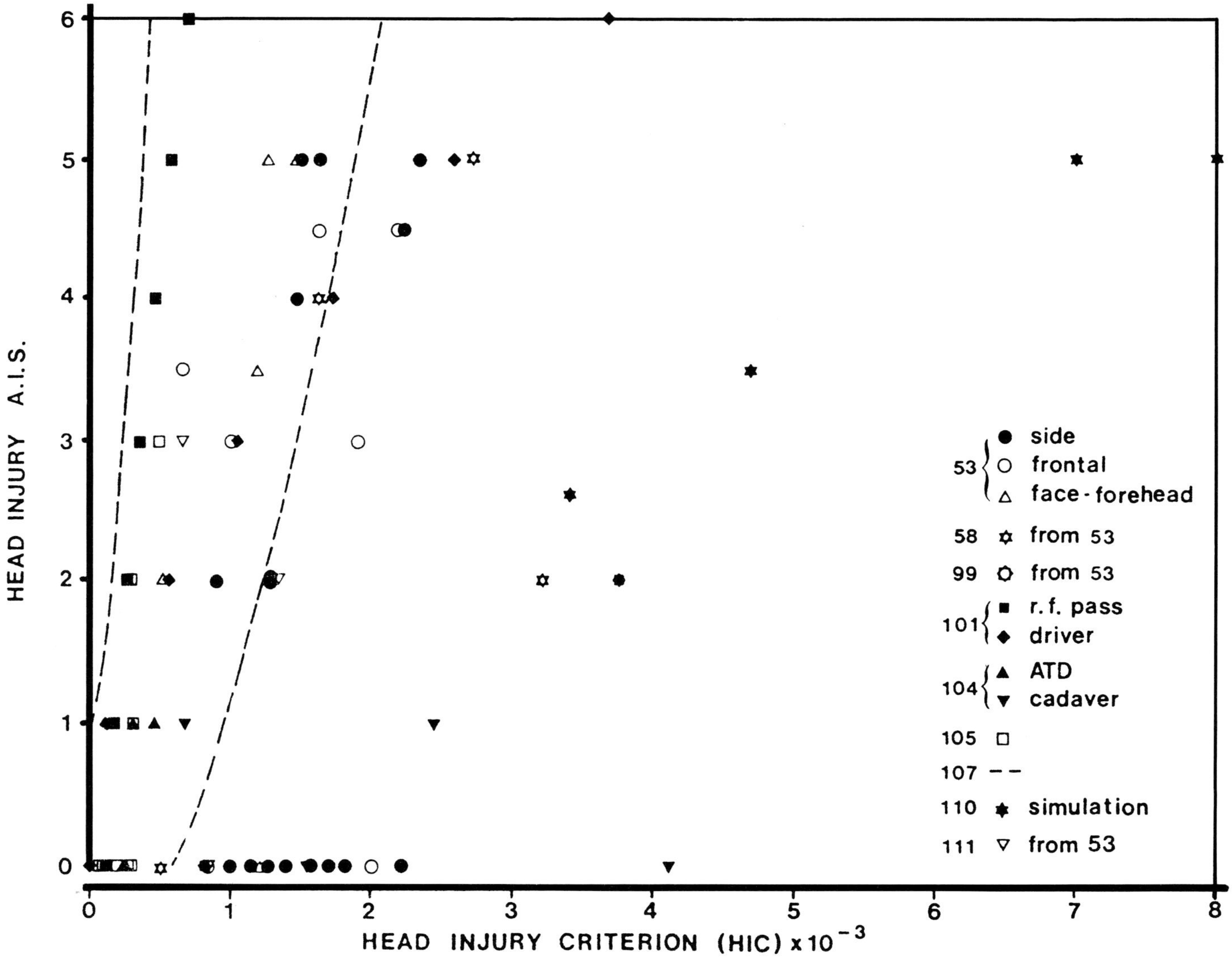

Figure 3. Head Injury Severity as a Function of HIC. Data from Various Sources J. Newman

tions, but for practical purposes a single, repeatable, transducer reading is needed which has been validated approximately over a broad range of conditions.

Variability in Strength of Biological Tissues

Research by the writer and numerous other investigators has shown that the resistance of biological materials or structures can vary by hundreds of percent. In spite of this, the "pièce de résistance" of Newman's presentations (Figure 3) purports to destroy the HIC simply by showing a large spread in HIC value obtained from various people's accident reconstructions. Nothing could be more misleading, since such a spread in HIC values is inevitable considering the great variation in the subjects involved (which include children in the plot of Figure 3) and considering the wide variety of accident conditions. The several highest HIC values plotted are not surprising since they represent the ultimate survivability under ideal conditions. Other injury hazard criteria would undoubtedly show large scatter as well. (A weighted-impulse criterion of course shows more spread at high values than would a simple "g" or pressure criterion, but this is not a mark against it; it is simply expressing the fact that damage to almost any material increases disproportionately rapidly as the danger level is reached.)

Physical Basis for an Injury Criterion

It has been suggested by Newman that the 2.5 power weighting is nothing more than a curve fit, and a poor one at that. One must agree that any predictor formula should have some physical basis rather than be nothing more than a curve fit. However a weighted impulse criterion does meet this requirement; failure of real-world materials generally becomes disproportionately more likely as imposed loading is increased. This has for a long time been known for both static and cyclic loading of solids, burn injury, loading of brain tissue and so on. Secondly, materials in general, even glass, are time-dependent in their failure properties, in that not just the peak, but the load profile as well, affect the strength.

In his early experiments with strain of brain tissue, Ommaya noted such effects, and this led R. Haut and the writer to propose (6) that a nonlinear viscoelastic model could serve as a reasonable physical basis for the reaction of the brain to accelerative loading. As shown in Figure 4 taken from this paper, such behavior leads directly to the same tolerance trend as portrayed in Figure 1.

Comparison of Some Differing Injury Criteria

In Figures 5 and 6 several different criteria including recent laboratory studies by a Japanese group

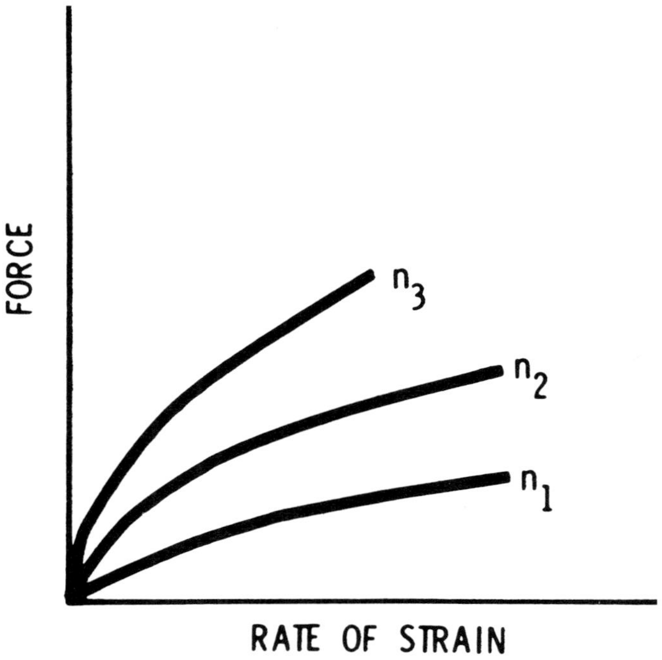

Pseudo-Bingham Behavior

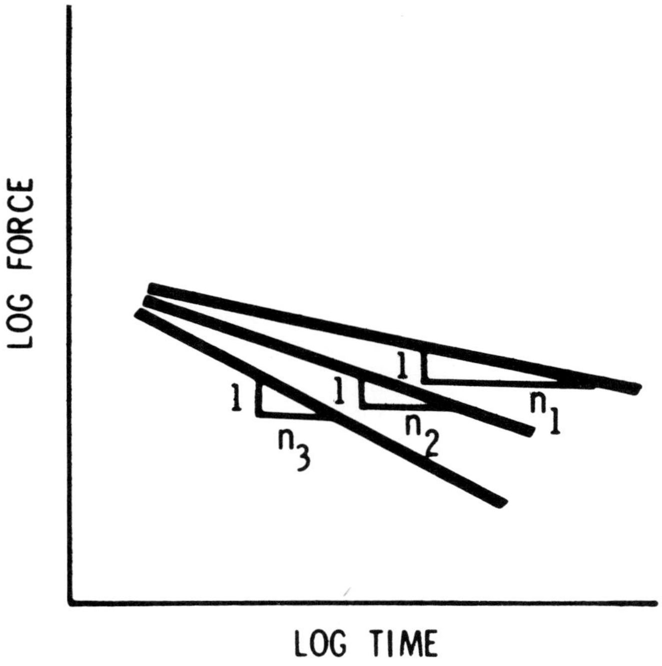

Figure 4. Log-Log Tolerance Plot of Fig. 6A

(9) and by Ward, Chan and Nahum (10) are compared with the older SI and HIC criteria. In Figure 5 it is interesting that the recent Japanese curves are very similar in character to the latter.

Figure 6 compares the SI and HIC curves for triangular pulses of varying duration. (The "g" levels for skull fracture may at first glance be in conflict with those of Figure 1, but this is because the latter are for square-wave approximations.)

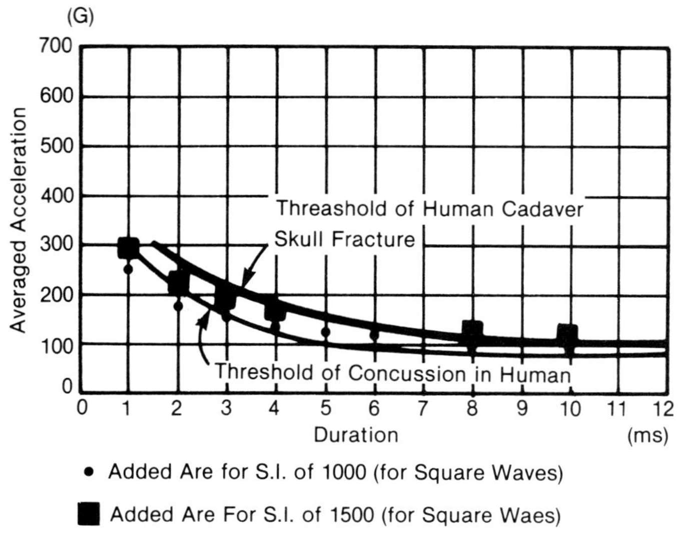

Figure 5. JARI Human Head Impact Tolerance Curve (JHTC)

The data points plotted at the right are for two of the airbag volunteer experiments, assuming triangular approximation. The lower circles represent the onset S's while the upper two combine the SIs for both onset and rebound.

By far the greatest discrepancies occur when comparing the recent peak pressure criterion of Ward, et al., for hard impact, with the HIC and SI. This interesting research with pressure measurement points to the need for further research into a number of things, including the great departure in curve shape compared with that of the work at Wayne State, the pressure tolerance at longer duration, whether a single point, that is, maximum pressure, will suffice, whether it is practical to do everyday sled testing with an array of pressure transducers in a simulated brain and whether it is practical to employ multiple criteria for several major modes of failure, as the authors suggest may be necessary.

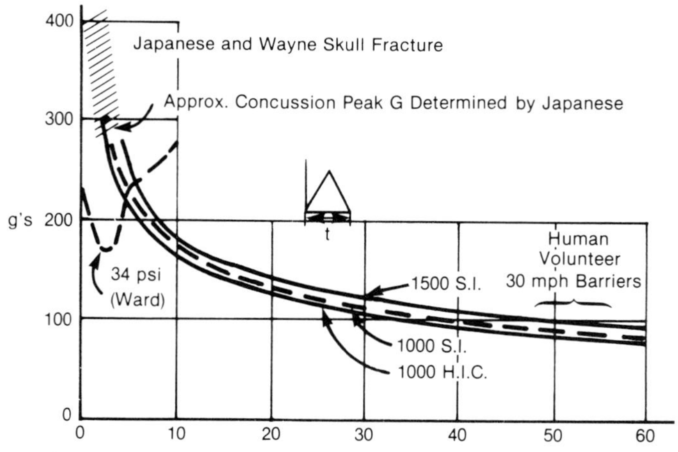

Figure 6. Pulse Width in MS

Speaking generally with regard to advancing the art of head injury hazard estimation, it is felt by the writer that a most easily accomplished objective for the near term would be to give recognition to the belief of a number of experienced specialists, that head injury is not a serious problem if the head merely swings freely but does not make hard contact with the vehicle interior.

Noncontact did not occur in vehicular accidents at the time the writer proposed the Severity Index in 1966 (1). At that time the simple straight line log-log approximation was felt reasonably accurate up to moderate duration of impulse. However, in that same paper the suggestion was made that for the future, consideration could be given to modifying the calculation to recognize the fact that as the pulse duration lengthens further, the straight line approximation becomes too conservative and that the tolerance tends to approach a horizontal asymptote even on log-log paper.

There should be ways in which such a modification could be worked out for the HIC as well. Such a modification should then allow the HIC to be computed over the entire head trajectory without undue penalty in a noncontact situation.

References

1. Charles W. Gadd, "Use of a Weighted Impulse Criterion for Estimating Injury Hazard," Proceedings of the 10th Stapp Car Crash Conference, SAE, 1966.
2. T. M. Fraser, "Human Response to Sustained Acceleration," NASA-SP-103, Scientific and Technical Information Division, NASA, Washington, D.C., 1966.
3. R. W. Sonntag, Jr., et al., "Use of Contoured Restraint Systems in Exposure of Large Primates to $-150\ g_x$ Impact," Proceedings of the 12th Stapp Car Crash Conference, SAE, New York, 1968.
4. J. P. Stapp, et al., "Analysis and Biodynamics of Selected Rocket Sled Experiments" Part 1, USAF School of Aerospace Medicine, Brooks AFB, July 1964.
5. G. R. Smith, et al., "Human Volunteer Testing of GM Air Cushions," 2nd International Conference on Passive Restraints, Publ. #720443, SAE, May 1972.
6. R. G. Hunt and C. W. Gadd, "Nonlinear Viscoelastic Model for Head Impact Injury Hazard," Proceedings of 16th Stapp Conference, 1972 and Transactions of SAE, 1973.
7. K. Ono, et al., "Human Head Tolerance of Sagittal Impact, Reliable Estimation Deduced from

Exp. Head Injury Using Subhuman Primates and Human Cadaver Skulls," Proceedings of 1980 Stapp Car Crash Conference, SAE, 1980.

8. J. A. Newman, "Head Injury Criteria in Automotive Crash Testing," Proceedings of the 1980 Stapp Car Crash Conference, SAE, 1980.

9. J. A. Newman, "Automobile Occupant Injury Criteria, Part 1: Head Injury," Automobile Safety Engineering, Road and Motor Vehicle Traffic Safety Transport, Canada, February 1980.

10. C. Ward, M. Chan, and A. Nahum, "Intracranial Pressure—A Brain Injury Criterion," Proceedings of the 1980 Stapp Car Crash Conference, SAE, 1980.

A Review of Research on Head Impact Tolerance and Injury Criteria Related to Occupant Protection

Robert L. Hess
Kathleen Weber
John W. Melvin

Introduction

Protecting the head from irreversible brain damage is one of the most critical tasks of the automotive safety design engineer and of the regulator who sets Federal Motor Vehicle Safety Standards (FMVSS). Both have based their work on human performance and injury data from a variety of sources. Although field accident data are available in large volume, very little have been able to provide the level of detail necessary to study actual mechanisms of injury. Regulators and engineers concerned with occupant protection have instead used the more scientific data coming from laboratory impact experiments with human volunteers to determine an acceptable level of protection and to measure whether or not a system achieves this level.

The intent of this paper is to review the development of biomechanical knowledge about skull/brain injury tolerance to impact and other accelerations, to examine the degree to which this knowledge has been used by the National Highway Traffic Safety Administration (NHTSA) in setting occupant protection standards, and to focus attention on that portion of the evidence that has not been effectively tapped. This latter body of information has been developed primarily in the period beginning 1972, the year in which the Head Injury Criterion (HIC) was incorporated into FMVSS 208 and a court decision was made requiring NHTSA to precisely specify its anthropomorphic test device. Finally, suggestions are made for further research that would enhance our understanding of head injury mechanisms and protection.

Early Period: 1960–1970

Wayne State Tolerance Curve

The Wayne State Tolerance Curve (WSTC), first suggested by Lissner, Lebow, and Evans (1960) (1) is the foundation upon which most currently accepted indexes of head injury tolerance are based. As originally presented, the "curve" included six points that represented the relationship between acceleration level and impulse duration (in the range of 1 to 6 ms) found to produce linear skull fracture in embalmed cadaver heads. Simply put, short pulses of high acceleration will cause injury, while lower acceleration levels require longer duration to do harm. The curve was later extended to pulse durations above 6 ms with comparative animal and cadaver impact data and with human volunteer acceleration test data. The details of the history of the WSTC are described in SAE J885b (1980) (2) and will not be repeated here.

The reader should be aware, however, of the physical nature of the experiments of Lissner et al. that produced the first data points to be used in the WSTC. Embalmed human cadavers were used as opposed to fresh cadavers or severed heads. Instrumentation consisted of pressure transducers in the right temporal and left posterior regions of the skull and an accelerometer on the center rear of the skull. The impact was on the forehead. The membranes surrounding lobes of the brain were mechanically punctured and torn to allow all parts of the cranial cavity to communicate. The impacts were accomplished by dropping the cadavers onto automotive instrument panels, damped steel plates, steel anvils, and padded steel anvils.

The important points for the present discussion are that (1) pressure change gradients in the region of the foramen magnum were understood to be the primary brain stem injury mechanism; (2) the original WSTC reported peak accelerations and peak pressures for translational impact with hard, flat surfaces in the anterior-posterior direction; (3) the authors cautioned that much data was needed to validate the curve; but (4) it was the first graphical representation of critical injury threshold based on impact conditions. The authors also provided insight into the goal for energy absorbing materials or structures:

> Any padding arrangement or reduction in stiffness of the [instrument] panel, or both, which increases the time duration of impact in an equal or diminished ratio to the decrease in acceleration or pressure produced, will be an improvement with regard to prevention of injury.

The relative decreases and increases necessary are described by a curved line, such as the WSTC.

Soon thereafter, Gadd (1961) (3) suggested plotting the injury threshold curve on logarithmic scales to achieve a straight line fit. The extent to which the slope of this line was steeper than -1 would indicate a greater dependence of injury on the intensity of loading, as opposed to dependence on time of loading. He also suggested that multiple impulses could be analyzed for injury potential by integrating the acceleration over the entire impulse profile, using the power weighting factor, derived above from the slope, on the acceleration portion of the profile. This fundamental engineering advice for those thinking of establishing an index of injury tolerance was later to be developed into the Gadd Severity Index, discussed below.

Before this index was finalized, however, changes were made in the WSTC. To make the triangular peak acceleration levels compatible with irregular wave forms and with the trapezoidal waves of human volunteer tests summarized by Eiband (1959) (4), the ordinate of the curve was changed to "effective" or average acceleration. A plot in this form appears in Patrick, Lissner, and Gurdjian (1963) (5). The asymptote of the curve, or the low-level acceleration threshold for very long time durations, was given as 42 g. The authors stated, however, that humans are known to have withstood considerably higher accelerations in cases where there was no impact. They suggested then a threshold of from 60 g to 80 g, and they themselves used 80 g as the upper safe limit on effective acceleration for impacts with a padded surface. This figure was later incorporated into FMVSS 201 instrument panel tests and an early version of FMVSS 208. It must be remembered, however, that for nonrectangular wave forms, peak accelerations can be higher than 80 g. The authors cited permissible peaks of 110 g for sinusoidal pulses and 160 g for triangular.

Other concepts coming from this paper that were to emerge later in standards were (1) the avoidance of high acceleration peaks lasting longer than 1 ms and (2) the use of interior impact test velocities of one half the probable vehicle velocity at impact. The reader is cautioned that the latter concept may not be valid in real crashes. Velocities chosen for impact tests should be reevaluated as occupant protection systems influence occupant kinematics and thus interior impact velocity.

Severity Index

At the Tenth Stapp Car Crash Conference, Gadd (1966) (6) brought to maturity the ideas presented in 1961. Although a log-log plot of the WSTC resulted in a somewhat curved line, Gadd felt his straight-line approximation was "insufficient at this time" because of the scatter of the data. The slope of his line was -2.5, and thus 2.5 became his power weighting factor. Using the Severity Index (SI) formula $\int a^{2.5}\,dt$, Gadd showed that a triangular pulse having the same area as a square pulse would have an injury potential 1.61 times as great. Near the end of his paper, Gadd returned to the question of his straightline approximation and suggested that, as more data became available, a curve of arbitrary shape could be constructed. He credited J. P. Danforth with the suggestion that the weighting exponent need not be constant but could vary as a function of acceleration.

FMVSS 201

On December 3, 1966, the proposed initial Federal Motor Vehicle Safety Standards appeared in the *Federal Register.** FMVSS 201, "Occupant Protection in Interior Impact," was among those proposed. Using the general test procedures and 15-pound, 6.5-inch-diameter headform from SAE J921 (7), 15 mph impacts with the "head impact area" of the instrument panel were to be performed.

The test criteria were as follows:

a) The deceleration of the head form shall not exceed 80 g for 1.0 ms or more; and,
b) The pressure in the area of contact shall not exceed 100 psi.

The proposed regulation did not apply to areas within 5 inches of the door nor closer to the windshield than could be contacted by the headform. It should be noted that the 80-g effective acceleration limit suggested by Patrick, et al. (1963) (5) was incorporated here as a maximum, except for peaks of very short duration that were also allowed by these authors. The pressure

* For regulatory details, citations to and excerpts from the *Federal Register* can be found in *A Review of Literature and Regulation Relating to Head Impact Tolerance and Injury Criteria,* July 1980, Report No. UM-HSRI-80-52-1.

limit of b) was included to control for impacts with protrusions that could be injurious at low acceleration levels. Two months after the initial proposal, the rule was issued with the same provisions, except that the concept of contact-area pressure was dropped.

At the request of petitioners, hearings were held in May 1967 regarding the provisions of FMVSS 201. The resulting revised regulation, issued in August, eliminated areas of the instrument panel below an upper lip from any impact testing and lengthened the duration of allowable deceleration above 80 g to 3 ms. Although no limit was placed on the peak allowable during the 3 ms window, it would be reasonably difficult to achieve an injurious level of acceleration during this short a period if the impacted surface were padded. Using current methods to calculate injury threshold (HIC < 1000, to be discussed below), a peak of 280 g would still be within the safe limit.

Injury Mechanisms

During this time, when tolerance curves and injury indexes were being developed and government standards were trying to reflect these developments, laboratory research continued to be concerned with the actual mechanisms within the skull that produce brain injury and with quantifying the mechanical properties of the skull/brain system. The eventual goal of this research would be the development of sophisticated analytical models to predict injury from impact and acceleration.

The WSTC was based on translational motion data, but rotation had also long been known to effect injury (Holbourn, 1943 (8); Gurdjian, Webster, and Lissner, 1955 (9)). Gurdjian, Roberts, and Thomas (1966) (10) observed that the "line of action" of a blow to the head had a significant effect on the resulting injury. If "an impact provides an unusually abrupt rotation of the skull, severe effects can occur in areas not immediately adjacent to the point of impact." Ommaya, Hirsch and Martinez (1966) (11) found that a cervical collar reduced the rotational acceleration of monkey heads and raised the concussion threshold for occipital impacts. The authors also found that abrupt rotation without impact could affect sensory responses.

A brief paper by Gurdjian, Hodgson, et al. (1968) (12) summarized the state of understanding at that time of brain injury mechanisms from head impacts. Specifically the paper mentioned (1) direct contusion from deformation at the point of impact; (2) indirect contusion produced by negative pressure on the side opposite the impact; (3) brain deformation as it responds to pressure gradients, causing shear stresses at the craniospinal junction; (4) contusion from movement of the brain against rough and irregular interior skull surfaces; and (5) subdural hematoma from movement of the brain relative to its dural envelope, resulting in tears of connecting blood vessels.

Mathematical Modeling

Early modeling efforts included the work of Hodgson and Patrick (1968) (13), who developed a simple one-degree-of-freedom model to predict the response of the occipital bone to frontal bone impact. The model was based on data from mechanical impedance tests of a human cadaver and two living human subjects in the range of 0 to 5000 Hz. Mechanical impedance measurements involve determining the ratio of a sinusoidal force, applied to a specimen, to a particular mechanical response of that specimen. As the frequency of the applied force varies, both the magnitude and the phase of the response vary. Once the impedance function is known, the impact response can be calculated. The results can also be used to develop and validate simple lumped parameter models of the head, both mathematical and physical, incorporating the same mechanical impedance in the frequency range of interest. The particular response used by Hodgson and Patrick was the amplification of acceleration at a point on the head opposite the applied force. This response of the cadaver head was found to be similar to that of a simple spring-mass system with an antiresonant frequency at 313 Hz and a resonant frequency at 900 Hz. At frequencies below 100 Hz, the response was that of a rigid body.

Another mechanical property important for head injury modeling is the dynamic complex shear modulus, G, of the brain. Technically, G is a vector quantity expressing two perpendicular components: G', the dynamic elastic modulus representing the springlike stiffness of the material under shear stress, and G'', the dynamic loss modulus representing the viscous losses in the material. This complex modulus is necessary for a numerical analysis of a viscoelastic material. Fallenstein, Hulce, and Melvin (1969) (14) studied this property as the initial phase of a larger program to completely characterize the material of the human head. In their paper, the authors discussed the work of others who provided guidance for the program and reported their own experimental results. The values obtained for *in vitro* human brain were just below those of *in vivo* human muscle tissue. Higher values were found in preliminary *in vivo* tests on Rhesus monkeys. The authors predicted that further tests and *in vitro/in vivo* correlations would help resolve questions about the effects of postmortem changes, blood pressure, and frequency on the dynamic properties of brain tissue.

Driving point impedance tests of the head were conducted by Stalnaker, Fogle, and McElhaney (1970) (15) on a human cadaver and on living and cadaver monkeys. The ratio of the driving force to the velocity at the driven point was measured over the frequency range of 30 to 5000 Hz. The authors' methods for attaching transducers and holding the subjects in place were an improvement over those used in previous impedance tests. A linear two-degree-of-freedom model was developed from the data obtained. The authors found the brain to be very nearly critically damped. Metz, McElhaney, and Ommaya (1970) (16) reported on a new method of measuring the elastic modulus of brain tissue. Values equivalent to G′ were found to be somewhat higher than those reported by Fallenstein, et al. (1969) (14).

The mechanical properties of cranial bone were studied by McElhaney, Fogle, et al. (1970) (17). This work, like that of Fallenstein, et al. (1969) (14), was part of a program to adequately characterize all the materials of the human head so that physical and mathematical models could be constructed for systematic study of head injury mechanisms. This work was sponsored by the National Institute of Neurological Diseases and Stroke. A variety of properties were reported in detail as well as the dependence of these properties on the structural arrangement of the diploe, a characteristic likely to vary considerably over a population of subjects. A model was developed to summarize the variations of mechanical properties with respect to the density of this region.

FMVSS 208

Getting out of the laboratory for a moment, it is appropriate at this point to discuss the developments in the area of regulation that occurred in 1970. In May, the first proposal to incorporate automatic (passive) crash protection into FMVSS 208 appeared in the *Federal Register.* To test the effectiveness of these systems, the standard was to establish "basic injury criteria with reference to an anthropomorphic dummy, expressed in terms of maximum forces and pressures on critical parts of the body." The dummy to be used was that described in SAE J963 (1968) (18). The occupant protection system would be tested the first year with dummies in a frontal fixed-barrier crash at 30 mph, and lateral and rollover tests would be added the following year. The proposal specified that "the resultant head acceleration shall not exceed 80 g for any continuous period of more than 3 milliseconds." NHTSA admitted that the specified dummy "may not provide totally reproducible results." There was, however, no easily available alternative at the time. It should be noted as well that the test criteria were based on the magnitude of the resultant acceleration rather than on its projection along a single axis, as was used in constructing the original WSTC. An interim option of manual lap/shoulder belts that had to meet the same test conditions was also included in the proposal. Comments on the proposal ensued. A presentation of the arguments on both sides concerning this and later proposals can be found in a report by the U.S. National Transportation Safety Board (1979) (19), and therefore only pertinent highlights will be mentioned here. The primary objection to the injury criteria measurements was that they were beyond the state of the art.

On September 25 a revised proposal was issued stating that "the resultant head acceleration shall not exceed 90 g, and shall not exceed 67 g for a cumulative duration of more than 3 milliseconds." These criteria differed from those of the earlier proposal and FMVSS 201 in that a peak acceleration was established and the 3-ms limit on high accelerations became cumulative rather than continuous. No explanation was given for the changes. The proposal also increased the number of interim options available. For fully automatic systems (first option) and semi-automatic systems in which a manual lap belt could be included (second option), the injury criteria above were to be met under frontal fixed-barrier test conditions. For manual lap/shoulder belts (third option), the test conditions remained the same, but the only criterion for passing the test was that the system "experience no complete separation of any element of a seat belt assembly." This option was given to reduce the cost of complying with interim improved belt systems.

To put FMVSS 201 somewhat more in line with 208, a proposal was made to increase the test velocity for the head impact areas and lower the allowable headform decelerations such that, when these areas were impacted at 25 mph by the standard headform, they could not cause a deceleration of more than 90 g for a cumulative duration of 1 ms nor 67 g for a cumulative duration of more than 3 ms. The proposal also sought to increase the size and number of impact areas covered. These changes, however, were never put into effect, and the current FMVSS 201 remains essentially as it was in 1967.

The first FMVSS 208 rule incorporating automatic restraints was issued November 3, 1970. The preamble read as follows with regard to permissible head accelerations:

> The levels proposed in the September 25 notice are adopted in this standard, with head accelerations changed from 67 g to 70 g, as the best available criteria for the quantities measured. Consideration will be given to adoption of a severity index or other criteria as further research results become known.

In the same issue of the *Federal Register,* amendments to the new rule were proposed. Stating that "biomechanical studies indicate that the lateral acceleration tolerance of the head and chest are significantly less than the frontal acceleration tolerance," a requirement was proposed that the lateral component of head accelerations could not exceed 40 g for a cumulative duration of more than 3 ms. The "biomechanical studies" referred to were not identified, but the data were presumably as yet unpublished results from NHTSA's contracted research project entitled "Door Crashworthiness Criteria." (The paper by McElhaney, Stalnaker, et al. (1971) (20) later presented the data base from this project.) The notice also proposed rollover and moving-barrier lateral tests.

A Period of Transition: 1970–1973

Alternate Views of Head Injury

While NHTSA was considering injury severity indexes and limits on lateral impact acceleration, interest continued in the contribution of rotational acceleration to head injury. At the Fourteenth Stapp Car Crash Conference, Hirsch (having joined NHTSA's research staff) and Ommaya (1970) (21) reported confirmation of their earlier findings (Ommaya, et al., 1966) (11) that rotational motion appeared to be more critical to the production of brain injury than translational motion. The authors further stated that "no convincing evidence has to this date been presented which relates brain injury and concussion to translational motion of the head for short-duration force inputs, whether through whiplash or direct impact." Caution was suggested when using "currently popular head tolerance criteria" based on translational head motion.

Other researchers, however, were using their own experimental data to develop head injury indexes that would approximate the WSTC. These were the J Tolerance Index (JTI) of Slattenschek (described in English in Slattenschek and Tauffkirchen, (1970) (22)), and the Effective Displacement Index (EDI) of Brinn and Staffeld (1970) (23). Both of these indexes were based on single-degree-of-freedom mass-spring-dashpot vibration models.

Stalnaker and McElhaney (1970) (24) further developed their two-mass model, based on data from their driving point impedance tests, and formulated an injury index called the Maximum Strain Criterion (MSC). This was presented in December at the ASME winter meeting. The MSC curve indicated a tolerance threshold significantly lower than did the WSTC, and injury tolerance was found to be dependent on the impact waveform. The MSC for human lateral head impact was also presented for the first time and was shown to be 50 percent lower than that for longitudinal impact.

Five years after Gadd's Severity Index had been adopted as an SAE recommended practice (SAE J885a, 1966) (25), and just as researchers were recommending the use of alternate criteria, NHTSA decided to adopt the SI as the head injury criterion for first and second options of FMVSS 208. In February 1971, a notice was issued stating NHTSA's intent to require completely automatic systems to provide "protection in frontal fixed barrier crash tests up to 30 mph, and up to 30 to either side of the perpendicular, and in lateral and rollover crash tests." The other two options were to be tested only in the frontal perpendicular configuration. The first and second options were to qualify under "a maximum head severity index of 1000, calculated according to SAE J885a." The third option (lap/shoulder belts) was again only required not to sustain structural failure. The rule appeared in March essentially as announced except that the third option was to be eliminated after August 1973. The preamble to the rule also reaffirmed NHTSA's opinion that the SAE J963 dummy specifications were "the best available." Research was being done, however, "with a view to issuance of further specifications for these devices." Soon thereafter Chrysler initiated legal proceedings that eventually ended the use of the SAE J963 dummy.

In October 1971, various amendments to the rule were issued regarding testing procedures. The preamble, however, responding to comments that the criterion for head injury was too stringent, restated NHTSA's belief that the SI$<$1000 was the most acceptable criterion at the time and that it would be retained. Responding again to comments that SAE J963 did not "completely define all the characteristics of the dummies that may be relevant to their performance in a crash," NHTSA accepted the validity of the comments but said,

> It would be difficult, if not impossible, to describe the test dummy in performance terms with such specificity that every dummy that could be built to the specifications would perform identically under similar conditions.

NHTSA thus declined to "freeze" dummy construction and performance specifications at that time.

Head Injury Criteria

The Fifteenth Stapp Car Crash Conference, held in the fall of 1971, included special sessions on head injury and became a forum for the discussion of head injury mechanisms, tolerance thresholds, and test criteria. Translation versus rotation was again discussed (Unterharnscheidt, (1971) (26); Gennarelli, Ommaya, and Thibault, (1971) (27); Gadd (1971) (28) suggested that, based on rocket sled experiments, the SI 1000 limit was much too conservative for non-contact, whole-body accelerations; and Fan (1971) (29) introduced the Revised Brain Model (RBM), a modification of the JTI) Versace (1971) (30) presented a mathematical critique of the SI and suggested an alternative method for calculating the index number, in which the effective acceleration, defined as $1/T \int a^n dt$ was raised to the 2.5 power and multiplied by the time duration. Versace argued the approach was still inadequate because of two factors: (1) biomechanical data were insufficient to accurately arrive at an appropriate exponent, and (2) the index represented only an intermediate stage in the injury chain of events. A measure of the actual response of the brain to head impact would be more relevant.

NHTSA liked Versace's formula because it was able to handle the seemingly high tolerance levels in cases of long duration, low-level acceleration, and in cases of two or more high peak accelerations associated with two or more impacts. In March 1972, a proposal was issued to replace the SI in FMVSS 208 with the following expression:

$$\left[\frac{1}{t_2 - t_1}\int_{t_1}^{t_2} a\,dt\right]^{2.5} (t_2 - t_1) < 1000$$

where a is the resultant acceleration and t_1 and t_2 are any two points in time during the crash. The decision to change was said to be based on research information that "head acceleration exposure is not always additive relative to head injury." Although not formally labeled at that time, the new index soon became known as the Head Injury Criterion (HIC).

In the month prior to the HIC proposal, NHTSA issued the FMVSS 208 rule that extended the injury criteria of automatic restraint systems to the manual lap/shoulder belts of the third option and added the ignition interlock. Vehicle manufacturers commented that, as long as the head does not contact anything, belt systems allow the head to flop loosely forward, creating a high SI value while not contributing significantly to injury. When the HIC was adopted as a rule in June 1972, NHTSA restricted the definition of t_2 and t_1 to be "any two points in time after the head contacts a part of the vehicle other than the belt system." This modification applied only to belt systems allowed under the interim third option. The issue was not resolved yet, however, and in October a further restriction was made to discount the effects of glancing blows. The regulation then specified "any two points in time during any interval in which the head is in continuous contact with a part of the vehicle other than the belt system."

Developments in Mathematical and Mechanical Models

Although the regulator had updated its injury criterion and testing procedures, research continued to better characterize and predict skull/brain injury and to use this information to develop test dummies having reasonable levels of repeatability and biofidelity. These issues were the subjects of several papers presented at the Symposium on Human Impact Response in October 1972.

At this symposium, McElhaney, Stalnaker, and Roberts (1972) (31) presented further refinements of the MSC and compared its injury predictions to those of the other indexes, i.e., SI, HIC, JTI, EDI, and RBM. The MSC was revised to represent the Mean (rather than maximum) Strain Criterion, where "mean strain" was defined as "the displacement of one side of the head relative to the other, divided by the distance across the cranium." Basing a tolerance curve on average rather than peak acceleration levels was more consistent with other criteria. The mean tolerable strain for human heads was calculated to be 0.0061 in./in. Comparing the MSC to other indexes for several simulated crashes, the JTI, EDI, and RBM predictions were similar to the MSC, but the SI and HIC were much more conservative. In the final section of the paper, the authors summarized data from human cadaver impact tests, undertaken to establish force- and acceleration-time histories of the human head, so that dummy head impact responses could be specified.

The discussion that followed the presentation dealt with the current state of understanding of brain injury mechanisms and the implications for head injury modeling. Part of this discussion is quoted here:

> J. H. McElhaney: The model we propose, which as we see predicts essentially the same things as many other models, is based on information from essentially rigid or almost hard impacts. Under these conditions we get a certain type of injury. We have certain injury mechanisms involved. We're starting to believe more and more, that this mechanism is cavitation whereas at one time we thought it might be just a gross deformation in the brain . . . We're still staying with a lumped-parameter model, but we're introducing many more parameters in an attempt to build into it the ability to consider different mechanisms of injury. We recognize particularly that as the pulse duration increases, there is a different mechanism of injury; and in fact, in the rigid striker impacts we see predominantly contracoup type injuries. When we pad this striker we don't see contracoup injuries anymore. We see minute hemorrhaging in much larger areas in the brain. Both of these injury types cause some difficulty in assessment. If the injuries occur in one region of the brain our pathologist tells us it's of no consequence; but if they occur in another region of the brain or tear a major artery, for example, it's very serious . . . When we go to long pulse durations where we have a lot of angular displacement of the head or high angular velocity, we see a completely different type of injury mechanism. We see subdural hematomas and brain stem involvement. What I think we will wind up with in the future is either several injury criteria, each relating to a specific injury depending on the mechanism, or possibly one injury criterion that covers all of the injury mechanisms . . . This is a difficult problem, and it's not going

> to be solved right away; but at the same time the automotive community is also faced with a difficult problem that they have to solve right away, and I don't have much more advice than to go slow until we learn more.

On December 5, 1972, the U.S. Court of Appeals, Sixth Circuit, ruled on the Chrysler suit challenging the automatic restraint regulations. The decision rendered the FMVSS 208 test procedures invalid because of an inadequately specified test dummy. In response to this ruling, NHTSA issued a proposal in April 1973 that introduced the General Motors Hybrid II Dummy, a highly repeatable test device, as the new test dummy for the first and second options. In June, a regulation was published that eliminated all dynamic tests for belt systems covered under the third option as a result of further court decisions on test dummy inadequacies. Dynamic tests for third option manual belts were never reinstituted. Automatic belt systems, however, would be covered under the first option test conditions.

In August, a new Part 572 was added to Title 49 of the Code of Federal Regulations that established the previously proposed dummy as NHTSA's test device. The dummy was specified with detailed drawings and performance criteria. The performance specifications of the dummy head were as follows:

> When the head is dropped from a height of 10 inches . . . the peak resultant accelerations at the head's center of gravity shall be not less than 210 g and not more than 260 g. The acceleration/time curve for the test shall lie at or above the 100 g level for an interval not less than 1.5 ms.

Except for minor problems with surface texture and accelerometer placement, these specifications were generally accepted by safety engineers.

During this same period, another dummy was being developed that had the joint goals of providing repeatable/reproducible results as well as having a biodynamic performance in frontal impacts closely matching that of unembalmed human cadavers. The dummy was introduced at the Seventeenth Stapp Car Crash Conference as "Repeatable Pete" (McElhaney, Mate, and Roberts (1973) (32)). The development process for the head and thorax of this dummy is significant in that it was the first time a laboratory had made mechanical measurements, designed a physical model, and evaluated the model using the same test equipment, instrumentation, and procedures. This closed-loop process resulted in the first demonstration of a repeatable test device that also had good biomechanical response.

At the same conference, Stalnaker, Roberts, and McElhaney (1973) (33) reported the results of new long-duration lateral head impacts to human cadavers and live infrahuman primates. Using dimensional analysis techniques, the animal data were scaled to estimate the side impact tolerance of the living human. The threshold of human closed-brain injury was reported to be 76 g for a 20-ms impulse. Autopsies showed that long-duration impacts most commonly resulted in brain stem and internal brain hemorrhaging in areas remote from the impact locations.

HIC Extensions

Returning to regulatory developments, the HIC was being extended into the test criteria of other standards. Shortly after the HIC was proposed for use in FMVSS 208, a proposal was issued for a new standard on motorcycle helmets. Initially, the helmets would meet certain peak and cumulative-duration g criteria, but eventually the standard would be upgraded to require helmets to meet the proposed HIC. When FMVSS 218 was issued in August 1973, however, the latter aspect was deferred pending further research and testing. A comprehensive review of head impact research and injury criteria as they relate to helmet standards can be found in Robbins (1980) (34).

A proposal for a new standard on school bus occupant protection was issued in July 1973. The proposal applied the HIC to the testing of head impact areas, such that when they were impacted at 15 mph by an 11.5-lb, 6.5-in.-diameter hemispherical headform, the HIC was to be less than 1000, using the resultant acceleration at the headform center of gravity. The proposal also described the force-time history on the headform by stating that the energy absorbed by the impacted material must be greater than 40 in.-lb before the force level on the impactor exceeded 150 lb; and it described the load distribution by stating that, at 5-ft/s impacts, the area impacted must be greater than 3 in.^{2}. In April 1975, the proposal was altered to limit the HIC calculation to the use of "axial" or translational acceleration of the headform in its direction of travel. In January 1976, FMVSS 222 was issued with the headform impact requirements included as proposed.

Later Period: 1974–1980

Finite Element and Kinematic Models

In the mid-1970's, new modeling efforts were launched using finite element analysis methods. Finite element models differ from traditional "infinitesimal models" primarily in the manner in which continuity is expressed. Generally, the former are more adaptable to digital computation techniques and more readily accept various forms of calculation tolerances. The ability of this type of approach to handle irregular shapes and inhomogeneous materials made it particularly suitable for modeling the mechanical structures and responses of the head. These efforts were hampered, however, by the lack of a complete set of data describing the properties of the various materials of the head.

Chan (1974) (35), following a discussion of shell models and a careful review of the continuum mechanics research on impact loading of headlike forms, presented a finite element model that predicted both shear strain and reduced pressure effects. The model was three-dimensional and had a symmetric axis of revolution. A more complex model, but still of idealized shape, was later developed by Khalil and Hubbard (1977) (36).

Two models reflecting the actual geometry of the head were developed under NHTSA sponsorship. These were reported to the Nineteenth Stapp Car Crash Conference. (Shugar, (1975) (37); Ward and Thompson (1975) (38)). The Shugar model concentrated on the mechanics of skull deformation and fracture, treating the brain as a homogenous, nearly incompressible material. The Ward model, on the other hand, assumed the skull to act as a rigid shell and only addressed the complex effects of impact and abrupt acceleration on the brain itself. For practical and economic reasons, these two approaches could not be integrated because each had several hundred degrees of freedom. Since the Ward model was more appropriate than the Shugar model for the longer-duration impacts experienced in crash environments having energy absorbing materials and structures, its further development was supported by NHTSA.

Mucciardi, Sanders, and Eppinger (1977) (39) demonstrated an interesting approach to predicting brain injury by analyzing head motion. Data from head impacts to monkeys performed by HSRI were used. Measured translational and rotational acceleration and velocity waveforms were treated by a nonlinear Adaptive Learning Network (ALN) program developed to produce empirically derived predictive models of head injury. The injury criterion was a special computed overall AIS. Time derivatives were used to create "jerk" waveforms to be used in addition to the measured waveforms. From thirty-four available kinematic parameters, the ALN model successfully predicted the observed integer AIS (using seven parameters), the unconsciousness AIS (using six parameters), and the time of unconsciousness (using seven parameters). The authors concluded that the overall AIS was a function of the total momentum transferred from the impact and the rate of momentum transfer. Their results suggested that rotational motion might be a prominent factor in causing unconsciousness, but that the overall AIS was primarily dependent upon translational motion.

Experimental Advances and Model Validation

More experimental data were still needed before brain injury could confidently be predicted, and experimental methods also needed to be improved. Nahum and Smith (1976) (40) made contributions to both areas. They performed experimental blunt impacts to the heads of human cadavers whose fluid pressures in the cerebrospinal fluid space and cerebral blood vessels had been raised to simulate realistic levels. Resultant accelerations were obtained from the signals of four head-mounted accelerometers and were used to calculate SI and HIC values. The time histories of the accelerations and impact forces were presented along with autopsy evaluations of the injuries produced. These experiments indicated that laboratory procedures could produce injuries similar to those seen in a clinical practice and that a rough correlation existed between currently used head injury criteria and the intracranial trauma observed.

In a continuation of their work, Nahum, Smith, and Ward (1977) (41) measured intracranial pressures arising from head motion during the impact and compared these to pressures predicted by the Ward model. Correlations were generally good, especially in the frontal region of the brain. Modifications to the damping factor and compressibility of the brain model were made to improve the correlations. Additional correlations of model predictions with live monkey tests at HSRI showed the same relationship as those for pressurized cadavers and thus indicated that the experimental procedures adequately simulated in *in vivo* state. This cooperative experimental/analytical research program was of benefit to both approaches.

Further contributions to experimental procedures were made by Stalnaker, Melvin, et al. (1977) (42). In a series of head impacts with human cadavers, head motion was measured using a new three-dimensional accelerometry technique that made the calculation of angular accelerations possible for the first time. These data were compared to brain motion observable using a new high-speed cineradiographic system. Brain vascular pressurization methods were also developed and used in some of the tests. Preliminary analysis of the data indicated that the brain was only partially coupled to the skull during impact, resulting in an effective head mass that varied with time during the impact. Pressurization was found to improve skull/brain coupling. In addition, the authors observed a degradation of brain stiffness as time after death increased.

Biomechanical data were also being used by those designing improved physical models. Foster, Kortge, and Wolanin (1977) (43) introduced the new General Motors Hybrid III Dummy, which had been under development since 1975. While retaining the repeatability of the Hybrid II, the Hybrid III provided biomechanical responses, including those of the head, consistent with responses found in published literature. Like "Repeatable Pete," however, biofidelity of this dummy was limited to the frontal impact direction.

In May 1978, a proposal was issued for an upgraded standard on child restraint systems, FMVSS 213. Dynamic tests were to be required for the first time using a "three-year-old" dummy to represent children between 20 and 50 lb in a 30-mph barrier crash. Lacking biomechanical data for child injury tolerance, NHTSA specified the same HIC threshold as that for "adult" dummies. Restraint systems for infants had only to meet certain head-area padding requirements, because the "infant" test dummies were not suitable for making acceleration measurements. The rule appeared a year and a half later with the injury criterion included as proposed.

In an attempt to determine the validity of the HIC threshold of 1000, Got, Patel, et al. (1978) (44) calculated the HIC for 42 free-fall impacts to the heads of human cadavers. Some were helmeted, some were not. Using their own method of measuring accelerations to calculate the resultant, the authors found that tolerance to head impact without fracture was much greater than the HIC would allow. They suggested that HIC 1500 was appropriate for both frontal and lateral impacts.

At the Twenty-Third Stapp Car Crash Conference, new head rotation experiments were reported, and further experimental validations of the Ward brain model were presented. Gennarelli, Abel, et al. (1979) (45) subjected monkeys to rotational head accelerations and found the threshold for frontal lobe contusion to be less than that for the temporal lobe. The authors attributed this finding to differences in mechanical input to the two regions rather than to differences in tissue properties.

Nahum, Smith, et al. (1979) (46) presented results of impacts to helmeted, human cadavers, finding that the protective device prevented high-magnitude, short-duration intracranial pressures for the first 8 ms. Positive posterior pressures, which seemed to be unique to helmeted-head impacts, developed after 8 ms and were not computed by the model.

Recognizing the fact that head impact tolerance of living humans would never be experimentally measured to the injurious level, Nusholtz, Melvin, and Alem (1979) (47) compared the head impact response of live and post-mortem monkeys and related the results to the earlier cadaver tests of Stalnaker, et al. (1977) (42). Differences in acceleration- and pressure-time histories were found between the live and unpressurized post-mortem states, the latter resulting in lower peaks and smoother waveforms. Comparisons with the human cadaver tests were complicated by differences in head size and head/neck muscle structure. The authors found, however, that by changing the data parameters from time to path arc length, the head response waveforms for monkeys and humans could be made more congruent.

The epidural pressures measured above were compared to predictions of the Ward model, adjusted for monkey head mass and geometry. The results, reported by Nusholtz, Axelrod, et al. (1979) (48), indicated significant differences between the live and post-mortem brain responses in terms of response time and magnitude, damping, compressibility, and coupling effects between the brain and cervical cord. The authors suggested that further tests and simulations of the impact response of pressurized post-mortem monkeys were needed.

In a paper presented at the Twenty-Fourth Stapp Car Crash Conference, Ward (1980) (49) indicated correlations between intracranial pressure magnitudes and brain injury severity. Based on specific levels of tolerable peak pressure, the paper compared various head injury criteria with the brain pressure tolerance (BPT) for different head acceleration pulses. For a triangular acceleration pulse of less than 5-ms duration, the BPT predicted lower tolerable peak acceleration levels than did either the WSTC or the HIC. The MSC was closer to the BPT in the 1- to 4-ms duration range. For triangular pulse durations from 5 to 10 ms, the BPT predicted higher tolerable accelerations than did either the WSTC or the MSC, while the HIC was in closer agreement.

Conclusions

Those who know the history and/or participated in the development of the Head Injury Criterion are the first to acknowledge its weaknesses: it was based on sparse experimental data, it is not actually a measure of injury, and it does not necessarily correspond to injuries produced under controlled laboratory conditions. Add to this the fact that the Part 572 Dummy, the test device used to produce the data with which the HIC is calculated, claims only to have repeatability and not biofidelity. Under certain impact conditions, the dummy head, because of its stiffness, produces higher accelerations than should be expected. The question then arises, just what is being measured?

It seems unlikely, however, that NHTSA will exchange the HIC for another index in the near future. Part of the reason for a reluctance to change may be that there is no other completely validated injury prediction tool available. Even though experimental techniques have been refined so that new and better measurements can be made, data analysis methods have been devised to deal with surrogate subjects, and mathematical models have been developed that incorporate the mechanical properties and responses measured in the laboratory, sufficient laboratory head impact research with human cadavers or with animals has not yet been done, and very little is currently being conducted.

Notwithstanding the advent of automatic restraint systems, the head will remain a critical area to deal with in any occupant protection system. Not only will there continue to be head impacts with various interior structures, but the effect of new systems on noncontact head accelerations must not be neglected. Proven laboratory techniques are currently available that can provide for significant progress toward meaningful understanding of human brain injury under impact conditions. In addition to techniques of subject preparation and parameter measurement, a variety of sophisticated methods of analysis have been created and tested. Research should be carried out during the next few years that would pursue a number of these techniques. Lateral impact studies and investigations into the relative influence of subject-to-subject parameter variability should also be conducted.

The question of the relative roles of pressure and shear strain seems answerable, at least for midplane impacts, and it is reasonable to believe that the variable relationship found between actual injury and HIC values can be explained to some extent. An evolutionary type of injury criteria for the head should then result, that can change as our knowledge and understanding change. The utility of the HIC as a reasonable tool for regulation would not be seriously threatened by such research, while the conditions for survival under impact loading of the head would be better understood.

References

1. Lissner, H.R.; Lebow, M.; Evans, F.G. Experimental studies on the relation between acceleration and intracranial pressure changes in man. *Surgery, Gynecology, and Obstetrics* 111:329–338.
2. Society of Automotive Engineers. *Human tolerance to impact conditions as related to motor vehicle design.* New York: SAE Handbook Supplement J885 APR 80.
3. Gadd, C.W. Criteria for injury potential. In *Impact Acceleration Stress Symposium, 27–29 November 1961, Brooks AFB, Texas,* pp. 141–144. Washington, D.C.: National Academy of Sciences—National Research Council publication no. 977, 1962.
4. Eiband, A.M. *Human tolerance to rapidly applied accelerations: A summary of the literature.* Cleveland: NASA Lewis Research Center. NASA Memorandum 5-19-59E.
5. Patrick, L.M.; Lissner, H.R.; Gurdjian, E.S. Survival by design-head protection. In *7th Stapp Car Crash Conference Proceedings, 11–13 November 1963, Los Angeles,* pp. 483–499. Springfield, Ill.: Charles C. Thomas, 1965.
6. Gadd, C.W. Use of a weighted impulse criterion for estimating injury hazard. In *10th Stapp Car Crash Conference Proceedings, 8–9 November 1966, Alamogordo, N.M.,* pp. 164–174. New York: SAE paper no. 660793, 1967.
7. Society of Automotive Engineers. Instrument panel laboratory impact test procedures. In *SAE Handbook 1966,* pp. 862–865. New York: SAE J921.
8. Holburn, A.H.S. Mechanics of head injuries. *Lancet,* 245:438–441, 1943.
9. Gurdjian, E.S.; Webster, J.E.; Lissner, H.R. Observations on the mechanism of brain concussion, contusion and laceration. *Surgery, Gynecology, and Obstetrics* 101:680–690.
10. Gurdjian, E.S.; Roberts, V.L.; Thomas, L.M. Tolerance curves of acceleration and intracranial pressure protective index in experimental head injury. *Journal of Trauma* 6(5):600–604.
11. Ommaya, A.K.; Hirsch, A.E.; Martinez, J.L. The role of whiplash in cerebral concussion. In *10th Stapp Car Crash Conference Proceedings, 8–9 November 1966, Alamogordo, N.M.,* pp. 314–324. New York: SAE paper no. 660804.
12. Gurdjian, E.S.; Hodgson, V.R.; Thomas, L.M.; Patrick, L.M. Significance of relative movements of scalp, skull, and intracranial contents during impact injury of the head. *Journal of Neurosurgery* 29(1):70–72.
13. Hodgson, V.R.; Patrick, L.M. Dynamic response of the human cadaver head compared to a simple mathematical model. In *12th Stapp Car Crash Conference Proceedings, 22–23 October 1968, Detroit,* pp. 280–301. New York: SAE paper no. 680784.
14. Fallenstein, G.T.; Hulce, V.D.; Melvin, J.W. Dynamic mechanical properties of human brain tissue. *Journal of Biomechanics* 2(3):217–226.
15. Stalnaker, R.L.; Fogle, J.L.; McElhaney, J.H. *Driving joint impedance characteristics of the head.* American Society of Mechanical Engineers Biochemical and Human Factors Conference, 31 May–3 June 1970, Washington, D.C. New York: ASME paper no. 70-BHF-14.
16. Metz, H.; McElhaney, J.H.; Ommaya, A.K. A comparison of the elasticity of live, dead, and fixed brain tissue. *Journal of Biomechanics* 3(4):453–458.
17. McElhaney, J.H.; Fogle, J.L.; Melvin, J.W.; Haynes, R.R.; Roberts, V.L.; Alem, N.M. Mechanical properties of cranial bone. *Journal of Biomechanics* 3(5):495–511.

18. Society of Automotive Engineers. Anthropomorphic test device for dynamic test. *SAE Handbook 1969),* pp. 977-980. New York: SAE J963.

19. U.S. National Transportation Safety Board. *Safety effectiveness evaluation of the National Highway Traffic Safety Administration's rulemaking process. Vol. 11: Case history of Federal Motor Vehicle Safety Standard 208: Occupant crash protection.* Washington, D.C. NTSB-SEE-79-5.

20. McElhaney, J.H.; Stalnaker, R.L.; Roberts, V.L.; Snyder, R.G. Door crashworthiness criteria. In *15th Stapp Car Crash Conference Proceedings, 17-19 November 1971, Coronado, Calif.,* pp. 489-517. New York: SAE paper no. 710864.

21. Hirsch, A.E.; Ommaya, A.K. Protection from brain injury: The relative significance of translational and rotational motions of the head after impact. In *14th Stapp Car Crash Conference Proceedings, 17-18 November 1970, Ann Arbor, Mich.,* pp. 299-328. New York: SAE paper no. 700899.

22. Slattenschek, A.; Tauffkirchen, W. Critical evaluation of assessment methods for head impact applied in appraisal of brain injury hazard, in particular in head impact on windshields. In *1970 International Automobile Safety Conference Compendium, 13-15 May 1970, Detroit; 8-11 June 1970, Brussels,* pp. 1084-1112. New York: SAE paper no. 700426.

23. Brinn, J.; Staffeld, S.E. Evaluation of impact test accelerations: A damage index for the head and torso. In *14th Stapp Car Crash Conference Proceedings, 17-18 November 1970, Ann Arbor, Mich.,* pp. 188-220. New York: SAE paper no. 700902.

24. Stalnaker, R.L.; McElhaney, J.H. *Head injury tolerance for linear impacts by mechanical impedance methods.* American Society of Mechanical Engineers Winter Annual Meeting, 29 November-3 December 1970, New York. New York: ASME paper no. 70-WA/BHF-4.

25. Society of Automotive Engineers. Human tolerance to impact conditions as related to motor vehicle design. *SAE Handbook 1968,* pp. 911-913. New York: SAE J885a.

26. Unterharnscheidt, F.J. Translational versus rotational acceleration: Animal experiments with measured input. In *15th Stapp Car Crash Conference Proceedings, 17-19 November 1971, Coronado, Calif.,* pp. 767-770. New York: SAE paper no. 710880.

27. Gennarelli, T.A.; Ommaya, A.K.; Thibault, L.E. Comparison of translational and rotational head motions in experimental cerebral concussion. In *15th Stapp Car Crash Conference Proceedings, 17-19 November 1971, Coronado, Calif.,* pp. 797-803. New York: Society of Automotive Engineers.

28. Gadd, C.W. Tolerable severity index in whole-head nonmechanical impact. In *15th Stapp Car Crash Conference Proceedings, 17-19 November 1971, Coronado, Calif.,* pp. 809-816. New York: Society of Automotive Engineers.

29. Fan, W.R.S. Internal head injury assessment. In *15th Stapp Car Crash Conference Proceedings, 17-19 November 1971, Coronado, Calif.,* pp. 645-665. New York: SAE paper no. 710870.

30. Versace, J. A review of the severity index. In *15th Stapp Car Crash Conference Proceedings, 17-19 November 1971, Coronado, Calif.,* pp. 771-796. New York: SAE paper no. 710881.

31. McElhaney, J.H.; Stalnaker, R.L.; Roberts, V.L. Biomechanical aspects of head injury. In *Human Impact Response—Measurement and Simulation. Proceedings of the Symposium on Human Impact Response, 2-3 October 1972, Warren, Mich.,* pp. 85-110. New York: Plenum Press, 1973.

32. McElhaney, J.H.; Mate, P.I.; Roberts, V.L. A new crash test device—"Repeatable Pete." In *17th Stapp Car Crash Conference Proceedings, 12-13 November 1973, Oklahoma City,* pp. 467-507. New York: SAE paper no. 730983.

33. Stalnaker, R.L.; Roberts, V.L.; McElhaney, J.H. Side impact tolerance to blunt trauma. In *17th Stapp Car Crash Conference Proceedings, 12-13 November 1973, Oklahoma City,* pp. 377-408. New York: SAE paper no. 730979.

34. Robbins, D.H. *Impact head injury data base.* Ann Arbor: The University of Michigan Highway Safety Research Institute for the National Institute for Occupational Safety and Health.

35. Chan, H.S. Mathematical model for closed head impact. In *18th Stapp Car Crash Conference Proceedings, 4-5 December 1974, Dearborn, Mich.,* pp. 557-578. Warrendale, Pa.: SAE paper no. 741191.

36. Khalil, T.B.; Hubbard, R.P. Parametric study of head response by finite element modeling. *Journal of Biomechanics* 10(2): 119-131.

37. Shugar, T.A. Transient structural response of the linear skull-brain system. In *19th Stapp Car Crash Conference Proceedings, 17-19 November 1975, San Diego, Calif.,* pp. 581-614. Warrendale, Pa.: SAE paper no. 751161.

38. Ward, C.C.; Thompson, R.B. The development of a detailed finite element brain model. In *19th Stapp Car Crash Conference Proceedings, 17-19 November 1975, San Diego,* pp. 641-674. Warrendale, Pa.: SAE paper no. 751163.

39. Mucciardi, A.N.; Sanders, J.D.; Eppinger, R.H. Prediction of brain injury measures from head motion parameters. In *21st Stapp Car Crash Conference Proceedings, 19–21 October 1977, New Orleans,* pp. 369–415. Warrendale, Pa.: SAE paper no. 770923.

40. Nahum, A.M.; Smith, R.W. An experimental model for closed head impact injury. In *20th Stapp Car Crash Conference Proceedings, 18–20 October 1976, Dearborn, Mich.,* pp. 783–814. Warrendale, Pa.: SAE paper no. 760825.

41. Nahum, A.M.; Smith, R.; Ward, C.C. Intracranial pressure dynamics during head impact. In *21st Stapp Car Crash Conference Proceedings, 19–21 October 1977, New Orleans,* pp. 339–366. Warrendale, Pa.: SAE paper no. 770922.

42. Stalnaker, R.L.; Melvin, J.W.; Nusholtz, G.S.; Alem, N.M.; Benson, J.B. Head impact response. In *21st Stapp Car Crash Conference Proceedings, 19–21 October 1977, New Orleans,* pp. 303–335. Warrendale, Pa.: SAE paper no. 770921.

43. Foster, J.K.; Kortge, J.O.; Wolanin, M.J. Hybrid III—A biomechanically-based crash test dummy. In *21st Stapp Car Crash Conference Proceedings, 19–21 October 1977, New Orleans,* pp. 975–1014. Warrendale, Pa.: SAE paper no. 770938.

44. Got, C.; Patel, A.; Fayon, A.; Tarriere, C.; Walfisch, G. Results of experimental head impacts on cadavers: The various data obtained and their relations to some measured physical parameters. In *22nd Stapp Car Crash Conference Proceedings, 24–26 October 1978, Ann Arbor, Mich.,* pp. 57–99. Warrendale, Pa.: SAE paper no. 780887.

45. Gennarelli, T.A.; Abel, J.M.; Adams, H.; Graham, D. Differential tolerance of frontal and temporal lobes to contusion induced by angular acceleration. In *23rd Stapp Car Crash Conference, 17–19 October 1979, San Diego,* pp. 563–586. Warrendale, Pa.: SAE paper no. 791022.

46. Nahum, A.M.; Smith, R.; Raasch, F.; Ward, C.C. Intracranial pressure relationships in the protected and unprotected head. In *23rd Stapp Car Crash Conference Proceedings, 17–19 October 1979, San Diego, Calif.,* pp. 615–636. Warrendale, Pa.: SAE paper no. 791024.

47. Nusholtz, G.S.; Melvin, J.W.; Alem, N.M. Head impact response comparisons of human surrogates. In *23rd Stapp Car Crash Conference Proceedings, 17–19 October 1979, San Diego, Calif.,* pp. 499–541. Warrendale, Pa.: SAE paper no. 791020.

48. Nusholtz, G.W.; Axelrod, J.B.; Melvin, J.W.; Ward, C.C. Comparison of epidural pressure in live anesthetized and postmortem primates. In *7th International Workshop on Human Subjects for Biomechanical Research Proceedings, 16 October 1979, Coronado, Calif.,* pp. 175–200. Washington, D.C.: Distributed by National Highway Traffic Safety Administration.

49. Ward, C.C.; Chan, M.; Nahum, A.M. Intracranial pressure—A brain injury criterion. In *24th Stapp Car Crash Conference Proceedings, 15–17 October 1980, Troy, Mich.,* pp. 161–186. Warrendale, Pa.: SAE paper no. 801304.

On the Analytical Approach to Head Injury Criteria

Christer Ljung
Sten Lindgren
Bertil Aldman

Abstract

Biomechanical research leading to head injury criteria is discussed. Special interest is given to the so-called analytical approach, which is founded on a good understanding of the basic physical injury-producing processes. It is maintained that this approach can be divided in four steps:

—A study of the well-defined pathophysiological and mechanical disturbances that can be produced under mechanical loading in a tissue with a distinct physiological function.

—A study, using various modeling techniques, of how intracranial deformations occur in reponse to sudden motions of the head.

—An interpretation of the results of the first step in the light of the second one yielding the kinematic parameter levels at which a certain injury is produced in a certain tissue.

—A process, where by consensus, different results from the third step are compiled to yield a detailed head injury criterion.

Introduction

A head injury criterion provides the link between the mechanical input to the head and the short- and long-term clinical outcome of the event. So far, it has been considered satisfactory to use a binary description of the outcome: injury above or below a certain level. However, as our knowledge of the various physical phenomena involved increases, our demands for more detailed information expand. It is obviously true that under certain circumstances, for instance involving calculated risks, we would be likely to accept a higher score on an injury scale than we would normally consider allowable. A possibility to judge safety margins is also needed. It might happen that a small increase in mechanical input to the head causes a drastic increase in injury severity. So, it seems that the tool we would really like to possess is the mapping of the space of mechanical events upon a continuous injury scale, and it is this mapping that would be called a head injury criterion.

Mucciardi et al. (1) have described an adaptive learning network which can provide the link between input and outcome on a solely empirical basis, that is, no knowledge of the physical processes which transform the kinematics of the head to a brain tissue injury is presupposed. The obvious disadvantage of the method is the problem to select representative experiments and representative parameters from the experiments. It is an empirical method, so that it is (normally) not possible to use the provided model for predictions outside the range of its generating experiments. The strength of the method, though, is clear since it provides the experimentalist with an organized insight in the outcome of experiments involving great numbers of parameters.

The analytical approach on the other hand is described by Mucciardi et al. as follows: "An analytical model is one obtained by 'reasoning from first principles'. That is, the investigator attempts to interrelate all pertinent physical laws thought to influence injury." Also, in this case, it is easy to pinpoint the disadvantages of the approach. It is difficult to establish which physical processes are pertinent to the problem and which are not. The choice of approximations made is usually only conjectural, and we certainly have to approximate. If, however, the reasoning behind the analytical model is correct, it should be possible to extrapolate results from the model beyond the range of experiments performed.

I think it must be clear that both of the above described approaches have to be used in order to finally reach the desired goal: a head injury criterion. The object of this paper is to describe the different steps into which the second approach, the analytical one, could be divided.

Step 1—Tissue Sensitivity

Consider a cell, a group of cells or a tissue with a distinct physiological function. In the simplest case of an essentially one-dimensional object, for instance a blood vessel or an axon, the stress-strain relationship in tension (possibly also compression) is obtained experimentally. Simultaneously, the physiological function is monitored for degradation or complete breakdown. The kind of result obtained is depicted in Figure 1.

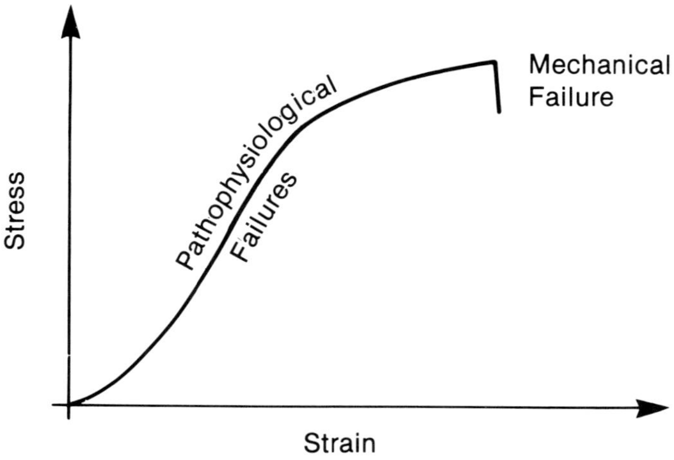

Figure 1. The Stress-Strain Relation for a One-Dimensional Tissue Also the Zone of Onset of Pathophsiological Failure Due to Mechanical Loading.

If the considered object does not fall into the one-dimensional category, the same kind of picture has to be obtained for other kinds of loading as well. Anisotropy would also have to be considered in such cases, and, to complicate things further, it is very likely that any biological material studied exhibits a strain rate sensitivity. Such a rate-dependence is, however, seldom of an extremely drastic nature when it comes to mechanical parameters such as ultimate strength, elastic modulus, etc. (Cf. for instance McElhaney and Byars (2) and Lowenhielm (3), which means that it would normally be adequate to obtain a few stress-strain relationships at different strain rates in the region of interest.)

Step 2—Models for Intracranial Deformations

In an injury causing event the head is acted upon by an outer load. It might be impact forces acting directly on the head or loads transferred from the torso via the neck. It seems that one way of accurately describing this outer action is by giving a complete kinematic description of the head motion as a whole during impact and stating all locally acting forces. The effects of location, direction and time history of those forces are omitted from the rest of the discussion since they, mechanically and clinically, pose a rather special problem. Its solution could, however, be accomplished along very much the same lines as those discussed.

The kinematic description is most conveniently given in the form of three linear and three angular acceleration time histories in a three-dimensional body fixed-coordinate system. Through a combination of modeling methods (finite elements, direct mathematical analysis, physical models, direct measurements, etc.) we obtain a picture of how the gross tissue motions inside the skull occur and from these we calculate how the strains are distributed. The idea in this step is that although the brain is nonhomogeneous in nature, it is often possible to use a fairly rough, bulk treatment of the different material involved and still get an adequate description of gross motion in any region of interest in the brain. Examples of such models are the ones proposed by Ward (4), Ljung (5), Hodgson and Gurdjian (6), and Pudenz and Shelden (7). The list of examples could be made much longer. The papers referenced here have been selected since they show the variety of methods that can be used.

Step 3—Interpretation of Results

It is now time to put the results from the first two steps together. That is, the strains calculated in step 2 are used together with the stress-strain relationship of step 1. So, for each of the six accelerations in the kinematic description, we can get a picture like Figure 2 for any cell, group of cells or tissue.

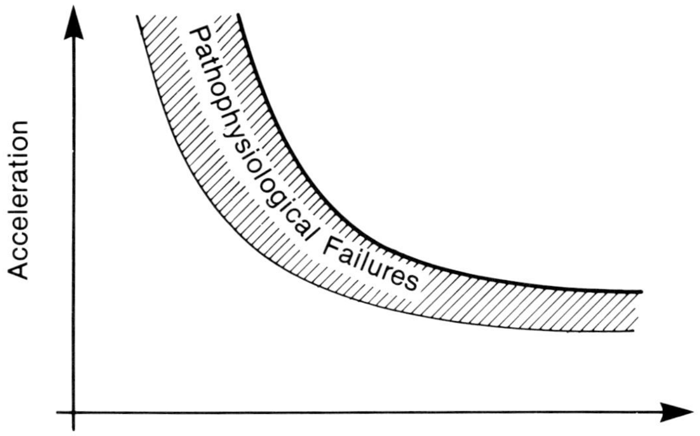

Figure 2. Pathophysiological and Mechanical Failures in a Tissue as a Function of Kinematic Parameters Related to One Mode of Head Motion.

Notice that when a diagram like Figure 2 is produced, several stress-strain relationships from step 1 might have to be used. Different kinds of strain occur and give, in a specific tissue, rise to pathophysiological failures of different kinds and locations. This means that depending on situation along the bold line of the diagram, different types of mechanical failure can occur. In a similar way, the shaded area may be subdivided into different kinds of pathophysiological failures. If, for instance, a nerve cell is under study, one might imagine areas representing transmission degradation and other areas representing synaptic malfunction.

Step 4—Head Injury Criteria

When a sufficient (from a clinical point of view) number of injury producing processes have been studied during steps 1 and 2, we proceed by isolating one of the six head response accelerations at a time and collect for that mode of motion information on the kinds of injury that can occur according to the previous work. This is diagrammatically represented in Figure 3, where results pertaining to three different kinds of tissue are superimposed.

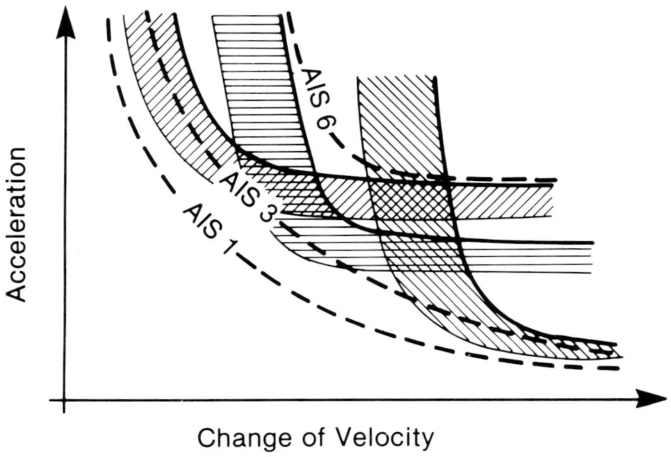

Figure 3. Combinatin of the Results Obtained in Step 3.

Since the shaded areas are subdivided into different kinds and degrees of injury it should be possible to construct tolerance thresholds in this mode of motion (and subsequently in the others) and label these thresholds by scores on an injury scale. The six resulting diagrams, one for each mode of motion, constitute the detailed head injury criterion needed (Figure 4).

Remarks and Conclusions

The above discussed four-step procedure is not necessarily to be performed in that order. From a practical point of view, it seems more feasible to study one particular injury at a time. An example of this is presented in a paper by Lowenhielm (8) concerning the so-called gliding contusions. In such a case, the step 3 results have to be compiled from the efforts of several research teams. Finally, the injury criteria are

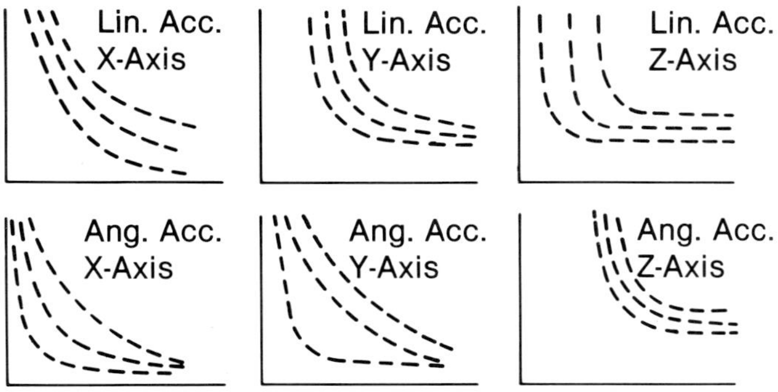

Figure 4. A Detailed Head Injury Criteron.

established by consensus. The only reason for isolating step 4 from step 3 is that it will probably be accomplished by someone else.

The outline given above is very much centered around the stress-strain curve of step 1. Intracranial pressure patterns have, for one thing, not been mentioned. This has been done to increase the clarity of the account and is not to say that pressure or pressure gradient cannot be correlated to injury. Displacements produced by steady acceleration pressure patterns inside the skull are negligibly small and noninjurious. The possibly injurious events such as cavitation and cavitation bubble implosion may secondarily cause large but very local strains. These local strains are, however, an impractical measure of the mechanical state of the system, and, consequently, the strain-oriented notation should be changed into a pressure-oriented one. It is, in this context, interesting to note the results by Hamberger and Rinder (9) on the succinoxidase activity of isolated neurons subjected to pressure pulses.

A problem which has also been omitted, again for reasons of clarity, is that of repeated trauma. This problem is perhaps most relevant to boxing injuries, but may have implications in other situations as well. In the literature has been described summation of damage at so-called experimental brain concussion (Rinder et al. (10)) and also adaption at repeated severe traumata (Unterharnscheidt (11)). This is a complication which should be borne in mind when injury criteria are proposed for use in situations involving repeated head trauma.

The phrasing "**the** analytical approach" has been used in the title of the paper. This simply reflects the belief that there is no other way to make ends meet using analytical tools. The possibility of constructing a complete mathematical model of head injury, complete in the sense that all kinds of injury and motion are incorporated at once, seems certainly to be a too overwhelming task.

In Figures 2 and 3, the kinematic description has been parametrized in terms of acceleration and change of velocity. Parametrization is certainly essential for reasons of clarity, but the actual choice of parameters could be a matter of taste. Nothing much would be lost, or for that matter gained, by using duration (as in the Wayne State Curve) instead of change of velocity. More essential then, is a uniform agreement on what parameters to use, and, above all, how they are explicitly defined in order to avoid confusion and misinterpretations. It could be argued that a two-parameter description of an acceleration time history is too simplified. It can, however, be shown to be adequate for prediction of mechanical failures in elastic systems, and there is much reason to believe that a two-parameter description is suitable compromise even in systems such as those studied here.

If one looks at what has been done so far along these lines, it is immediately clear that most of the effort has been put into development of the kind of models used in step 2. This is, of course, very natural since they provide us with a deeper understanding of what physical processes are at play and how and to what extent they take part in producing injury. The big vacuum of knowledge is associated with step 1, especially as regards the so-called pathophysiological failures. In consequence, this is a field where efforts ought to be concentrated in the future. Today, we could probably only produce a head injury criterion with respect to the resultants of the three linear and three angular acceleration of the head. There is much clinical evidence to show that impact location and direction influence the outcome of an accident. This is a problem related to model refinement during step 2, which means that better three-dimensional models shall have to be procured.

References

1. Mucciardi, A.N., Sanders, J.D. and Eppinger, R.H. "Prediction of brain injury measures from head motion parameters." Proc. 21st Stapp Car Crash Conf., New Orleans, 1977.
2. McElhaney, J.H. and Byars, E.F. "Dynamic response of biological materials." Paper 65-WA/HUF-9, ASME Winter Ann. Meet., Chicago, 1965.
3. Lowenhielm, C.G.P. "Dynamic properties of the parasagittal bridging veins." *Z. Rechtsmedizin* 74, 55–62, 1974.
4. Ward, C.C. "Analytical brain models for head impact." Proc. IIId. IRCOBI Int. Conf. Impact Trauma, Berlin, 1977.
5. Ljung, C. "A model for brain deformation due to rotation of the skull." *J. Biomechanics* 8, 263–274, 1975.
6. Hodgson, V.R. and Gurdjian, E.S. "Experimental skull deformation and brain displacement demonstrated by flash X-ray technique." *J. Neurosurg,* 549–552, 1966.

7. Pudenz, H. and Shelden, H.C. "The lucite calvarium—a method for direct observation of the brain—II. Cranial trauma and brain movement." *J. Neurosurg,* 487–505, 1946.

8. Lowenhielm, C.G.P. "Mathematical simulation of gliding contusions." *J. Biomechanics* 8, 351–356, 1975.

9. Hamberger, A. and Rinder, L. "Experimental brain concussion: The early effects of sudden increase in intracranial pressure on the succinoxidase activity of isolated neurons and glial cells from the lateral vestibular nucleus of the rabbit." *J. Neuropath, Experim. Neurol.,* Vol. XXV, No. 1, 68–75, 1966.

10. Rinder, L., Olsson, Y., Lindgren, S. and Stalhammar, D. "Comparison of effects from single and repeated trauma to the animal brain." *Scand. J. Rehab. Med.* 4:97–99, 1972.

11. Unterharnscheidt, F. "Die gedeckten Schaden des Gehirns. Experimentelle Untersuchungen mit einmaliger, wiederholter und gehaufter stumpfer Gewalteinwirkung auf den Schadel." *Monographien aus dem Gesamtgebiet d. Neurologie u. Psychiatrie,* Heft 103, 1963.

Head Injury Criterion (HIC)

Claude Tarriere

Relationship Between HIC and AIS

Analysis of the synthesis by Newman (1)

A consideration of Newman's data (Figure 1) and the sources of these data (Figure 2) reveal extremely variegated origins. It is not surprising that there is no particular relationship between HIC and cerebral AIS on the basis of such a gathering of data. We must separate the human tolerance data where HIC is a human tolerance level and the dummy data where HIC is a protection criterion for a dummy.

From Newman's paper, if one considers only the human head tolerance by eliminating the dummy results, the mathematical model results, the facial impacts of cadavers, and the single cadaver test because of its very weak and fragile skull bone, there remains cadaver head impact (Figure 3).

If one uses the AIS=3 as the cerebral injury limit (50% of subjects having an AIS<3 and 50% of subjects having an AIS≧3), it appears that the limit is very close to HIC=1500.

Among the two worse cases here available, one cadaver (HIC 1500, AIS=4) wore a helmet and fell from a 2-m height onto a rigid hemisphere with a 10 cm diameter: such test conditions are very seldom observed in actual head impacts and can be considered as the most severe testing condition: The other case (HIC #600 and AIS=3) is outside of our own sample, and more details are needed (skull characteristics, etc.).

Of course, even if there is no correlation between the HIC and the AIS, it is possible to use the HIC as a human head tolerance criterion, because, below an HIC value very close to 1500, the probability of finding a severe brain injury is lower than 50%.

Again from Newman's paper, if we separate the side impacts from the frontal ones, we obtain (Figure 4) the distribution of HIC versus AIS in side impacts (including impacts against the rigid hemisphere) and, on Figure 5, the HIC versus AIS in frontal impacts.

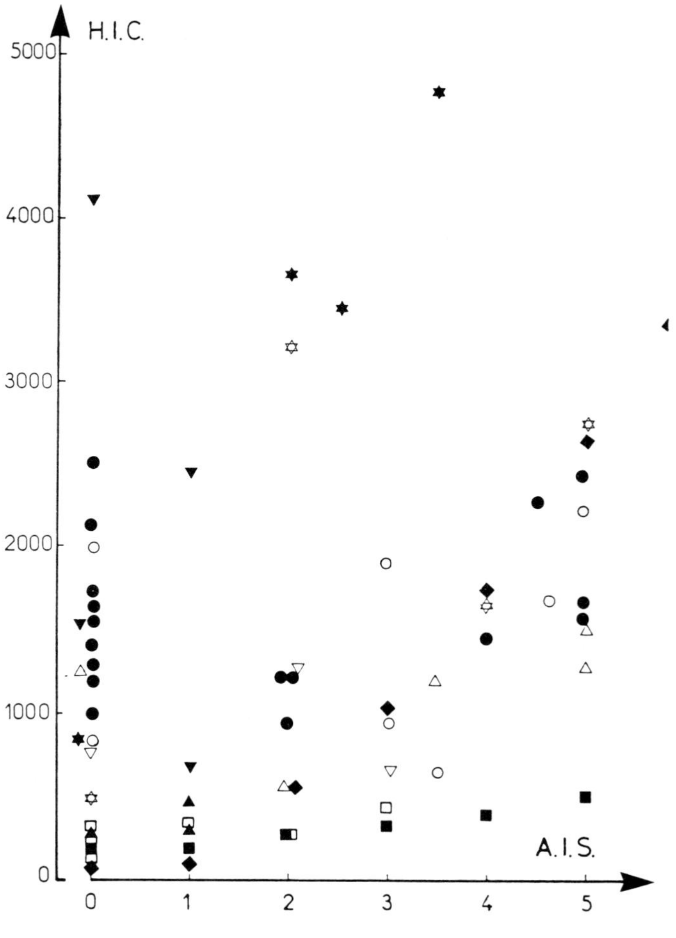

Figure 1. H.I.C. Versus A.I.S. - Reference: Newman 24th Stapp.

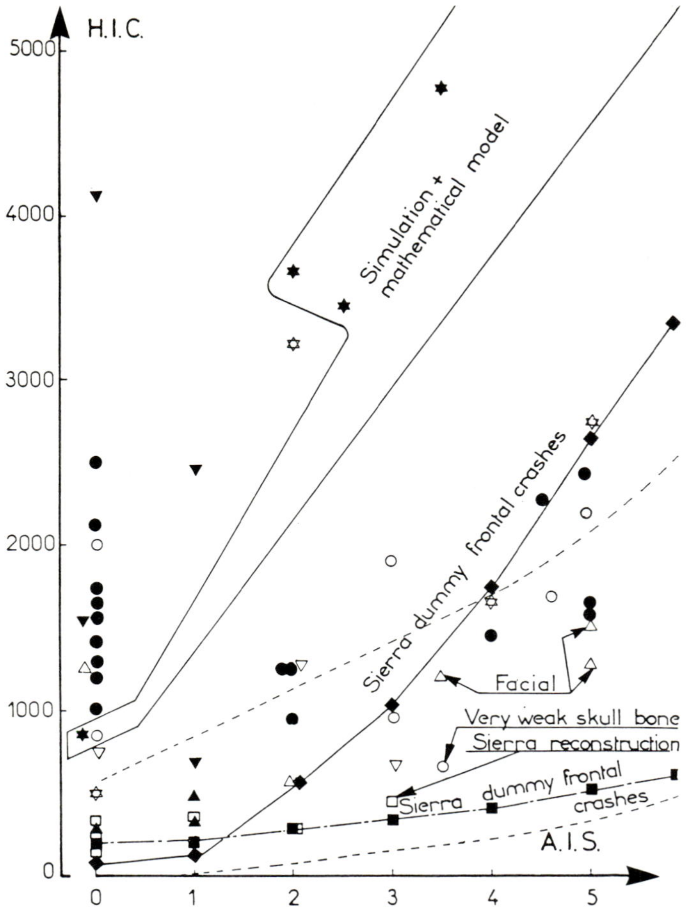

Figure 2. H.I.C. Versus A.I.S. - Reference: Newman 24th Stapp.

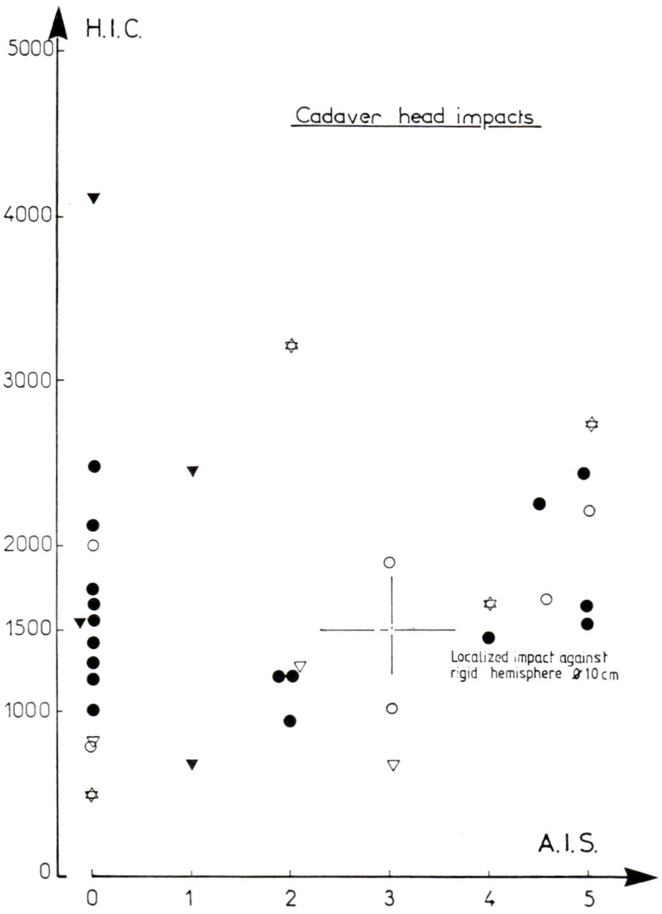

Figure 3. H.I.C. Versus A.I.S. - Reference: Newman 24th Stapp.

New Results

During the past year, we performed new frontal and side cadaver head impacts. In Figure 6, one can see Newman's references and nine new results concerning side impacts. The new results are represented by black triangles. It appears that the new results confirm the previous conclusion on HIC=1500 value. Likewise, in frontal impacts, we obtained 12 new results which also corroborate the previous conclusion on HIC=1500 (Figure 7). All the data are assembled in Figure 8. One can see, on the basis of 53 cadaver head impact results, the application of 50% of AIS<3; 50% AIS≧3 leads to a tolerance level >1500. That means that, even though the HIC is not perfect for many reasons, it is possible to use it as a tolerance criterion.

On the basis of the relationship between HIC and AIS described above, the level is conservative because, generally speaking, the cadaver tolerance is an underestimation of the tolerance of the population at risk.

Without head impact

In frontal collisions, with cadavers retained by a 3-point seat belt, we never found cervical or cerebral injury, although the HIC reached a high level (1000≦HIC≦2000).

In lateral collisions, we twice observed a large magnitude flexion of the head, associated with cerebral injuries (class AIS≧4). The corresponding HIC value was about 100 for Citroen LN case.

These two results confirm the accidentological data. The conclusion is that—without head impact—HIC is not a significant parameter to predict brain injury.

Dummy's Head Protection Criteria

It is possible to establish a relationship between cadaver HIC and dummy HIC when both are tested under the same test conditions; such is the case for the results presented in Figure 9 (head impacts of cadavers and dummies wearing helmets).

Generally speaking, with regard to dummy problems, biofidelity must be sufficient in the case of the considered impacts. With such a dummy, it will be possible to measure an injury criterion close to the tolerance level.

Concerning the HIC, for a belted occupant in a frontal collision, it is important to separate the values obtained during the head impact alone from the value

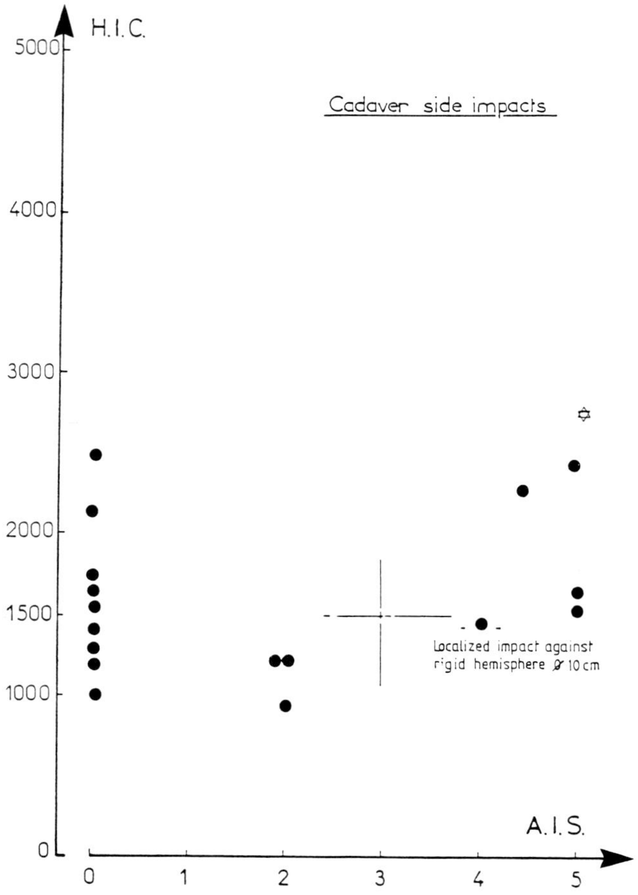

Figure 4. H.I.C. Versus A.I.S. - Reference: Newman 24th Stapp.

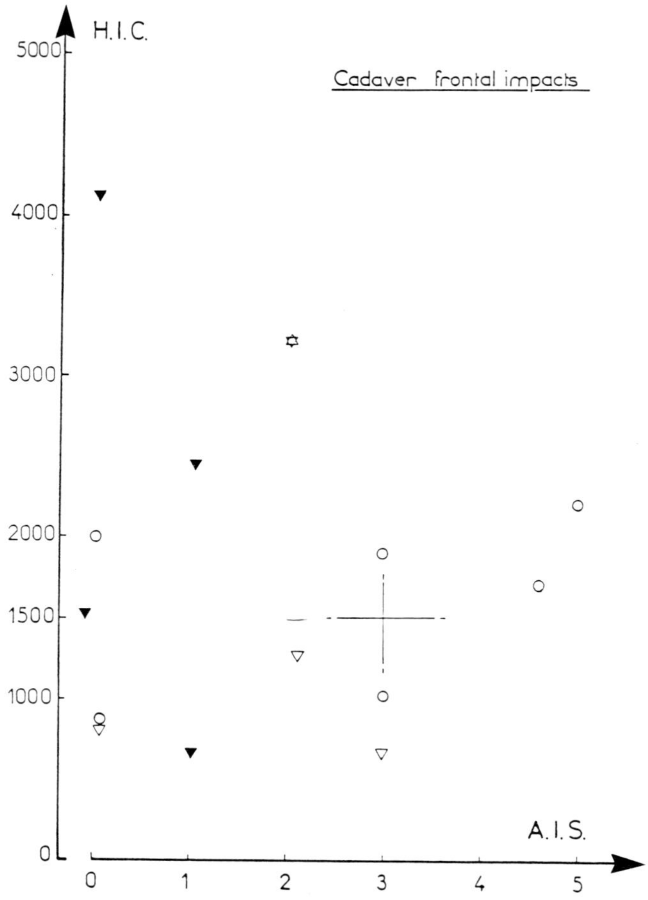

Figure 5. H.I.C. Versus A.I.S. - Reference: Newman 24th Stapp.

obtained from the complete head motion for the two following reasons:

1. With cadavers, and in real-world accidents, without head impact, we never found a cervical or cerebral injury, although the HIC value was at a high level.
2. In a dummy test, the only head rotation case led to a HIC close to 800 or 1000. In order to rate more accurately the impact, one has to select the period during which head contact occurs.

Important Remarks

One could note previously that it was justified to compute the HIC within the head impact time interval. A complementary remark has to be made.

The acceleration recorded on the skull C.G. of a dummy restrained by a seat belt is defined by the forces acting on the head. These forces are due to the impacts and to the neck. When a slight impact occurs while the restraint is effective, the HIC is very high, even if it is calculated during the only impact duration. If the same impact, which is supposed nonhazardous, is associated with a poor restraint, the HIC is noticeably lower.

Therefore, the HIC value is not more linked to the likelihood of injuries, as long as an infinite number of neck forces—head impact forces, give the same HIC value. Furthermore, it prevents using effective restraints when low HIC values are planned.

Theoretically, it seems possible to take into account the forces applied to the base of the skull, if convenient measurements are provided. The head impact forces could then be calculated, and two separate conditions might be established. The first condition would limit the severity of the head impact, and the second condition would be related to the neck forces. Such a study appears possible, but it requires time and further research.

Reference

1. Newman, James A., "Head Injury Criteria in Automotive Crash Testing," in Proceedings of the 24th Stapp Car Crash Conference, October 1980. (SAE Paper 801.317)

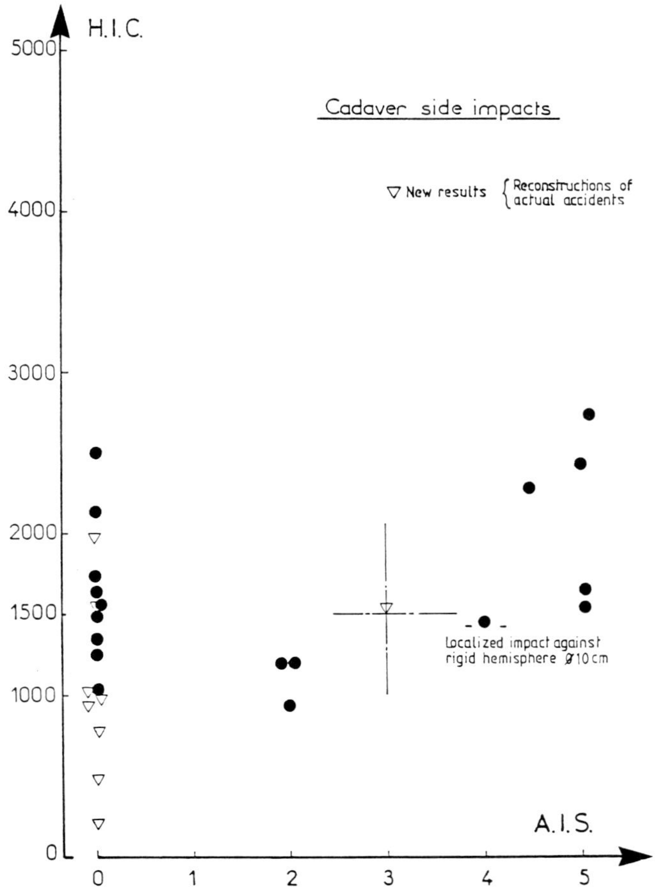

Figure 6. H.I.C. Versus A.I.S. - Newman + Reconstructions:

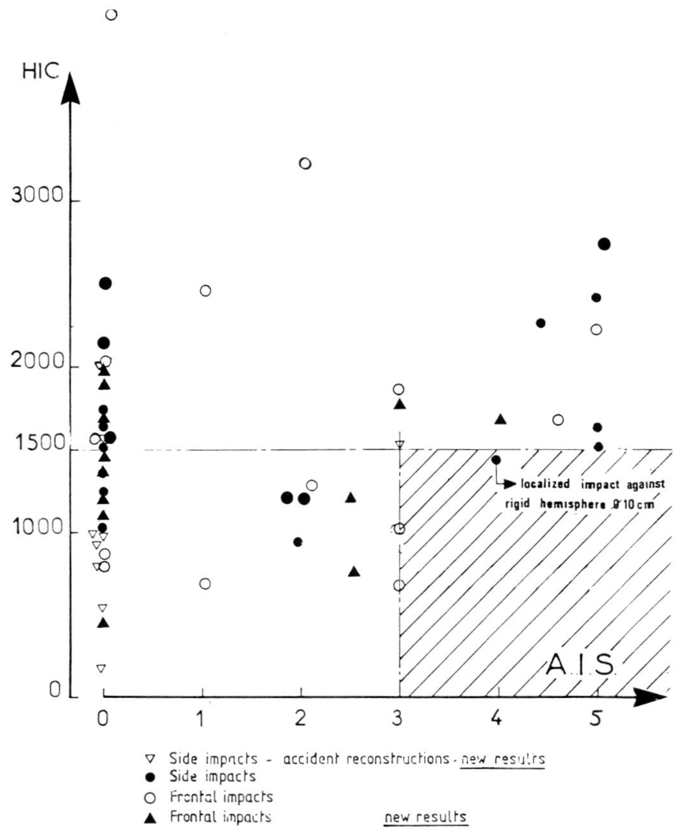

Figure 8. Human Head Impact Tolerance Synthesis

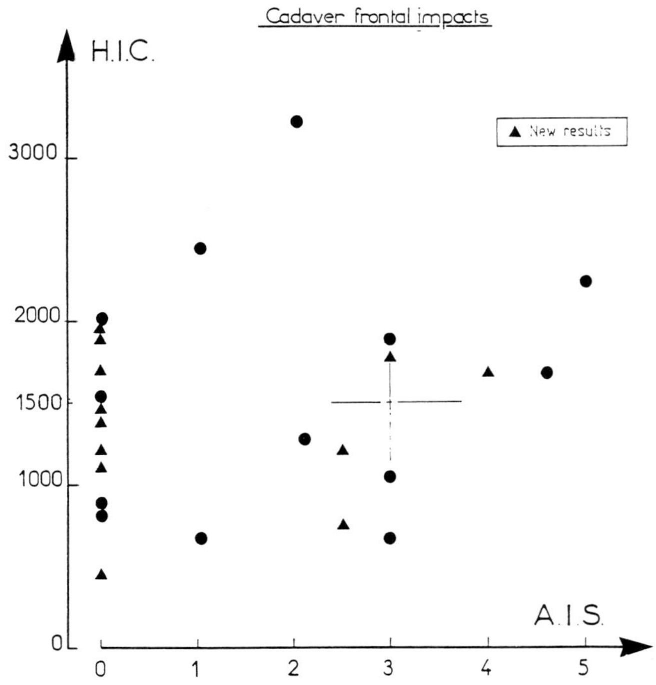

Figure 7. H.I.C. Versus A.I.S. - Newman + New Results

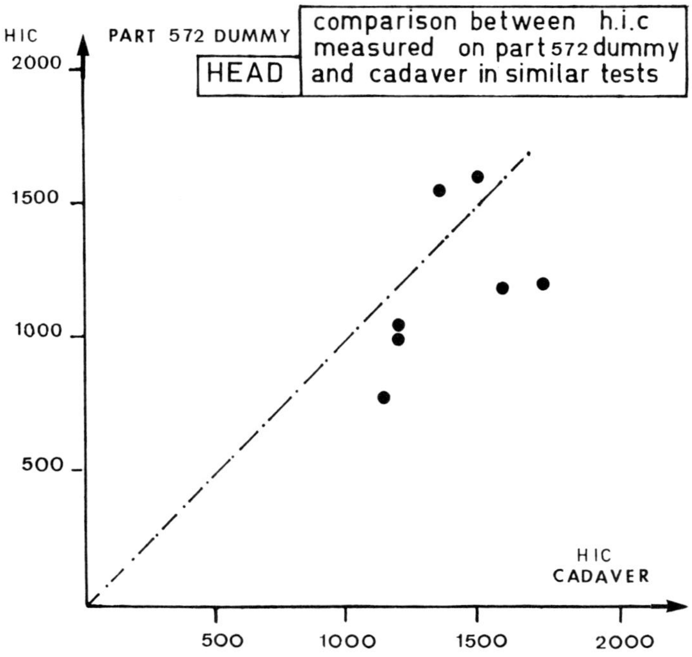

Figure 9.

Review of Neck Injury Criteria

Dr. Albert Burstein

The whole problem of neck injury criteria, as you recognize from the speakers today, is an extremely difficult one simply because, for one thing, we're talking about: A) a wide variety of injuries; B) a wide variety of structures; and C) a wide variety of loading conditions. In order to make some sense of it, at least in my own mind, I have tried to divide the problem and simply come to some conclusions as to what a logical approach might be to the problem of describing neck injury criteria.

The first thing that I wanted to organize is a description of what the problem is. As we have seen, it is much different than the problem of head injury. We are dealing with a multi-segment structure in terms of its bony configuration. We would have to consider at least nine elements, including the skull and T–1, and these elements have variable geometry. Now, the fact that it has variable geometry makes it much different than head injury criteria and head injury testing because, as we will see later on, we are going to have to include a geometric vector in our description of an injury criteria.

Also recognize that unlike the head, where you can preserve the essential properties for some time after death and even reconstruct the essential properties in the model, it is virtually impossible to reconstruct some of the essential properties, or save some of the essential properties in the cadaver. Those properties, of course, are of the muscles, and, as we saw so vividly demonstrated this morning, the forces generated within the muscles are certainly capable of causing injury to the muscles, and, as was at least alluded to, forces that are applied to the skull through the muscles somehow are causing skull fractures, at least in some of the animal models that have been looked at.

Nobody mentioned the fact that there are muscles attached to some of those portions of the skull as well, and it's my intuitive feeling that some of those muscles forces will be responsible for some of the damages that we see. Clearly, in the patient or in the victim who has been in an accident where the nervous system is functioning and the muscles are intact, any criteria for injury has to take into account the two factors, that the muscles can: 1) inflict injury upon themselves; and 2) put loads into the system such as they will influence the injury criteria to a very great extent.

So the third item in the description of any model ought to be the variable internal load time history that can occur.

The second major point that I would like to clarify is what injury modes are we going to discuss? Now, there were several brought out this morning, and I'm sure there are a wide variety of injury modes. There are probably as many injury modes as there are accident configurations. But it is pretty clear we ought to try and tackle those that occur most commonly and those that have the biggest clinical interest. From my point of view, I suggest three modes of loading that ought to be attacked using some sort of at least common form of criteria. These three modes are:

The compression type injuries in which loads are either essentially axial or have a large axial component, so we might consider them as concentric and eccentric axial loading conditions.

Second, are those that essentially cause shear damage, and we saw some illustration of those. Those are commonly the high-speed transverse loads.

And the third classification we saw this morning, the tension type injuries, that which we saw are the results of the inertial properties of the head under high trunk acceleration/deceleration conditions.

As I say, those are tension, off-axis tension but very different in mechanism than the previous two.

Any criteria that we come up with is going to have to be based on some set of what I would consider to be controlling variables. We have heard several of them for the head and brain injury models, we have talked about stresses within the brain, we have talked about displacement criteria, and we have talked about load distribution over area. There are acceleration time histories that have been brought into load distribution as well.

Those factors which seem to control neck injury are somewhat different. I have broken them up into, again, three classifications, and they follow the descriptions that I've previously given:

First of all, the geometric variable. I think it is necessary for us to consider a vector description of the geometry. I think this will work as some spatial description of the major elements over time. This would include the muscle deformations as well.

It is clear that there are certain geometries which have associated with the failure modes and certain geometries which have not.

The second one would be the external loading variables, as functions of time again. These can, of course, include the inertial terms or they can include the externally applied loads; the third one is the internal forces, also as a function of time.

You see, this is a rather different track than we do with head injury, and it's also different than considering the single-element criteria that we have used in the past when trying to reconstruct injury criteria for the neck. We recognize that certainly there is some data, some was just presented, as to how much force it takes to crush a vertebra, how much force it takes to take an individual vertebra and cause failure due to torsion and due to bending; and yet these are single elements. They do not portray the interaction between the elements, and they do not take into account some of the types of injuries that can occur with elastically constrained structures as opposed to single-elastic elements, and so I suggest that we consider all three of these, including the geometry, as vectors and look at this problem as a coupled problem in its entirety.

These variables are, of course, very general but we have gotten a lot of insight this morning and this afternoon as to how these variables would interact in various types of modes of failure and for this we can go back to very classical engineering definitions and perhaps propose that we look at some of the classical combinations of these variables for the various types of failure analysis.

For example, as a fundamental form for compression failures, we would look at a dot product between the geometry vectors and position vectors as a function of time. We could then construct similar types of dimensional formulations for shear vectors which would be cross-products between the geometries and the forces perhaps divided by the absolute forces, and for the moments that might reproduce, of course, we could go to a cross-product formulation.

We have included all of these factors as functions of time. It is pretty clear that they are not going to be smooth functions of time, especially if we want to do any realistic modeling with the muscles, and I don't propose that any of this is linear. I go along with the concepts that we're talking about nonlinearities; but I think, if we have an overview of which way we want to head with the injury criteria, we can simplify from that point down.

I'm not proposing that we start off with the most simple criteria, since I don't think that's truly useful in some of these systems. I think we have to take one or two steps above the most simple form of criteria.

I also want to emphasize that the loading function should always consider some function of muscle force over time, that the magnitude of the muscle forces and the damage that is produced by the muscle forces has been made evident today. To eliminate the muscle forces and their time functions from the criteria may actually destroy the usefulness of some of these criteria. You may be overlooking the major form of loading, especially when we start getting into the large displacement models.

I think the indication was that in the experiments we are getting into larger displacement models rather quickly, once we get into some of the longer time pulses. We have been told this morning that a lot of these injuries occur with long-duration time pulses, for example, football injuries or those injuries which don't involve direct head contact; and so I suggest we very quickly look upon this additional muscle force in its appropriate physiological form in our loading criteria.

Now, it is very easy to say we are going to develop a criteria for failure; and yet, if we reflect back on the simpler structure of the head, we recognize that the discussions simply as to form of the criteria have been debated long and hard and with good reason.

I think it is important that we consider the nature of the form of the criteria that we want to use initially. It seems to me that most people in their studies, as reflected in the literature, have taken a simple, one-dimensional form of criteria, be it maximum load or maximum strain, for the elements of the cervical spine. Neck criteria, as far as I can determine, have been mostly of this one-dimensional type, and, whereas, I think it's acceptable to use discrete criteria of failure, I certainly don't think it's an end point or even necessarily a starting point, if there is going to be a concerted effort to get failure criteria.

I suggest that we might want to go to some more integral type of failure criteria in which we take into account the immediate history of what is happening. I would also like to suggest a second possibility which might be useful, especially in the types of multiple trauma or complex trauma that is looked at, and that is a probabilistic approach in which you can describe some of the events with some degree of certainty and lack description of some of the other events.

In that case, then you can use theories of probability to describe the likelihood of some of these events or the product or cross-product of some of these events happening simultaneously. Therefore, put some probability as to the occurrence of a failure based on this criteria rather than an absolute statement as to whether or not that failure would have existed.

The reason that we want to develop failure criteria, at least as I reflect upon it, is so that we can have a useful statement at the end of an analytical exercise or that we can look at an experimental result; be it planned experiment or any one of the millions of unplanned experiments that we discussed before, and talk about the likelihood of such events or the likelihood of such models predicting failures or occurrences of failures.

Because of that, I feel that a statistical approach or the probability approach is actually, although the modeling may be a little more difficult, much more cost effective. If I could use that word now, since for each exercise you get not simply a yes or no answer, but a prediction as to the likelihood of the event occurring, given similar types of circumstances.

There are a lot of other scientific disciplines that use that approach, and they use it to good advantage. I don't think we have taken up that methodology and used it to good advantage in our own particular studies.

Discussion of Injury Criteria

Dr. Eppinger: We now have arrived at the point where I would like to open up the floor for discussions. I believe we could range over the entire topics.

Dr. J. Newman: I would like to make a comment I would like to compliment Mr. Gadd quite honestly for two things. First of all, his ability to continue to perceive the nature of the problems that we are still faced with and, secondly, for his truly pioneering efforts in attempting to get some rational tools together in the form of the severity index. It is without question it was a major contribution in this area, and his efforts are still very noteworthy.

I would like for the record, though, to note that I, in spite of Mr. Gadd's remarks, have never personally in any writing or publication criticized his creation of the severity index. I have admittedly reiterated the concerns that others expressed.

I have, for example, not commented on the use of the severity index concept in football helmet testing procedures. In fact, it is obviously a very valid and worthwhile tool. In that sense, take a look at football helmets since that stand has been implemented. But that by itself, of course, doesn't prove that the severity index concept is valid or true; but it works. It does serve that purpose.

My concern has been and still is not with the Gadd severity index but with the head injury criteria as it is presently formulated in the DOT 208 standard. It is not the same as was conceived by Mr. Gadd. It invokes elements and ideas and thoughts which are not as soundly based as his original analysis of existing data and, indeed, observations which have subsequently been made in my view shed considerable doubt on the validity of the HIC, and that's all I try to restrict my remarks to. Thank you.

Dr. Eppinger: Allow me to take a Chairman's prerogative at this moment to give you a possible physical meaning of what HIC represents. If we examine the HIC formulation as it is usually written, i.e.,

$$HIC = \underset{t_1, t_2}{Max} (t_2 = t_1) \left[\frac{1}{(t_2 - t_2)} \int_{t_1}^{t_2} a_R(t) dt \right]^{2.5}$$

we note that it operates on the measured resultant acceleration of the head and searches over all possible integration limits, t_1 and t_2, to find the maximum value of the function. If we assume that this maximizing process has been performed, a more physical form of HIC can be derived by redefining a few terms. That is, by making the time interval over which HIC is maximum, t_2–t_1, equal to T and the intergral of the resultant acceleration with respect to time between t_1 and t_2 equal to V (a reasonable assumption if head rotation is minimal and translation is essentially along a straight line) HIC becomes,

$$HIC = T\left[\frac{V}{T}\right]^{2.5}$$

$$= T \frac{V}{T}^{2.5}$$

$$= \left(\frac{V}{T}\right)^{0.5} \frac{V^2}{T}$$

This can then be interpreted as a measure of the rate of change of specific kinetic energy (the second term) modulated by the square root of the average acceleration over the interval T.

If the 2.5 power in the HIC function were instead 2, the function would represent directly the peak average specific power delivered to the head. Therefore, in practice, the act of limiting the HIC to be below a certain maximum, limits the peak average specific power delivered to the head. Stated another way, it suggests that the head is capable of undergoing a certain maximum rate of change of energy and if circumstances cause it to exceed this limit, injury will result.

Prof. Goldsmith: But in the case you are taking the absolute value of the acceleration, isn't that right?

Dr. Eppinger: Yes, the process of calculating the resultant does produce a scalar which is the absolute value of acceleration.

Prof. Goldsmith: But acceleration is per se a vector quantity and when properly integrated could give a different value than the integral of its absolute value.

Dr. Eppinger: That is correct. However, since the time interval that is finally considered maximizes HIC, it cannot occur during a period when the direction of the acceleration is reversed. Therefore, in practice, the maximum HIC is found at the same time interval as would a HIC calculation where the direction of acceleration vector is preserved.

Dr. Gennarelli: I would submit that our ability to generate computer models and sophisticated mathematical analyses has far exceeded our ability to do two things which I think are going to—if not solved—continue to cloud this issue.

One of these is to talk about specific types of head injury. I think one cannot continue to talk about severe head injury in general without specifying what that means. The mechanisms are different and so on. So I think one has to talk about specific types of head injuries before one can start developing criteria for tolerance.

The second relates to injury severity. I think better mechanisms to define injury in a very clean fashion are needed before these kinds of correlations can be made between some mathematical function and injury severity.

As Dr. Lindgren pointed out earlier, the AIS has some problems for him. The AIS 80 has approached those problems in the head section to some degree and perhaps will continue to improve as time goes on; but I think, if one mixes all types of apples and oranges, even though they occur in the head, one is never going to get a good correlation and if one has an imprecise mechanism to determine severity, it's going to only compound any injury severity system, tolerance system that we try to achieve.

Dr. Ewing: Along much the same lines, I really think that there is some problem with definition of head injury and/or neck injury because most of the injuries that have been discussed have been the sorts of injuries that the pathologist detects, injuries measurable on the cadaver, bony injuries, so-called hemorrhages resulting from impact acceleration.

I would like to submit that I'm not sure that the present AIS scale takes into account transient modifications, physiological functions in the central nervous system. I made this same point at the last head injury conference. I still think it. I may be wrong. I've been wrong before, but I earnestly request that you consider the problem of including transient changes in neurophysiological function in your injury codes.

Dr. Eppinger: Various neural reflexes, durations of concussion and other types of neural dysfunction, are these kind of measures that we should include?

Dr. Ewing: Changes in function is what I'm talking about. One way of measuring them is by noting the absence of reflexes. Another way is by measuring cortical-evoked potentials or efferent-evoked potentials in the cord.

Dr. Eppinger: If we're talking in detailed clinical study, that is one thing, but if we looked and tried to categorize the total automotive environment, I think that's an impossibility. We attempt to incorporate these things, the cross-clinical manifestations of head injury within the AIS, and I believe the AIS 80 has addressed these things in greater detail.

Tom Gennarelli has published a paper on what I believe is the stronger correlation with clinical versus the AIS ratings itself to demonstrate that it is indeed a more viable, more rugged approach to determining the overall threat to life.

Prof. Goldsmith: I would just like to say one thing about the use of properties of the human system, the brain, the skull and so on and so forth. Much of the original work on this was done under the old head injury model construction committee. What was done there was that certain tests were conducted and the mean value was given and also a spread, plus or minus. In some cases the standard deviation was 50% of the mean value. But what was not given, which I think would be extremely interesting, would be the 10 percentile and the 90 percentile values of a particular parameter.

No, I don't think we know anything about that sort of thing, and I would suggest that some effort ought to be made to get these data.

Dr. Eppinger: You should forward that suggestion in our discussions tomorrow. That's the entire purpose of the discussion groups that we have scheduled; and I hope they will truly be working groups where we can come back with the consensus, both from the experimental side and from the clinical side, to determine what we should be doing, what we should be measuring, what we should be looking at on the clinical side in the detailing of the pathology, what is necessary in sufficient instrumentation from the experimental side. I bring your attention to this final thing: injury criteria is the offspring of a shotgun marriage between the engineer and the physician, and you cannot have bad information on one side of the equation and great detailed information on the other side. You have to obtain a balance in the quality of the physiological aspects and the mechanical aspects of this problem.

Prof. Goldsmith: I had attempted to address it to the establishment of a criterion. That is what I would like to see done but I wanted to mention it now, in the context of, let us say, an HIC value of 1500, because that's intimately related, I believe, to that sort of thing.

Dr. Eppinger: I believe in any of our use of an HIC you must understand the regulatory process it goes through. We can go back down and establish a mean value and we are fully cognizant of the fact that there could be a noninjurious situations or elements of the population that could experience an HIC of 3000 without any visible signs, as well as somebody could have an HIC and suffer injury, therefore, the choice of a value, say 1000 or whatever the value would be, is also a mean representative. When you finally promulgate a rule, the lawyers in this process do not allow you to say it's going to be a mean value of such and so. They want exact value.

We have to come up with it through a process of understanding that it is a mean value, some idea of what the spread is, and make a determination of what is the maximum allowable value that we promulgate within the standard and so, if you put yourself into the position that we're in, the ultimate user of this, first off, you have to put it into a physical manifestation of a human; therefore, you have to avoid undue complexity because there's a myriad of other complications and requirements that are placed upon you to design this physical surrogate and then also the requirements of what is the actual operating level.

We have many other choices or decisions we have to make. What is the collision speed we test at? What is the crash mode we test at? All those things all feed into this. What we're addressing now is just the first aspect and to understand mean value is what we do use.

Dr. Tarriere: Perhaps we should have two parameters one for the direct head impact, and something for what passes through the neck to see if the restraint is efficient or not. Maybe it's too complicated, maybe it's not ready for our talk today or for tomorrow. So the solution might be to increase the HIC value to 1500 or something like that.

Dr. Eppinger: I would like to comment on the use of the evidence from field data that head and neck injuries do not occur in situations without head or neck contact to put forward the argument that HIC calculation should be eliminated for noncontact situations. First, I believe that it can be easily shown that when testing current production belt systems at high crash intensities, that there is a high probability of always having a head strike into some structure within the occupant compartment. In other words, present belt systems are not designed to preclude head strikes at high intensities. This fact would imply that the field data has also very few occurrences of high intensity loading to the head or neck without concomitant contacts with the compartment. Therefore field data cannot be used to preclude the existence of a noncontact injury mechanism since the environment of the field data does not have that type of situation within it, and also, it cannot be used to imply that better performing belt systems (those that prevent head contacts in high-intensity crashes) would not excite this injury mechanism.

The argument, albeit a subjective one, for maintaining the HIC calculations over the entire crash event could be as follows. Since, in the high-intensity, noncontact situations, it is centripetal acceleration component of the head that causes HIC to exceed the allowed maximum, one can envision that by limiting HIC to a certain level would limit neck tension to below a certain maximum and eliminating a very probable cause of injury in that mode. Therefore, speaking very loosely, the HIC is also a neck injury criteria.

Dr. Newman: On that very same theme, I think that there is something of a danger in the constant and ongoing use of the term of the words: the HIC.

Dr. Eppinger: It's defined very nicely in the government regulations.

Dr. Newman: Right. So, therefore, it is cast in stone. The point is, if it is only the HIC, then anything else has got to be something else, and I think it's probably time to think in terms of head injury criteria in whatever forms they may take. For example, that function squared might even be better, the same terms and the same general relationship holdup.

As another example, Dr. Tarriere's final slide which showed the blank spot down in the righthand corner, no AIS–3's at HIC's less than 1500. If you take the same datum points and change the ordinate to maximum g's, they all move around a little bit but the window's still blank. You don't find, for example, any AIS–3's with a peak g over 200. In other words, the data doesn't necessarily support HIC. They show that HIC works, it gives a little window and provides you with a number, but we could also. By using your data, get the same kind of window with peak g.

There may be others, too, so, if we are going to make any attempts to search for some other head injury criteria, it's probably appropriate to give that another name or something.

Dr. Eppinger: We're open for suggestions.

Dr. C. Ward: I would just like to repeat that although we don't know the tolerance to head rotation and shear strain, because the head is attached to the neck, maintaining the HIC limitation may actually be protecting the neck. I think we have to determine that before we can be overly critical.

Research Planning

Prof. Goldsmith: There are approximately 30 people signed up for this committee and that's too many for one committee, so we were splitting up the group into two, one under the direction of Larry Thibault, the other under the direction of Albert King.

I think perhaps we should address ourselves first to what we know, sort of make a general statement of where the state of the art is, and in particular what areas, while not perhaps satisfactory, do not need first-order priorities for further research.

Then the second thing that we want to do is decide what does need intensive attention and provide a listing of what is most important, what is less important and so on down the line so that we have some kind of recommendations to make which involve priorities of funding, priorities of attention; and both of these should include not just the subject and the methodology, but it also should include a timespan. In other words, whether or not you can think that you can accomplish something in two years, in three years, in five years, or that you don't think you can accomplish it in an eternity.

So together with concrete recommendations of the work to be done and the level of priority, we would like some kind of time scale that you feel is feasible in terms of the accomplishment of this goal.

And then the third thing that needs to be addressed is how this fits in with DOT objectives and with such things as standards and public policy, et cetera.

Dr. Melvin: This group is to consider four subsets of human surrogates: animals, cadavers, physical models and theoretical models. We were concerned that if we were to break into four small groups, on the one hand we would be too fragmented and not be able to get the viewpoints across. On the other hand, if we were all to stay in one large group, we might not make good progress either. Therefore, we would like to separate into two groups, one dealing with cadavers and physical models, the other dealing with animals and theoretical models.

That may sound a little strange at first but the key issue is that you cannot solve our problem with any one of those approaches, concerted use of all is required. The physical model in many ways is going to be an end product, if we're talking about an improved dummy. The mathematical models, theoretical models may supplant the physical some day but certainly not in the near future. So that all of these four methods have to interact to get the answers we're after, in our view, and it's probably most likely that the animal work will be related through theoretical models to the final product which is the prediction of human response in injury, because the animals can be tested throughout the range of physiological and nonphysiological situations, whereas, at least as far as this group is concerned, our human testing is always going to to be nonphysiological because it is the cadaver.

So we felt that breakdown had some logic to it, hence we would like to have you in these two separate groups. They will be subchaired, by Albert King and Larry Thibault in order to insure that we keep things moving in those two groups while Werner and I will interact with both. This is the way we would like to try to approach this.

Albert will be chairing the subcommittee on Animals and Theoretical Models and Larry Thibault will be in charge of Cadavers and Physical Models.

We've stirred things up a little bit in doing this because we would like to have a cross-fertilization in this process. I think it is very important that the people that are involved in, say, cadaver testing and animal testing, are aware of the needs of the models, both physical and theoretical, and because of the problem of measuring things that can't be modeled or modeling things that can't be measured. It's a very important question, and we have to keep the two in communication.

So that is the way we would like to approach this and then bring it back together. Don't forget that our goal is a written product outlining our feelings of where the state of the art is. We want to answer some of those questions. All of this relates to the list of questions that you have. Some of those are not pertinent to this group directly, many of them are, the ones that Ken Digges posed to us. We would like to at least be able to give some indication of the group's feelings regarding those questions.

Dr. Goldsmith: I think I will call on Larry Thibault to announce the members of his group.

Dr. Thibault: Tarriere, Gadd, Alem, Stalnaker, Aldman, Bohlin, Lee, Fozzati, Henson, Marcus, Goi, Backaitis, Saul and Niederer.

Dr. King: For the Animal and Theoretical Models I have Lennox, Huang, Nuscholtz, Ljung, Thomas, Privitzer, Ward, Prasad, Morgan, Haley, Nahum, Kulkarni, Kotwick and Newman.

Dr. Thibault: I wish to make a brief summary of the major areas of that so they may be included for discussion and perhaps if applicable proposals for a consensus attack may be generated.

First: General lack of funding basic research and the consequent inability to conduct adequate studies is resulting in irreproducible, unreliable kinds of measurements or at least measurements that are more difficult to interpret.

Second: There is a need for standardization, in test methods and reporting of data. The DOT could contribute very largely in this area; for example, by providing some kind of standard reporting sheets or methods that everyone agreed were useful.

Third: Characterization of cadaver and physical models. Cadaver models more specifically in order to get some feel for the range of variability that we've been working with and, if we get lucky and find out that we can treat that variability statistically and develop a mean standard deviation and have some confidence in that, provided we describe the condition of the cadaver, it would be a useful way to tighten up our results. Again, it implies doing some basic work that hasn't been done.

Fourth: Neck development be given the highest priority item in terms of modeling specific components.

Fifth: A study of muscle mechanics is important, in so far it is yet to be determined how muscle mechanics modifies the kinematics.

Sixth: That our injury criteria should now become much more specific. We wouldn't be talking about head injury, we should be talking about vascular disruption and maybe even specific anatomical vascular disruption versus brain tissue primary neurological lesions versus secondary phenomena brought on by either of the above. We must become much more specific in terms of injury, because the implications of injury mechanisms are more specific.

Seventh: The interagency coordination, should move into the area of prevention and not just the area of reconstruction. There may be a terrible amount of duplication of effort and we want to avoid that. We should pool resources and take advantage to any data base that might exist that we don't have access to right now.

Eighth: With regard to instrumentation; there is a need to be able to measure angular acceleration.

Are there any words, key words or ideas that I didn't extract from my notes that were made or that don't fit into one of these categories?

Mr. Backaitis: Somehow I fail to see a reflection of what has been discussed in relation to what is going on in the real-world accident system. It's fine to talk about lesions, and it's fine to talk about various types of injuries; but we must concern ourselves with those events that are occurring in the real world, not something that perhaps can be obtained only at the laboratory level.

Dr. Thibault: I think along that line of relevance, if you will, the point also that Mark Hafner made, that in developing model systems it should be kept in mind that somehow this work is to eventually reflect itself in an advanced dummy and, if you have options at different points in experimental work, to choose that option that may be extrapolated to the dummy, incorporated into the dummy system rather than a more abstract measurement.

Dr. Tarriere: Could we say something about the head protection criteria. I think that we could criticize the present usage of HIC by regulation 208, for instance, when the HIC is measured even if there is no head impact. I think that now, through the real-world investigation of accidents and also from cadaver testing, it is well established that there is no brain injury and no neck injury received except the muscles injured, minor injuries on the AIS–1 level. But there is no brain and neck injury with AIS higher than 2 when there is no head impact in frontal collisions.

Mr. Backaitis: We have one case with AIS–4.

Dr. Tarriere: One with 4, you say, one case.

Mr. Backaitis: One.

Dr. Tarriere: Okay, one. And maybe we have to see this case and to discuss what happened. So through the real world I think that's something well established and a proposal could be to measure the HIC only when there is an impact and during the impact as a contact interval. That's a very practical proposal.

And a second proposal, more difficult for application, is how to split the part of HIC coming from the restraint through the neck and the part of the HIC from the direct impact. Maybe a proposal could be to measure the force at the neck level with a device, with the same device on Hybrid III. There is a device to measure something on the restraint on the neck. So maybe it could be a means, a way to improve the significance of HIC.

Prof. Goldsmith: I'd like to add two things to this that I don't think are reflected in what you have right now.

First: We need further data on the distribution of properties and geometries within humans. Now, maybe that's characterization but I would like to be more specific than that and, say, talk about a 10 percentile or a 50 percentile or 100 percentile or 90 percentile individual, and for perhaps even subdivisions into males and females and conceivably even further subdivisions by regions of the world. That gets into detail.

Second: I think measurement of contact phenomena is something that is not encompassed within your program.

Dr. Thibault: Yes. I had that, but I guess I missed that.

Mr. Haffner: Presser distribution.

Prof. Goldsmith: Yes. In head impact.

Dr. Stalnaker: Maybe just to add to that, I was at an SAE subcommittee meeting last week on dummies and the number one item that we wanted addressed on the new dummies was head contact, direct head contact. We talked about forces and ways of measuring it and the number one priority was a way of measuring localized loading to the head.

Prof. Goldsmith: The instrumentation on that particular one has not been solved. I mean, you talk about the solution of instrumentation but not for that point.

Dr. Alem: That gets into the time frame that we were asked to consider. Will it take two years or ten years?

Prof. Goldsmith: Yes.

Mr. Gadd: I agree with that but just to step back to Tarriere for a second, from what I've heard in the last couple of days I think there is a consensus on this idea he just expressed of not requiring HIC if there's no contact and will that be written down as one of the consensus items?

Dr. Thibault: Unless there's objection to that. The statement was that in the absence of impact that perhaps the HIC not be used.

Mr. Backaitis: I remember Dr. Ewing's movie in which he showed that if you have a 120-g level of fairly long duration in monkey tests, that you do have transection of the neck occurring. This might create a problem.

Mr. Gadd: There could be some—We could just suggest there is a consideration given to some kind of measurement to estimate neck hazard if we propose eliminating the head contact situation.

Mr. Backaitis: Yes.

Mr. Gadd: The nonhead contact. The corollary to that would be to give consideration to some kind of neck measurement.

Dr. Aldman: Is it that easy to define head contact? A head contact with an airbag, for example.

Mr. Gadd: Normally you think of some kind of colored material that would show a pretty definite contact.

Dr. Stalnaker: But the problem is you have to start reading the HIC, don't you, at the point of contact.

Dr. Thibault: I think the distinction there is whether or not you're talking about distributed forces versus concentrated focus loading and I think all of that's impact.

Mr. Gadd: Why not read the HIC over the whole thing just as you have been doing right along, if there's contact, but, if there's no contact, then don't read it. That would be easier, wouldn't it?

Dr. Stalnaker: Yes, but what if you just barely touch it with the top of the head? Then you get a little smudge on the thing and then all you've got to think of is a HIC of a few thousandths and you can't do that.

Mr. Haffner: It seems to be you need HIC to talk about the inertial problem. Then you need some type of pressure sensitive mask or something, coating, that will indicate where the pressure goes when it's rather severe.

Mr. Gadd: At a significant level.

Mr. Haffner: Yes.

Dr. Stalnaker: That gets us back into some way of measuring contact.

Mr. Gadd: Yes.

Dr. Stalnaker: Localized contact.

Dr. Alem: That's right.

Dr. Stalnaker: You can use the HIC for inertial contact.

Mr. Gadd: Part of the recommendation could be, to find a way to define head contact or nonhead contact. That would have to be studied a little further. We can't solve it today.

Dr. Alem: That's right.

Mr. Gadd: With all of the measurements.

Dr. Alem: We're really not here to solve problems, I think.

Dr. Thibault: No, that's right.

Dr. Alem: We are recommending that we study those problems. We all agree it seems to me, that HIC cannot be used universally.

We agree on that. So the recommendation ought to be, Okay, let's find out, what are the limitations, where can you use it? If you cannot use it in some cases, what should we use? These are the questions that DOT should address. We're not here in the position to—we're not trying to say, Okay, under this condition and this condition we're not going to use HIC, under this condition we can use HIC. All we should say in this forum is there is a problem.

This follows what you are saying, that we have to be specific about injury criteria, where they apply and how to.

Dr. Thibault: Yes, that's correct.

Dr. Aldman: But I think that the problem of head contact is not that simple, actually, because I'm not convinced that it's localized force that is important. It might well be the change in kinematics of the head at that contact that is important. So I think we should be very careful here to know what we are saying when we say head contact.

Dr. Tarriere: We say head contact with the rigid, part of the vehicle. But there is a problem, you are right, is it possible to have the same protection criteria using both for each kind of test and so on? I don't think so, and my proposal is especially for belted occupants and for the airbag maybe it could be another thing.

Dr. Alem: Larry, can we take those items that you have in here in brief to go over them—to summarize our feelings?

Dr. Thibault: I think there's a consensus with regard to the need for funding more basic research. It comes out of discussions on a certain degree of variability associated with experimental models, be they cadaver or physical models, and uncertainty associated with ranges of variation in those parameters. We feel that there is a need to fund more basic research in these areas, even though there is no immediate payoff. If we don't do it now, we're eventually going to pay the price.

And there is a general agreement that standardization in a variety of forms would be valuable in helping to tighten the data that are being reported in the scientific literature, and the Department of Transportation could make major contributions in that area by providing consensus, standardized experimental protocol report forms, if you will, anthropomorphic, anthropomorphic kinds of data recording sheets and whatever else may be agreed upon in the future.

Characterization, especially in the case of cadavers, in order to develop confidence intervals to see what the range of variability is. On the one hand, variation in the state of the cadaver as a physical model, also the type of characterization, as Dr. Goldsmith pointed out, the range of normal human variability in some parameters which may have surfaced more recently that we consider to be important and to find out what that 10- to 90-percentile variation is.

I think we have agreed that a very high-priority item in terms of future development, is the neck and that along that same line to elucidate by testing the role of muscle mechanics and the modifications that they may make.

Dr. Alem: That would be the same. I would probably lump it into the neck.

Dr. Thibault: In addition, we should become more specific in describing injury mechanisms rather than to call them head and neck injury. There are very discrete types of injury mechanisms that may be produced by greatly different types of mechanical insults.

Dr. Aldman: Is there a scaling problem involved there or do we have enough data to scale the various injuries?

Dr. Thibault: I think there is basic work needed to define the envelopes within which these specific injuries occur and in light of the epidemiological evidence to look at the tradeoffs. Is subdural hematoma important from an outcome point of view and where does subdural hematoma occur in some physical variable envelope? Is there a specific domain within which subdural hematoma occurs? And then you could talk about mild head injury and where does that occur, but is mild head injury important from the outcome point of view? What should we really be protecting against? And go after the most difficult and most significant problems.

But to start handling them as if they are in fact different entities, which they are, that there should be within the interagency coordination effort existing under the Office of the President, which presumably involves DOT, NIOSH, the Department of Defense and some other government agencies, there should be a parallel effort in the area of prevention which apparently does not exist at the present time and through that mechanism take advantage of the multiple resources of these agencies and try and develop, for example, data banks or pools of information that all of us can have access to.

Mr. Backaitis: How about mentioning international?

Dr. Thibault: And perhaps expanding that into the international scene, yes.

Contact phenomena, load distribution is an area where future development should be placed. I'm not sure it fits into the instrumentation category or just in general in technical problems associated with basic research to give us better understanding of the loading conditions of the system.

A study of some type should be undertaken to elucidate where the limitations arise in application of the head injury criteria as it exists, to look at questions of applying HIC with and without impact, supplemental injury criteria that may be necessary. We should try to define in general where head injury criteria as it exists now is applicable and can be used. There is a development effort under way which should be supported to develop angular accelerometers and angular acceleration measurements that can then be incorporated into advance dummies.

Mr. Gadd: In this regard a couple of people mentioned that they didn't feel the state of the art on instrumentation and the background information on rotational tolerance were such that we're ready to incorporate those.

The present state of the art doesn't look, from what I hear said, as though we can work with large quantities of pressure or rotational accelerometer instrumentation right now. In other words, we're not ready to incorporate an additional criterion of rotational acceleration and pressure at this juncture at least, that more development is needed. That's the impression I get.

Dr. Alem: There is something else, I think will need talking about, instrumentation as related to the head injury per se rather than head and neck. The neck we haven't touched a whole lot upon. The idea is to develop criteria, can we come up with criteria, so toward that end what should we be looking at in terms of injury criteria for the neck.

Are we looking for parameters or quantities, physical quantities, measurable quantities that are related to muscle, muscle-ligament injury, soft tissue injury? Are we talking about the measurement of quantities that relate to bone fracture? This is all within the spirit of leading to neck injury criteria. Is deformation, deflection of a bone, rotation or displacement very important, in, head impact? What happens to the neck?

Prof. Goldsmith: Do you know of any other criteria besides the Mertz corridors that define supposed tolerance?

Dr. Alem: That's a limit of motion and not an injury.

Prof. Goldsmith: It's a response.

Dr. Thibault: I think it's an injury. Head injury criteria are much further along than neck injury criteria.

Dr. Alem: That's right.

Dr. Thibault: And I think you mean from the outcome point of view.

Dr. Alem: Are we at the basic research level as regards the neck?

Dr. Thibault: Absolutely, I think it's almost at the beginning stages, to define, set up definitions for neck injury criteria in general.

Dr. Alem: So should we define at this time what are the quantities that should be measured?

Mr. Haffner: I think we've got to go into the field and accident files first. I think, as you had said before, we should in this form point out the need for work in that area and not attempt to try and answer the question.

Dr. Thibault: I don't think we can at this stage.

Mr. Haffner: No.

Mr. Gadd: Al Nahum and I ran a study and published the results. It was just a short study, in which the neck of fresh cadavers was bent over in the two planes to see what angles it stiffened up and began to show ligamentous damage. Of course, that was only for elderly, and it's naturally a lot more for youngsters; but a more comprehensive study along that line of actual measurements—on fresh cadavers—would be logical, I think.

Dr. Thibault: Yes. But, as I say, too, supplemented with the appropriate failure criteria. In other words, cord transection, vertebral body fracture, and break those out as elements the way I think we're moving and in direction in head injury and talk to them as discrete injury mechanism forms, some of which are important, some of which are not terribly important.

Prof. Goldsmith: In both the head and the neck I would worry about the limits of physiological damage as opposed to the limits of mechanical damage.

Dr. Thibault: Right.

Prof. Goldsmith: And I don't know whether we understand that adequately.

Mr. Gadd: It's complicated.

Dr. Thibault: That's right. At Penn we have a study underway now looking at that question.

Dr. Aldman: Isn't it also a question that the HIC, for instance, is measured in the head on a very bad representation of the neck?

Prof. Goldsmith: I think perhaps the physiological versus the mechanical damage is another topic that ought to be looked into, especially in the neck.

Dr. Alem: I think that would be a higher level analysis of research from animal.

Dr. Thibault: Actually, what we're doing, at Penn is operating on the philosophy that, it's difficult to design and build a bridge if you don't understand what the strength of the bolts are. So we're working with a single neuron, a single axon that we can subject to high strain rate loading conditions, actually our loading conditions have a very broad dynamic spectrum, and study the physiology, electrophysiology of that cell.

When did it stop working as an active electrical elementary system? In fact that does occur at levels below those at which structural, presumably irreversible damage occurs, but nevertheless leads to functional impairment. As you heard Joe Tory say yesterday, he sees transient quadriplegia, which we believe to be somewhat analogous to cerebral concussion, in that there is loss of function that presumably is fully recoverable in a time cycle. It varies. In his case it's from 10 minutes to maybe weeks but there is this consideration of functional versus structural which is a non-normal-engineering consideration and I think one that will be receiving more attention in time.

Prof. Goldsmith: I think this is a point that has not been sufficiently developed. The original intention of the head injury model construction committee way back 15 years ago, was to try to define the mechanical involvement and then go to the physiologists and ask them, given a certain force history at a given point, what is the physiological reaction of the unit and that question as far as I know, has still not been adequately answered.

Dr. Thibault: Virtually unanswered.

Dr. Aldman: It's biomechanics by the cell.

Dr. Thibault: It's biomechanics of the cell and that's what you have to do, you have to stress single cells and ask the question of when does their physiology change. When it is reversible and irreversible and it can be irreversible without irreversible structural damage, according to some evidence we have.

Prof. Goldsmith: Are there any other topics that you wish to bring up within this framework? Because I do want to say something about what we ought to do with these, namely, we ought to talk now about the second thing, priorities, time scales and methodologies for all of these. I don't know whether we can do that in half an hour.

Dr. Thibault: A draft of that is going to be typed up and I think the only thing you need to do now is cover the details of rank ordering, the priority and establishing to the best of your ability the time frame.

Dr. Aldman: Can I ask a question first?

Prof. Goldsmith: Yes.

Dr. Aldman: About facial injuries.

Prof. Goldsmith: I think in a sense that's a separate issue because we're talking about primarily lacerations.

Dr. Aldman: No, no. What I mean is if you hit something with your face that would change the input to the head actually.

Prof. Goldsmith: Yes, but when we talk about head impact, we talk about loading at any point of the face and skull and so on. I know of a case where a person was killed by being hit by a horse right on the chin.

All right. Basic research is obviously a number—Maybe we should talk about categories one, two and three in terms of priorities, rather than trying to list all of these in some different order, one being the most important. Basic research is clearly one and it's clearly definite.

But number two, standardization, what is the methodology, what kind of priority should it have, what is the timespan for reasonable—Does anyone care to comment on that?

Mr. Marcus: Before we leave number one, before we leave the basic research, I think we should conclude the basic research.

Prof. Goldsmith: All right. Category one, time scale? I think we should look at something like two years, five years and ten years as a reasonable. . . .

Dr. Alem: Can I say something about the standardization and the time scale? By standardization I think what is meant by it, is to set up a framework within which the rest of the work can be done so you've really got to do it immediately. It is not a time-consuming thing at this time, just to set up forms, what needs to be done and then require that everything else follow that standard more or less whenever appropriate, a protocol.

Prof. Goldsmith: Now, who do you think should do this? Set up these protocols, set up forms? Somebody is going to have to do it.

Dr. Alem: Name me, I'll do it.

Dr. Aldman: I think it should be done in different places and then compared.

Prof. Goldsmith: All right. Say 3 to 5 locales plus a meeting afterwards for uniformity.

Dr. Alem: I think you have to recognize on this issue that many of these protocols are already set up, are defined. All you have to do is gather and unify all the procedures that are the state of the art and put them in one document.

Prof. Goldsmith: But somebody has got to do it. Now, who is the best person to do it? Would NHTSA do this? And I don't think that NHTSA can do it alone. I think they're going to have to talk to other people.

Mr. Backaitis: I think there is some activity at the International Standards Organization going on right now.

Dr. Tarriere: Working Group 108.

Mr. Backaitis: Yes. Another organization that should be getting into this is the Society of Automotive Engineers, SAE.

And then certainly NHTSA should get involved.

Prof. Goldsmith: What about the working group of the National Academy, for example?

Dr. Tarriere: But it's important to do this work at the international level.

Mr. Backaitis: Yes.

Dr. Tarriere: It is not sufficient to do that in the United States, because we need to have comparable and additional data for the world.

Prof. Goldsmith: Does anybody know if the United States has something like that?

Mr. Backaitis: ISO.

Dr. Tarriere: I think ISO is good. I would think so.

Prof. Goldsmith: All right.

Dr. Tarriere: And they're working on these problems. With push from DOT this working group could have the standardization in 6 months or 1 year.

Dr. Stalnaker: Just one word. I don't think it can be done that way. To me the scope of the whole thing is such that it will take 20 years and still you'll never get anybody to agree. The problem is that we're all doing this on a voluntary basis. If you're going to get it done, it has to be done by somebody at DOT, through a contract, with some travel money, and a time limit and they are forced to bring in other people and they would be forced to do it. But that's the only way you're ever going to get it done right.

Mr. Backaitis: The problem is that the contractor doesn't have that kind of liberty to call in an international set of experts.

Prof. Goldsmith: I'm noting down that there is disagreement.

Mr. Backaitis: I realize this but, you know, if you wait for ISO to do it . . .

Dr. Stalnaker: It will take 20 years, yes.

Prof. Goldsmith: Let us go on to the next item "characterization." For example, human range of variability. Definition of cadaver geometries, properties, human geometries, properties. What priority should we assign this?

Mr. Backaitis: One.

Mr. Saul: I was going to say two. You really get that after you've got your standardization.

Mr. Gadd: I think these are all going to be one unless we're hard-nosed about this thing.

Mr. Backaitis: It should be one.

Prof. Goldsmith: All right, one.

Time Scale?

Mr. Gadd: I think it's a long range, perhaps five years.

Prof. Goldsmith: Five years, nobody is going to hold us to this. This is our best estimate at this point. Let's proceed to Methodology. How do we go about doing this?

Dr. Aldman: I think there are different methods here. You characterize a human being by different methods and then different types of each body risk, and then you go down to tissues and to the cell level.

Mr. Marcus: I think the first thing we probably need to do with this is to decide what variables among the variability we want to look at and that's tied back in with standardizing the protocol. A longer-range problem would be to decide on additional measurements we want to look at. After that, we would probably try to collect additional data or use the existing anthropometry basis.

Dr. Stalnaker: If I can add to what you're saying, DOT is already paying HSRI to do this, to determine what kind of dummies we need and how they can be characterized. They're going to come up with a bunch of measurements and from the set of data that they use to define the dummy we can take a subset to characterize. Let them do the legwork, let them set the protocol more or less and then adapt it to what we're doing.

Prof. Goldsmith: Are you talking about both geometry and properties?

Dr. Stalnaker: Only the geometries.

Prof. Goldsmith: The geometry only. Well, what about properties?

Mr. Haffner: That's a separate issue. That's another problem.

Prof. Goldsmith: But is this not part of characterization?

Dr. Stalnaker: I understand but for that part they are already doing a lot of it. For example, they've dropped the terminology 50th percentile, which is the right thing to do. You can't talk about a 50th-percentile person. He doesn't exist.

Mr. Backaitis: That is the contractor's recommendation. That is not necessarily official.

Dr. Stalnaker: Officially they may not have dropped it but you can't talk about a 50-percent person and say you're talking about a medium-sized person as opposed to a 50-percentile person. It has very little scientific meaning.

You just can't do it. Every time you go to do a study with volunteers you measure a 50-percentile arm, and 50-percentile shoulder and it doesn't add up to a 50-percentile total limb and it never will.

Mr. Backaitis: Dick, again, that's your opinion.

Dr. Stalnaker: That's a fact.

Mr. Backaitis: That is not necessarily an international agreement.

Dr. Aldman: There's another problem to this and that is the mass distribution. I think in the current dummy that you have most of the mass in the skeleton and nothing in the subparts.

Prof. Goldsmith: The mass distribution in the dummies?

Dr. Aldman: Yes.

Prof. Goldsmith: Now, let me ask this. What can we do, if anything, about properties?

Mr. Marcus: Do we have enough properties available to go through and try to look at variability?

Prof. Goldsmith: In my 1971 paper on head injury I summarized the work that was done by the groups in West Virginia and Michigan among them. McElhaney came up, as a typical case in point, with 10,000 psi for the radial compression of the skull, plus or minus 5,000 psi. Now, that's a mean and a range, I guess. It's certainly not a standard deviation. The question is did he have enough test material available? And this is for an adult cadaver skull. We're not talking about living. We're not talking about living. We're not talking about children. We're not talking about people in far distant parts of the world.

What I'm asking is do we need more information on properties measured not just in the research laboratory but locally by whatever means we can do it?

Mr. Gadd: That would be one of the subheadings under your number one, which is more basic research needed, I would stay.

Mr. Marcus: I think that any future research also needs to spend a considerable amount of time looking at past efforts in the variability and before you go into the laboratory and identify what was causing the variability as well as measuring the properties.

Prof. Goldsmith: Some of this material will not be available that hasn't been measured.

Dr. Stalnaker: Yes. But that's important.

Dr. Aldman: I think the question of vasculature is another thing that has to be explored more thoroughly.

Prof. Goldsmith: The vasculature needs to be explored. In terms of what? Properties and strength and things like that?

Dr. Aldman: In terms of properties and strength, yes.

Prof. Goldsmith: When you talk about brain properties, Dr. Aldman, you know a lot of people have tried to measure them and not very successfully, especially the failure modes.

Dr. Stalnaker: That's a lifetime of work.

Prof. Goldsmith: Well, that's perhaps something we need to say.

Dr. Stalnaker: Probably that would come out of Thibault and Gennarelli's book, a lot of that. They are looking at what kind of injuries they really see and then once they figure out what's happening then you can address it. They decided to start with. So it has to be tied in closely to what we're looking at. What kind of failures we see and then address yourselves to what vascular system circuit is important, tissue, gray matter, white matter, something about that, that is important.

Prof. Goldsmith: Properties of strength. What were we talking about the vasculature? Strength and also mechanical properties.

Dr. Stalnaker: Mechnical properties.

Mr. Marcus: Also, on these properties the question of the changes, post mortem changes.

Prof. Goldsmith: Anything else on properties?

Mr. Saul: Somehow these need to be tied in with the animal type studies and be consistent with them.

Mr. Gadd: Some of it will have to be done on animals, the immediate fresh properties of the brain.

Prof. Goldsmith: Well, how do you do it? I mean, methodology.

Dr. Stalnaker: Again, I think it's all tied in together. We're talking about characterization of these properties and we'll have the properties plus or minus something and that is going to be from various cadavers and give you some range.

Prof. Goldsmith: I would like to put down that the methodology needs to be addressed but has not yet been sufficiently defined. How is that?

Dr. Stalnaker: Sounds good to me.

Dr. Tarriere: I come back to the characteristics. I think that it's not sufficient to have characteristics form the experiments on cadavers. We need characteristics of the population at risk. These data could be gotten from road accident victims. If you do, you have to have the same characteristics for this population as for the cadavers.

Prof. Goldsmith: We need proper correlation of accident history. How's that?

Dr. Tarriere: Yes.

Dr. Stalnaker: When you do these properties you're not restricting yourself just to the cadavers that you have, you're supposed to draw in all sources, operating room, etc.

Prof. Goldsmith: Neck development. Item priority number 1–A?

Dr. Niederer: Think this is a two-stage process. For priority that could be muscle mechanics of the neck region, and priority two than the actual development of the new neck surrogate.

Prof. Goldsmith: All right. So muscle mechanics is item one.

Mr. Marcus: Why don't we just cut that back to mechanics of the neck, instead of muscle mechanics?

Prof. Goldsmith: Soft tissue mechanics?

Mr. Marcus: I don't think it should be just soft tissue.

Prof. Goldsmith: Mechanics of the neck?

Mr. Marcus: Of the neck, yes.

Prof. Goldsmith: And then two, development of a model, is that what you were talking about?

Dr. Neiderer: A neck surrogate.

Mr. Gadd: The musculature, the thing that we thought was the top priority, we don't know how to cope with just yet.

Mr. Haffner: I think that's part of the mechanics.

Mr. Gadd: Yes, but the mechanics is everything.

Prof. Goldsmith: All right, with particular reference to musculature.

Mr. Haffner: I'd just like to throw in the opinion that it might be wise to develop the head and neck physically as a unit together, for practical purposes.

Dr. Stalnaker: I don't think you can do the head and neck separately, put them together and have it come up with properties.

Prof. Goldsmith: It's been done though.

Mr. Backaitis: Yes, but it didn't get us far.

Mr. Haffner: It's a chance to talk about how to do the problem up front.

Prof. Goldsmith: Then neck development is tied in with the head-neck system.

Mr. Backaitis: Tie it in.

Prof. Goldsmith: Time scale?

Mr. Marcus: You want a time scale for each of the two?

Prof. Goldsmith: I think so.

Mr. Marcus: I think it should be more like 4.

Dr. Stalnaker: Yes, but if you say 4, then it's going to be 10, you know. Say 2. Let's push for everything in 2 years.

Prof. Goldsmith: Two years for the mechanics of the neck with particular reference to musculature and say another 3 years for the development. Everything depends on the funding.

Dr. Stalnaker: If nobody pays anything for anything, it never gets done.

Prof. Goldsmith: But you know, of course, it depends on the funding but no matter how much money you have you're not going to get results in a period of less time. How long to develop a neck surrogate that we can start using?

Dr. Tarriere: Two years.

Prof. Goldsmith: Priority one for the muscle mechanics, the mechanics of the neck and priority two for the development of the dummy. Now specific injury criteria. Anyone care to comment on that?

Mr. Gadd: Several people suggested that for the near term maybe the quickest thing that could be done would be to recognize what a lot of people have said, that is for a noncontact, maybe the HIC isn't needed.

Mr. Backaitis: I don't consent to that.

Prof. Goldsmith: Maybe we should, first of all, separate noncontact and the contact.

Dr. Niederer: Right.

Mr. Marcus: You also want to consider the input of the head, over and above contact, with rotational versus side versus direct. Some accommodation of side movement.

Prof. Goldsmith: Rotational versus translation. Well, that's not an input. You're not going to talk about an input of a rotation. That's the end product.

Mr. Gadd: There was a suggestion made that more research is needed before we could actually implement the rotation or the pressure. . . .

Prof. Goldsmith: The rotational injury criteria.

Mr. Gadd: Yes.

Prof. Goldsmith: Is that what you meant?

Mr. Marcus: Right.

Dr. Stalnaker: I'd like, if I could, just to add to that. I don't see how you can just set the HIC over here and say we need to do more work on pressure and on acceleration. I think you can forget about the HIC. We need to do a lot more work on head injury and specific types of head injury, as we discussed earlier, in developing it into some kind of criteria we can use.

I'm not satisfied with the HIC and I'm not ready to put any other.

Prof. Goldsmith: Yes, I understand and I agree with you. When I'm saying—I guess what most everyone agrees with is that there is a need for a better definition of a criterion but we don't know what that is yet.

Dr. Stalnaker: Right.

Prof. Goldsmith: A need for better definition of criteria. Specific criteria. But are not ready yet to implement.

Dr. Stalnaker: Where HIC is being used, fine.

Prof. Goldsmith: And that I think in my mind is extremely important.

Time scale? I think some of this can be done within 2 years. Some of it will take a lifetime.

Dr. Alem: It will depend on the outcome of a lot of other things.

Prof. Goldsmith: I would say that, for example, the noncontact versus contact can probably be addressed in 2 years. In other words, to try to make a separation there as to what happens. Beyond this, the type of injury, I think that's going to take a lot longer. That may even take 10 years.

Dr. Tarriere: For what?

Prof. Goldsmith: For separating, let's say, a contact injury into its separate effects like, epidural, skull fracture, coup, contrecoup injury, the various kinds of physiological results or end products that we get. I would say that may very well take 5 to 10 years.

Dr. Tarriere: A long way.

Prof. Goldsmith: Yes.

Let's see. Rotational injury criterion development. I think that possibly can be done within 2 to 3 years.

Dr. Aldman: I don't think so.

Prof. Goldsmith: No? Longer?

Dr. Tarriere: Longer?

Dr. Aldman: You have got to do the instrumentation.

Prof. Goldsmith: Two to three years beyond instrumentation. And, finally the need for better definition of specific criteria. I think that's open ended. You know, that's never going to cease, I hope.

All right. Next. Interagency coordination. Very important but really out of the hands of this committee. I mean this group.

Mr. Backaitis: Just a suggestion.

Prof. Goldsmith: Yes. Interagency coordination must be done. I'm not even going to give that a priority or a time scale.

Angular accelerometer. That I will put in the appropriate place, but it has a high priority.

Mr. Backaitis: The contact phenomenon.

Prof. Goldsmith: The contact phenomenon is something else. I want to address that.

Dr. Stalnaker: Localized loading.

Prof. Goldsmith: All right. Localized loading measurement. I hate to call it just pressure. It may be other things. I mean, pressure clearly is one of the features, but it may also be deformation.

Dr. Alem: I think you could lump them all into one word, instrumentation development, for the measurements of quantities that we need.

Prof. Goldsmith: Except that Larry said that the one area he is satisfied with is instrumentation.

Dr. Alem: There is also in terms of neck, in terms of bone injury, bone cervical vertebrae fracture from motion or dislocation motion. How are you going to observe that, with material properties, with pressure transistors?

Prof. Goldsmith: Okay. Instrumentation development for neck phenomena.

Contact phenomena. Now, the HIC without impact is not valid but consideration be given to neck injury. I think we've covered that.

We talked about specific injury criteria and the HIC is under that.

Mr. Backaitis: I still disagree with the concept that the HIC without contact is not valid.

Prof. Goldsmith: All right. I will make a note to this effect. I will make a note to the effect disagreement re. applicability of HIC for noncontact. This is a consensus and so people are allowed to disagree.

Are neck injury criteria needed?

Dr. Alem: Yes. We don't have any.

Mr. Gadd: That should be of top priority then, I guess.

Prof. Goldsmith: It is, top priority. There is almost nothing that is not top priority.

Dr. Stalnaker: They're all in the same category.

Prof. Goldsmith: I may just leave out the priority from the report. I was hoping we could get some differentiation but apparently that's not possible.

All right, neck injury criteria. We should separate that too into, A, physiological, and B, mechanical.

Dr. Alem: How does cadaver testing correlate with the living?

Prof. Goldsmith: Cadaver testing. All right. Does anybody have any ideas on what kind of experiments should be conducted here? We have the human volunteers of Chan Ewing, of course, but that's pretty limited.

Mr. Backaitis: It's better than having nothing.

Prof. Goldsmith: Yes, but I'm afraid of extrapolations in nonlinear situations, especially linear extrapolations.

Mr. Gadd: No, you can't. No.

Dr. Alem: With cadavers, what data measurement you could make would probably be in dislocation observation.

Prof. Goldsmith: Dislocation of the vertebral bodies.

Dr. Alem: Skeletal measurements.

Prof. Goldsmith: Dislocation of vertebral bodies.

Dr. Alem: You have a problem with muscles, you have a problem with physiological.

Mr. Backaitis: Dislocation and fractures.

Dr. Alem: Fractures and dislocation. So that's the type of measurement you could get from cadaver testing.

Mr. Gadd: Subluxation, at the lesser level.

Dr. Tarriere: Nervous system injuries.

Prof. Goldsmith: How are we going to get nervous system injuries out of a cadaver?

Dr. Tarriere: Out of the brain.

Prof. Goldsmith: What I'm saying is out of cadavers. What would worry me is the extent or the range of the physiological versus the mechanical damage. I can see that we can get the mechanical damage all right.

Mr. Marcus: I think the physiological damage is going to have to be restricted to animal head studies and some attempt to scale those for humans.

Prof. Goldsmith: Physiological damage.

Mr. Backaitis: Or observations of the real-world injuries, the physiological outcome.

Dr. Stalnaker: Something like this thing that Prof. Thibault is doing.

Prof. Goldsmith: Animals.

Dr. Tarriere: X-ray, x-ray cinegraph, x-ray movie would be helpful.

Prof. Goldsmith: What I have on the neck injury criteria is, A, physiological, B, mechanical, C, how does cadaver testing correlate. We can do this by human volunteers, get fractures, dislocation and subluxal location of vertebral bodies from cadavers and physiological damage restricted to animals.

Then there is the reconstruction of accidents. I think I have one more point that needs definition. It involves a question of functional versus structural failure. I don't know what that means.

Mr. Marcus: I think it's what we were talking about before with the physiological versus the mechanical.

Prof. Goldsmith: Oh. Okay. That's been covered. Gentleman, have you anything else?

Dr. Tarriere: The face. That's a part of the head and there are two sides for this question. The problem of the brain injury leading to a facial. You said that's the face impact, one among an infinity.

Dr. Aldman: Contact.

Dr. Tarriere: There is also the problem of face injuries for themselves, their own soft tissue and so on.

Dr. Stalnaker: I think we covered that. That was under the facial contact. We were talking about loading of the skull, direct loading of the skull.

Dr. Tarriere: Maybe. That is a problem for the physical model for that.

Prof. Goldsmith: Okay. It will be mentioned.

Human Research Group Proceedings

Dr. Ommaya: As I see it, the key things we want to pin down are the type of data we can obtain from the human injury situation and to determine which aspects of human head and neck injury should be modeled. While we discuss these issues, colleagues on the Human Surrogate Research Subcommittee will be talking about what types of models are available and which may be systematically used.

Dr. Gennarelli: A lot of work by neurosurgeons is trying to define outcome from injuries and the work of the Glasgow Group has led to a formulation known as the Glasgow Coma Scale which evolved from earlier work by others and is now generally accepted as a useful predictor of injury outcome. While opinions about the validity of using such a scale differ, this Coma Scale has successfully served to gather groups of patients who have suffered relatively the same head injury severity. I think one of the problems we have had in head injury research—and I am sure the neck suffers from the same thing—is that if I have a series of patients from my hospital and you have one from your hospital, it has been very difficult to tell how comparable those groups of patients are. We are now much more aware of different kinds of injuries, but also of different severities of injury of the same kind.

Many neurosurgeons have been working on these two questions in the last few years and at least we now have an idea of how to classify our patient groups. We could start out with various people's ideas of how to classify head injury patients. Phil, do you have problems with the Glasgow Coma Scale?

Dr. Gildenberg: Yes. I think it was perhaps unfortunate that the Glasgow Scale was adopted by so many people, somewhat prematurely. My criticism is that the scale differentiates fairly readily between people who are at the very minor end of the range of head trauma and very poorly between patients in the in-between range, and only grossly at the more severe end.

Basically what is done when the Glasgow Coma Scale is used for statistical purposes is as follows: There are three categories of information that are used: eye opening, verbal response, and then the best motor response. In anyone who has more than a mild head injury, i.e., a coma, the eye opening is invariably one; the verbal response is one, that is, no response, or else the patients are intubated, so you end up with a scale of only five degrees of freedom. Once you start working with this scale in patients with significant and severe head injury, it turns out you have just insufficient categories that don't differentiate nearly well enough with enough sensitivity.

We have started to use another scale, which we call the Houston Coma Scale, which is a continuum of some 15 different levels, which is based on two questions. One question is: What is the least stimulus required to get a response from the patient? The second question is: What is that response? Which is actually what people do automatically when they look at a patient. You look to see if the patient is spontaneously awake. If not, you call their name and if they don't respond to that, you pinch them or apply a painful stimulus. So "What is the least of these stimuli to get a response?", then just a description of the response gives you a lot more information than artificially separating verbal and eye opening as criteria.

In addition to the problems we have with the Coma Scale being perhaps too rough an index of severity, we also, because of ignorance of knowing how better to classify patients, have a few very specific criteria. Penetrating wounds could be accompanied by subdural hematoma which it may or may not be possible to classify at the moment as subacute or acute, or there may be an epidural hematoma or other associated lesions in other types of patients. The most challenging group of patients are these "others" and yet we don't have the means to ferret them out. It is more likely that this will depend on physiologic parameters rather than an analysis of the biomechanics of the injury itself. But we do need more information about what really is the nature of the injury in order to classify the trauma better. Certainly the CT scan has been a tremendous help in that regard in that we now have some direct anatomical means or direct means of seeing anatomical disruption prior to autopsy.

So I think that adding CT criteria to the list in order to subclassify these "others" will be very helpful. For different purposes it is sometimes better to lump and sometimes it is better to split. I think in most of the things that we are doing right now, we are erring in the direction of lumping perhaps too much. This "other" group, the closed head injury or the diffuse head injury group, is really a group of very different entities that we are just classifying together at the moment. And I think we have to split a little more finely in order to start to investigate the differences in the outcome in the different groups of patients.

Dr. Ommaya: Can we agree roughly, before we go into the details, that—it seems that we would all agree that we need two kinds of scores, at least for head injuries, and maybe two separate kinds of scores for neck injury. One would be a clincial score and it would be some variant of either the Glasgow Coma Scale or Houston Scale or the duration of coma or the old amnesia plus coma. In response to Dr. Gildenberg I would like to remind you that many years before the Glasgow Coma Scale I had proposed a system of coding Head Injuries for identical scoring needs—perhaps in too much detail! There would be also a CT scoring of some kind. We need CT scan for this and the clinical data will have to be correlated in a well-designed prospective study.

Dr. Gildenberg: We are talking really about one score being a rough index of severity so that patients can be classified according to severity, both for statistical and outcome purposes, and another, a finer definition of the actual nature of the injury.

Dr. Ommaya: Yes. What I was trying to get at was the practical method. In other words, if you have a patient and you want to get one index, should that index be the result of a clinical plus CT examination, and then you come up with a score and say, this patient is type XD, and give some kind of score? And, like for a neck injury, you would give clinical plus an x-ray study and say, this is it.

Dr. Levine: An existing scoring method which is useful in many areas is the AIS. Those of us who use it in cadaver research can attempt to compare an AIS from our cadaver lesions with that for people in real-life accidents.

The AIS method is well accepted by the automobile impact people and I think it is a scale which we could probably try to correlate with the other scales that exist now and are being used by treating physicians. It is based on survivability, although I think it has weak areas in neck and head injuries and limb injuries also because it doesn't talk about long-term morbidity. But it is also a survivability scale.

Dr. Ommaya: Yes. Actually the AIS grades the severity at the time of the accident but really doesn't tell you too much about the subsequent outcome.

Dr. Levine: No.

Dr. Ommaya: So if we could somehow link the medical scales such as the Glasgow score and tie it into the AIS we would have the advantage that the AIS is in place in terms of accident investigation. This would greatly simplify our research efforts.

Dr. Gennarelli: Dr. Rehman.

Dr. Rehman: I think in reference to the point being raised about CAT scans for detail, right now under the direction of Professor Hurt, as you know, we are carrying on a program of comparison between CAT scan and detailed layer by layer autopsy in fatal motorcycle accident cases to see whether the CAT scan gives us enough detail so that the information gained would be adequate.

I don't think we know at the moment what the comparative results are, because that data hasn't yet been resolved? Has it, Harry?

Dr. Hurt: No. It so far is very indefinite. The description of the aggregate of injuries is fairly good, but that composition is just almost impossible to define.

Dr. Levine: Is anyone using the injury coding book that has been published by NHTSA for head injuries?

Dr. Ommaya: Yes, there is an ongoing study funded by NHTSA in Philadelphia.

Dr. Gennarelli: We have used it in Philadelphia to classify CT scans but with some modification. And once you convince the neuroradiologist that it is not quite so cumbersome as it looks, it is workable. I don't know if anyone has used it for pathological studies.

Dr. Levine: There are parts of that study that were fairly well worked out, that we really haven't tested.

Dr. Gennarelli: I think some of the problems from NHTSA's viewpoint of the situation are that we have two varieties of problems, things that we can see with the CT scan, the subdural hematomas and the big hemorrhages and so on inside the brain. Those are relatively little problems because they can be well defined, either by anatomy if the patient dies, or by CAT scan if the patient survives, and one sooner or later can study those phenomena and develop mechanisms for them and failure criteria, if you will, somehow, with some sort of research project. The other problem, as I see it, is, as Phil said, with the "other" group, the things that we call diffuse injuries, which really means that there is nothing to see either at autopsy or in most CT scans; the CAT scan is often normal or virtually normal. Unless very detailed pathology is done in the nonsurvivors, very little may be seen. And yet in automotive accidents, those lesions comprise a high percentage of the cases.

Dr. Ommaya: That is correct, and in addition such diffuse lesions are probably the major determinants of one outcome.

Dr. Rehman: I think that this is one of the things we have been finding in our study. Our autopsies show that there are many significant lesions that you can't pick up on x-ray. We normally x-ray the individuals, both A/P's laterals, and pillar views and so on, and you see nothing there. And, as a matter of fact, in the 30 or so cases with CT scans there was also a difference of opinion between the results of one layer dissection at autopsy and the CAT scans. Thus you couldn't pick up the injuries on the CAT scans. It is not unreasonable to say that in patients with such soft tissue injuries, who survive, the morbidity is going to be very high. But we don't know exactly how to pin-point what will be happening clinically on the basis of what we have been finding.

So I think the point you are bringing up, which is certainly more than valid, is that we have these so-called diffuse injuries that in themselves may not be sufficient to cause death but can cause a considerable posttraumatic sequalae.

Dr. Ommaya: And that brings us back to the point that Phil raised, that you have to be concerned with the clinical classification because it really wasn't detailed enough for research purposes. On the other hand, the Glasgow Coma Scale is quite well established as a clinical tool. In the process of collecting the Houston score data, for example, could you relate it to the Glasgow Coma score data?

Dr. Gildenberg: Well, actually one of the things we did when we designed the Houston Coma Score— was to define our categories in such a way that we can ask the computer to turn them into the Glasgow Scale for statistical purposes.

Dr. Ommaya: At the present time you are recording the AIS score on these patients as they come in?

Dr. Gildenberg: No, we are not.

Dr. Ommaya: I think Dr. Gennarelli's group is probably the only one who has done that with NHTSA support.

That is the kind of thing which I think would be very important to do in order to obtain valid data relating accident injury severity and outcome.

Dr. Gildenberg: One of the things that seems to be evolving as a suggestion that might come directly from this conference is to survey those people who are keeping head trauma data and to see if such things as the AIS score or the categories from the NHTSA CT scan head injury coding book might be used as a guideline for the manner in which the information is accumulated.

For instance, we have six or seven head injury centers supported by NIH which are putting together information which includes CT scan data and, as far as I know, there is not really a well thought out data base for using that CT information, and yet there is one available that has not been disseminated to each of the centers.

Dr. Ommaya: That is a very good point. I think that is something which you might want to make as a formal recommendation, i.e., how we can tie in

NHTSA's efforts to the existing NIH head injury centers.

Dr. Levine: This meeting has made me realize some of us who have been in NHTSA-supported impact research should really try to get together with you guys who are supported by NIH so that we can talk together. I think there hasn't been enough communication between the automobile impact workers and other workers in biomechanics interested in the physiopathology and impact injury.

Dr. McLaurin: Tom, I would like to complicate the problem just a little bit further. The only things that have been mentioned this morning so far as tools for obtaining injury criteria are the Glasgow Coma Scale and the CT scan, which I agree are the most common methods of assessment at the moment. Whatever we decide in terms of those are going to be complicated a year or two down the line by further observations on what happens to intracranial pressure monitoring, what happens to recording of various kinds of sensory evoked potentials and probably other things such as cerebral blood flow. There could be many other criteria that are going to be added to the mix.

Therefore I think we should recognize at this point, that there are many other methods of clinical assessment, that are being introduced and are going to be introduced that will sharpen our focus on the intracranial pathophysiology as we go down the line.

The second thing that I wanted to mention is that we seem to like to make an observation at one point in time and then try to predict everything in relation to an observation made at that one point in time, whether it is the Glasgow Coma Scale on admission or the CT scan on admission, or whatever. I think that we have to keep in mind that there may be some merit to sequential observations and that the time element should be considered in our clinical assessment.

Dr. Levine: I am going to jump back to the AIS. It sounds like the AIS is a scale that is really a summation of many things, and we might be able to do a sequential AIS day by day and say, okay, we will take all this data we have and convert it to an AIS.

Dr. Ommaya: This would mean expanding and modifying the present way that you obtain the AIS score. If we expand it to include neurophysiological, neuropsychological and CT scan we would certainly get a very superior AIS score related not only to the initial injury severity but also a better predictor of outcome. However, I doubt whether this can be done without changing the idea of the AIS score that we would create a totally different entity.

Dr. Gennarelli: I agree. The AIS is conceptually a different kind of scale. It is designed as a global severity measure, that is, it is determinable only once in any one patient. Your particular injury is either an AIS-1, 2 or a 3 and so on. Whereas the Glasgow Coma Scale is designed as a sequential system. Thus Glasgow Coma score measures what I would call instantaneous severity indices, as opposed to global, like the AIS.

The problem is that there aren't many other scales that are global like the AIS, and I think it is not going to change substantially in the near future, since it has just been revised, at least in terms of adding in other factors right now. But it can be used in order to compare with these other instantaneous scales, the Houston Scale, the Glasgow Scale, etc.

Dr. Gildenberg: Before one can define what a good scale would be, one has to define the purpose for which it is going to be used. For instance, a six-category scale is really ideal for statistical purposes. It has enough degrees of freedom to be able to differentiate patients, if the six categories are reasonably equally weighted. But it is absolutely inadequate, for instance as far as defining groups of patients on a clinical basis to determine eventual outcome.

So I think we have to remain flexible enough so that we can, for different purposes, rely on different scales. Now, the AIS may be part of this clinical scale which eventually will be used for outcome. But more than that would be needed for other purposes.

Ms. Pedder: Can I just back up that comment? I think the problem with the AIS is the fact, that in a way, it is often an anticipated outcome scale. When you are asking, what are you going to use the scale for, the main answer is for economic purposes. The outcome, in my opinion, is one of the primary interests, as a nonclinician, in terms of all the road trauma. Speaking economically that is in fact what you need to know in order to improve existing legislation, regulations and various other matters too. The best argument is often to say how much it is going to cost. In order to do that, you have got to not only look at the outcome, but also at the length, the extent of treatment, and the type of treatment required.

I agree that the AIS certainly is very short on this. Personally I think, from our own experience, there is no way that we can relate real outcome back to the AIS score that was given at the time of treatment.

Dr. Gildenberg: Well, actually there is no real way to devise a scale in anticipation. One has to test different means of scaling and validate that against recognized outcome in a fairly large group of patients before a scale could be used for such purposes.

Ms. Pedder: Yes.

Dr. Gildenberg: If one is to use a scale to assign priorities for allocation of resources, that has to be a proven and accurate outcome scale.

Ms. Pedder: Yes. I think there has been one developed called the Comprehensive Road Injury Scale or CRIS. This has in fact got a treatment period scale in it, which in fact we have been checking against, and it looks pretty good. I feel very strongly that one should not only assess the injury as it comes in to the Emergency Room but I feel strongly one should have a follow-up.

Dr. Gildenberg: This is one of the things that we are right in getting a daily data base on patients and looking back as to what is the earliest time that we can accurately predict outcome at a given confidence level.

We had one project going where the Glasgow Scale neurological exam was done hourly after the patient arrived to see if maybe the second hour or the fourth hour might give us a better index than on arrival.

What we found was that the patients were so involved with having other things done during those first six hours that it just wasn't possible to assess the patients after the second hour. By the second hour, they were maybe in CT, possibly sedated for their CT, possibly in the operating room, not yet upon the monitor. So that it may be that a 24-hour scale would be the ideal scale.

Dr. Lindgren: May I draw your attention to this chart which follows Dr. Ommaya's suggestion that we need a classification as well as a more detailed description of the focal injuries. By the way, Teasdale and Jennet have pronounced the Glasgow Coma Score as the best, ten days ago in Rotterdam. Firstly the clinical scales such as the Glasgow Coma Scale assess the severity of disturbance of consciousness. Assessment of focal lesions can be done by CT scan and by pathoanatomy when available. The secondary lesions which are initiated by the trauma, but do not become evident to the clinician until later on, cannot easily be assessed by the clinical methods.

Dr. Lindgren's Chart

Kinematics	Intracranial Mechanics	"Primary" or Immediate Input Lesions	"Secondary" 6 hours (Expansive lesions)
Assessment	Specific?	Diffusive damage Clinical scales (Unconsciousness)	Clinical signs Intracranial pressure (ICP) CT
		Focal damage —clinical features —CT scan — Pathoanatomy	(operation) (autopsy) More influenced by nonimpact factions—med. care, transportation, etc.
Existing Head Injury Criteria Approaches			

I don't think that it is possible today to come to an agreement about the intracranial mechanics, for instance, to construct head injury criteria based on the kinematics as I have shown, nor is it possible to obtain agreement about the secondary complications; you have to go to the immediate impact damage and assess it clinically as well as with CT scan and the pathoanatomy.

So if we have to try to make a start, we must go into the two middle columns and utilize the third column to understand a second.

Dr. Gennarelli: How serious are the individual injuries? I think if one would start with that, we would certainly be a lot further along. The cost of treatment is often dependent on all of the factors we have mentioned. For instance, the length of hospitalization as a first cut may be a reasonable measure of injury severity, although there are many noninjury factors that would go into that. In terms of global epidemiological studies, if you are talking about hundred of thousands of patients, some of these factors may smooth out. But for individual patients, I think we would be pretty inaccurate in terms of describing severity if we confined ourselves only to the primary injuries.

Let's say we can solve the problem of classifying injuries and attributing some severity to them, is the outcome that we see going to relate to that in any way, or is it going to relate to all these secondary factors?

Dr. Ommaya: The best hypotheses are those which can be most easily tested and refuted if inadequate. I would therefore suggest that we take the data now available from the Coma Scale studies, e.g., by Overgard and by Jennet et al. which suggest a major influence of the primary factors as indicated by Dr. Lindgren and only a minor effect by the secondary factors—I would suggest the figure of 80% for Primary Injury effects and 20% for Secondary Injury effects on outcome and proceed to test this prediction.

Dr. Hurt: I see a conflict there, because in the motorcycle injury cases that we have looked at in the last couple of years, the outcome has been fairly sensitive to the management. So that there is a great disparity in some of the cases by comparison.

Dr. Ommaya: Yes, but please note that your cases were selected for fatality, i.e., at the most severe end of the scale.

Dr. Gildenberg: When we include outcome, we really have to relate to everything that is going to influence the outcome, which must include the nature of the injury, the secondary complication factors, the speed at which treatment is begun, the type of treatment, and then all of these factors together are going to determine what the outcome is going to be. So if one starts to assess outcome, one has to consider everything that leads up to it, some factors, of course, being much more important than others.

There is a certain group of patients that are going to die, no matter what is done. There is another group that is going to do fine, no matter what is done. And then for the big group in the middle, they may go one way or the other, depending on the intervention.

Dr. Ommaya: I would question the sizes of these groups. Perhaps the group in the middle—significant modulation of the outcome by our interventions may be true only for a minority, i.e., not more than 20%.

Dr. Hurt: In the **individual** case it may be a very strong effect, for example, we have an accident notification and the the victim goes to Martin Luther King Hospital in South LA and we know that is going to be the most likely case for our fatality study. And then we have another accident notification and the victim goes to Huntington Memorial and we know that he will most probably survive, i.e., very marked difference in outcome according to the treatment.

Dr. Ommaya: Again, I would like to remind the audience that Dr. Hurt is talking about mortality and not quality of survival.

Dr. Gildenberg: This also illustrates another factor that concerns outcome, just where the patient is referred and the manner in which the decision is made.

Dr. Ommaya: I would like to reiterate that in terms of both quality and extent of survival the effect of treatment as a major influence on outcome is not suggested in the epidemiological data I have seen so far. I mean to say that what you are talking about may be to emphasize that type of management affects **individual** treatment of patients and their outcomes very significantly, but when you look at large numbers of patients, for example, in the book on Epidemiology of Head Injuries in England and Wales, management seemed to make no difference in terms of the mortality. I am referring to the Field Report.

So on this in-between group, Phil, that you are talking about, I am questioning how big is that group.

Dr. Gildenberg: I think that the data that you are referring to may be coincidental more than anything else. Very often a group like that is looked at as far as over-all mortality is selected by relatively arbitrary means. The patient referral system will determine how the—the composition of the group and, consequently, what the outcome may be, as, for instance, may occur in LA, depending on—if you look at the outcome figures for those two different hospitals, you will find much different outcomes.

Dr. Ommaya: But how do you explain the data on outcome from the three centers that were compared, in Glasgow, California and the Netherlands which also came out with fairly equivalent figures for outcome in terms of initial assessment of the primary injury?

Dr. Gildenberg: Yes, but again, the pattern of referral to those three centers was so different that one can't conceive that they are the same group of patients. One of the things that we are finding in Houston is an example of the effect of treatment. Our hospital is a private hospital and it turns out that we have the helicopters and next door to us at the Ben Taub County Hospital, they rely strictly on ambulances. Our patient profile, the group of patients, is just completely different. If you look at the types of injuries, they are different; if you look at the severity of injury, they are much different.

So I think one can't look at just raw outcome figures and say, well, they are the same. There is a narrow group of patients in the middle where management does make a difference. If you dilute that with the big groups of patients on either end, if you have a 50-percent decrease in mortality in just that middle group but that only constitutes 10 percent of the entire group, it is going to be hidden in all the static.

Dr. Ommaya: I agree that the group of patients in which management is critical may be a small proportion submerged within the large and small group.

Dr. Gildenberg: I think that is true. The treatment group is a relatively small group hidden within the overall group. If you have a hospital that admits everyone who had just transient loss of consciousness after a head injury, that may make up half of their head injuries.

Dr. Ommaya: Right.

Dr. Gildenberg: So you have 50 percent as a group that is going to survive and do well, with no treatment at all.

Dr. Ommaya: Right.

Dr. Gildenberg: Another hospital may admit very few of those patients. And consequently the group of patients where treatment does make a difference may constitute a much larger portion of that group.

Dr. Ommaya: That is a very critical hypothesis. Because it would be very important for NHTSA to know that we do have an outcome measurement index that would be very sensitive to overall management. This is something that the AIS cannot give us.

Dr. Eppinger. I agree, we want the global outcome. If there are hospitals that don't provide good care and there are hospitals that do, we want the average. Given that somebody comes up with this, we want to see today what kind of trauma should we go after, what kind of trauma should we prevent? We cannot at this stage make the management of head and neck injuries uniform.

Dr. Gildenberg: Well, that's the problem, that you can't take an average and find out the truth about the efficiency of management.

Dr. Eppinger. But that is what is happening in the real world now!

Dr. Gildenberg: That's right. But in order for us as neurosurgeons to advise the government of the best policies for patient treatment we have to determine the truth in comparable patient groups and not lump all groups together.

Dr. Ommaya: What I am also concerned about is the discrepancy between AIS scores and ultimate outcome. Dr. Gennarelli has done a study showing that there was good correlation between initial injury severity, AIS score, and cost. The higher the AIS score, the higher the cost. Another study by one of the NHTSA scientists gave different results for **outcome.** This study included family factors, the long-term psychological effects of trauma, and the data suggested an **inverse** correlation of injury. In other words, with AIS the ones who had lesser injuries ended up costing more to society because there were more chronic problems as compared to the ones who died and had more severe injuries, probably because the management of their problems was settled earlier.

Dr. Graham: You could start by comparing clinical management between different hospitals and institutions. But I think you must have some index of what the cause of death is.

Dr. Ommaya: Yes. I think that is very important, as well as developing indices for the causes of mortality.

Dr. Graham: And I think this has been totally ignored up to date. We talk about outcomes or predictions, but we ignore actually from what the patient has eventually died.

We recently started doing this in Glasgow, and it is amazing in fact how good the correspondence is between clinical and ultimate pathological details. But there is a group of about 10 percent where the two data sets are so divergent that we need other indices, be it clinical or pathological or whatever, in order to get some assessment as to why the patient has actually died. When you actually get people to commit themselves as to why they think someone has died, it is very different.

Dr. McLaurin: It seems to me that we should at this point define really what our purpose is in the prediction of outcome.

Admitting that there is a difference in quality of care, the input that is going to come from this group and our immediate associates, is going to be, one, the value of better quality of care, two, the immediate effects of the trauma, not what may develop five years down the line, i.e., what the psychological family costs, unemployment rates, etc., are. We are not going to get that type of outcome predictions from this group. On the other hand, if you want to know what the outcome will be in the immediate future when the "ideal" treatment has been applied, then I think you can get it from this group. And maybe that is what our objective should be, because that is what we can do to improve the quality of care by developing standards of such care for national use.

But we must recognize that this will be the opinions of Gennarelli in Philadelphia, me in Cincinnati, Phil Gildenberg in Houston, Ayub Ommaya here in Washington, D.C. and so on. We are only going to be dealing with a set of very idealized settings in which we treat patients using an idealized method of treatment.

If we are talking about trying to represent the overall impact of treatment across the nation, forget it. We are not going to get it from this group.

Ms. Pedder: I don't know. I tend to disagree with you there. We are not only seeking to know about **care**. I think I agree with you in terms of maybe not clearly knowing the longer-term outcomes. I have used the word "economic" perhaps wrongly and been misunderstood. What you said concerning the long-term psychological effects is very possibly true because they are very illusive and hard to quantify.

But we certainly learn a lot about the overall outcome from the detailed clinical data. I am with the Accident Research Group in Birmingham (England) and I assume that Dr. Ommaya has the same understanding, that we certainly do see the immediate effects, at least we receive the immediate clinical information as it is interpreted for us by a clinician. Now, what we in fact are very aware of is that, especially with the young seriously injured patients, e.g., the motorcycling population, there is a very significant effect which is indeed the immediate effect of the trauma on such person's prognoses, e.g., their ability to continue their job, to be able to take care of himself, etc. Now, I am not talking about the truly long-term effects, e.g., whether the patient is going to be able to cope maritally and I am not talking about what I think are the more elusive things such as the quality of his future contributions to society. But I would consider it very important to know the immediate effects as described in any consideration of a scaling system to assess head and neck injury severity.

Dr. McLaurin: But you have heard at least two examples already this morning, of the significant differences in the standard of care between hospitals in the U.S. Would that not have a major effect on outcome?

Ms. Pedder: Yes. That is obviously a problem, maybe more so in the U.S.A. than in England where the standard of care is more uniform. Perhaps the gentleman from Glasgow would know more about that.

Dr. Ommaya: I would propose that because the **existing data** comparing mortality and morbidity outcomes from countries (U.S., England, Holland, and Scandinavia) are so similar that it is reasonable to hypothesize that "quality of care" differences may **not** be a significant **issue**, at least for the more severe cases.

Dr. Eppinger: I would like to make a point. Consider this problem not to be an open-loop function where we have to have the absolute answer out at this point. I will give you an example. The old AIS scale was instituted maybe 8, 10 years ago, and we collected lots and lots of accident data to do that. And by one of our definitions the most severe level of injury, AIS 6 is defined by death within 30 days. So as you would read that scale and assign a less severe case and AIS 3 you may say there is **no** chance of death. It is just a moderate injury. But as we go back into the accident data, there is a **certain probability** of death from an AIS 3. It might be an elderly patient that had a leg fracture, a fatty embolism or pneumonia, some subsequent secondary effects of the initial trauma. But there is a certain portion of our population that dies from that type of trauma. That is what we would like to see come back to us in our follow-up data. So what started out as a consensus of opinion of **risk** of this type of trauma would be supplemented by feedback from our actual data to tell us that although initially we thought nobody would die or that the risk is low, would then be calibrated by the true risk of the measure or scale assignments.

Dr. McLaurin: Okay. But what is your original contact with the individual who has been injured?

Dr. Eppinger: By our accident teams.

Dr. McLaurin: Okay. You see, if you pick them up at that point, then you can follow it. If you pick it up when they arrive in the intensive care unit, that is a totally different population.

Dr. Eppinger: I understand.

That is why I would like to describe this new system that we are putting into effect. This National Accident Severity Sampling or NASS System has 57 teams strategically located over the total United States, where they go in to attempt to get detailed accident data so we know what is happening with vehicles and also the victim follow-up.

Dr. Gennarelli: There is a problem with that. I would like to see that this problem be advanced as one of the recommendations of this Consensus Workshop. The problem is that there is a gross mismatch in the NASS data between the amount and quality of medical data. It is almost a 100-to-1 mismatch. I don't know if the clinicians here are familiar with the kind of engineering detail, which is obtained on these accidents, e.g., the measurements of deformations and computations of the weight of the vehicle and the speed, etc.

Dr. Ommaya: I agree that the NASS obtains superb data from the accident on the vehicle and its mechanical behavior but does not contain equivalent quality of medical data.

Dr. Gildenberg: Not only does there appear to be a mismatch between the amount and quality of data from the engineering and medical aspects, but also there is a mismatch between the location of the NASS teams and that of physicians collecting medical data. It would seem that if there were some coordination between the location of these 57 NASS centers and those centers that are collecting physiologic data, e.g., the Head Injury Centers and the Spinal Cord Injury Centers supported by the NIH . . . it would become possible to put together these two huge masses of data and start looking at possible correlations.

Dr. Ommaya: This discussion addresses very precisely the question No. 8 in our preliminary charge as presented by Dr. Digges. How are we going to effect this dialogue, which is very much needed?

Dr. Gennarelli: I don't know if you saw the recent HSRI summary of the NASS system. Did you go through it?

Dr. Ommaya: Yes.

Dr. Gennarelli: There is very little **useful** information in there because of the lack of detail in the medical information. I am not sure what to do about that, short of having physicians on each of the NASS teams to quality-control the medical data so that it is uniform.

Dr. Levine: But breaking that data out even by a physician looking at the medical records is not the answer.

Dr. Gennarelli: Yes, that is true. You cannot extract this kind of information from the face sheet of the standard hospital record.

Dr. Gildenberg: Standard hospital records are useless, absolutely. But there are Head Injury Centers where they are collecting a lot of data. I don't know how good it is, at any rate, they are collecting a lot of data. But these data are not related in any way to the NASS data. It is as if there were two separate groups of patients. If the two data sets could be brought together, there would be a tremendous advance in the utilization of these two resources.

Dr. Rehman: I think in all this discussion the points you have just raised cover really two points, the accident, the collection of data at the scene, and the clinical data. Now, I would suggest adding an additional factor to that, and that is the autopsy data.

Dr. Levine: There is also the quality of autopsy. We have to standardize our autopsy data. Maybe it might take a pilot research project in selected areas to make sure that we are getting a high-quality autopsy and a high-quality medical injury evaluation of patients who survive and really set the format of how we want it done and then advance into a prospective study to look at every accident in epidemiologically selected areas.

Dr. Graham: As you know, Glasgow has been associated with detailed autopsies and neuropathological reports from head injuries for the last decade. But it has been absolutely dependent on an agreement with the Crown Office. In other words, the lawyers are happy that we do this and we provide reports which they subsequently use for medical-legal purposes. And without their backup and willingness, this would not take place. We have endeavored to get other centers in Europe and North America to join us in this venture. The medical-legal considerations are so overriding in the U.S. that this may not happen.

Dr. Ommaya: It can happen if we somehow could arrange a marriage—of convenience between at least some of the head injury and spinal cord injury centers that are doing the detailed kinds of medical research like Phil Gildenberg and Tom Gennarelli are doing and NHTSA. We do have a working relationship between Philadelphia and NHTSA; and it has really been very effective for some kinds of data. If this mechanism of the NASS teams could somehow be linked—and it should be obviously a two-way link; it can't come all from NHTSA. It has to come from NIH as well. Somehow these two groups have to get together so that this kind of dialogue—and probably we shouldn't make it too rigid. I think there should be comparability in some way, but there should be the ability, for example, for Phil to do **his** kind of scaling but be able to talk to the other centers in an agreed scaling language.

Dr. Gildenberg: You are proposing a marriage where both partners have a job.

Dr. Ommaya: Right.

Dr. Gildenberg: So that each works independently, but yet at the end of the day they come home and have dinner together.

Dr. Ommaya: Exactly.

Dr. McLaurin: I hate to be repetitive in this question. But I agree that a marriage is probably a good thing, whether it is arranged or shotgun or whatever. But I am still a little bit vague in my own mind and I would like for some of you to sort of define for me what the purpose of this marriage is. Because I think that the mechanics of it will be very much related to the purpose of it. And I am not clear in my own mind what you see as the purpose of the marriage.

I can see several different possible purposes, all of them good: prevention, treatment, outcome, predictability, economic, etc. I can see a lot of different purposes.

But I think that we should really define what our main purpose is in order to try to establish the best possible relationship to achieve that purpose. And I am not quite sure what that is.

Dr. Ommaya: I think the main immediate purpose would be to correct what Tom pointed out, and that is the mismatch of data, to have a better match, so that useful correlations between the mechanical input and the biologic response can be made.

Dr. Levine: If I may, isn't it accident, morbidity and mortality reduction on the highways?

Dr. Ommaya: That is the long-term goal, which can only be reached if first we succeed in our immediate purpose.

Dr. Levine: Well, this is still our main purpose.

Dr. McLaurin: I hear one person talking about prevention. I hear a lot of different things being discussed, and it seems to be that we—that until we define in our minds what the short-term and maybe the—long-term objectives are. . . .

Dr. Ommaya: Let me suggest one way to see these objectives. The long-term goal of NIH-supported research in head and neck injury is to improve the quality of care, and secondarily to improve prevention, because that is not their main goal in trauma research. NHTSA's goal is primarily to improve prevention and secondarily to improve care by understanding the **mechanisms** of such injuries.

Now, I think these are overlapping goals. And what impedes us in reaching these overlapping and mutually complementary goals is a crucial short-term problem, i.e., a complete mismatch of data, like Tom Gennarelli was pointing out between detailed mechanical data for the input based on accident data up to the entry into the hospital and the detailed medical data maintained separately from the accident data by two sets of investigators only vaguely aware of what the other is trying to do.

Dr. McLaurin: But then you have to define for me what the purpose of matching the data is, what the purpose of achieving a good match is.

Dr. Ommaya: Okay, I thought I just did that a little while ago but I will do so again.

Dr. Liu: Can I speak to that briefly?

Dr. Ommaya: Yes. Go ahead.

Dr. Liu: What it is, purely from the researcher's point of view, that right now the biomedical data that is gotten is a very detailed sort of output data, and that data somehow is not correlated to the input data, which is the accident investigation, you see. In order to bring a functional relationship between these two things, that is why the marriage in a sense is necessary.

Phil may have a patient whom he monitors for the coming six months with all sorts of data, but if we don't have any idea concerning the type of injury or even the possibility of an accident reconstruction in the case, the ability to be able to relate what caused this injury, what were the mechanical problems that caused the injury, and the outcome, there will never be a chance to learn that functional relationship. But if we put it together, there will be that chance.

Dr. Gildenberg: And this might help define, then, this "other" group much better?

Dr. Ommaya: Yes.

Dr. McLaurin: I'm way down the road a little bit further than that, though, and I still am asking, having correlated all this, what do you see as the ultimate objective?

Dr. Eppinger: We put out a safety standard. From the NHTSA point of view, that is our sole way of utilizing the results of such studies. We build that into standard test devices and we put out a rule and after considering other economic and cost factors we can turn to the auto manufacturer, and indicate to him the speed at which crash testing is required and also which engineering measurements are to be made and provide the level of the indices below which the measures must read. This implies that the trauma produced in that situation on the average will be below a certain level.

Dr. McLaurin: Okay. So you are really looking at it from the standpoint of prevention, then.

Dr. Eppinger: That's correct.

Dr. McLaurin: But, you see, other people are looking at it from the standpoint of "What is the ultimate outcome, the accident having occurred. . . .

Dr. Eppinger: Wait. Let me explain further. That is how we measure the outcome of how effective we should be or where we set out limits. If I can advise automobile manufacturers that by altering the mechanical environment from what it is today to another level, I would reduce the probability of your becoming an injury statistic or fatality—or the total fatality rate nationwide would be reduced from the present level to a lower level. That might ultimately be calculated as an economic effect, by putting a dollar worth on a life. It might even be a distribution over age, or it might indicate reduction of expenditures for health of unnecessary highway injuries.

We also can go back and ascertain the economic costs through each one of the, let's say 4 or 5 severity rankings—that eventually if a person is in the hospital 60 days and has another recovery period of 60 days, we end up by estimating that severity ranking X costs in X dollars, etc. So to find out what the ultimate outcome is, it is a measure in dollars of the effect of our standards on injury prevention. But we have to go through this very tenuous link of some sort of impairment and so forth. What is a 10-percent impairment, dollarwise? What does a 10-percent impairment mean?

Ms. Pedder: I think the other point also is that perhaps even before you make those safety measures, having a common basic information source enables one to identify the problem and thereby to formulate **new** protective measures, safety measures.

Dr. Eppinger: Let me describe how we function: We look at our data, and classify the types of automotive crash events, by direction and so forth. And then we establish priorities by asking—How many people get killed in frontal crashes, how many get killed in lateral crashes, how many in roll-overs? This classification of the mechancial event, because when we promulgate a standard, we have to make a physical test of the system, the car. So we say, if 50 percent of the people are killed frontally and only 2 percent are roll-overs, of all fatalities, and we are trying to reduce fatalities, it is best to go after frontal accident. Therefore we will focus on that. This will also affect our test devices and planning of tests to simulate all the types of trauma that are produced in these frontal impacts. How do injuries occur? Is it because occupants are thrown around, or whatever? And we sift down all this data until we get a handle on the mechanism of injury.

When we finally put out a regulation, it has to be very, very specific. The car goes down straight in here, it runs into some type of collision barrier exactly at 30 miles an hour, and the dummy readings have to be calculated this way, the dummy's position is specified etc. But we need to have good medical data for injury severity **and** injury outcome correlated with mechanical input data which have been analyzed and on which judgments are made, before we come down to that final test point.

Dr. Gildenberg: What we are talking about really is—that basically we don't know enough about the mechanisms of head trauma and spine trauma.

I am sure if that data base correlating injury input and injury outcome were today available, one could go around this table and have every person at the table use that data in a different fashion for some particular end, the clinicians to improve their treatment and the engineers to improve design standards.

Dr. McLaurin: I agree with that up to a point, Phil. But I get back to the point that I raised a while ago, and that is that if you are talking about **national** data on the outcome of injuries you are not going to get it from what we are going to put in, because our management of injuries is done in an idealized setting. And that is not going to give us a true picture of the average management effect or outcome when diluted by cases treated in a less than ideal circumstance.

Dr. Gennarelli: I don't think that is the point, though. I think the situation, at least as I understand the problem, is that you are at an accident scene, let's say, or you are in the emergency room, and five patients come in with head injuries or spine injuries and you evaluate them and you say, this guy has a very bad injury and I really don't think he's going to make it and this one over here, it looks like he can go home in five minutes, and the other three in the middle have moderate injuries. I think the whole problem is to try to put that kind of clinical judgment, with everything that goes through the process, into some sort of quantitative fashion so that we can say, "Yes, this is a severe injury because . . . ." and it is not necessarily dependent on whether that patient lives or dies. But you see that patient and you know if he has a bad head injury or not.

It is in some ways related to your statistical evaluation that you make grossly in your mind of what the outcome would possibly be, at least at the bad end of the spectrum **before** management has begun. Next, we make assessment of outcome after management has begun.

Dr. Eppinger: With regard to the question of quality of medical care as it affects outcome after accidental injuries we have to take the **mean** medical care that everybody would receive, not the best or worst, but the mean. Now, let's say five years from this time for a particular trauma, some great miraculous clinical technique comes out that "cures" the effects of that injury, we would have to go back and say that that particular trauma now has much lower risk and therefore we don't even have to put out a rule that addresses that particular trauma. Or if we happen to eliminate alcohol and the spectrum changes. But at this time we have to assess what is the environment today and what are the highest priorities that we should go after.

Dr. Ommaya: We are probably getting away from the main point which is **how** to correct the mismatch of the medical and engineering data.

Dr. Levine: I wonder if we really should consider a different input. You know, we're talking a lot about using the crash as the starting point of the system. Maybe we should use the injury, that we are going to look at all head injuries that come into a given hospital and then backtrack and look at what caused this head injury, be it an automobile crash, football injury, or whatever, and then use that for the base of the system for analysis and then look from the injury to the outcome, and then go back to the cause, so that you get both the mechanical from going backward and the outcome from going forward.

Dr. Rehman: I think what you are saying is what we seem to be doing at the University of Southern California in the program that Professor Hurt is directing under the sponsorship of NHTSA. His crash investigative team is sent out after an injured patient is recovered and they get all the details regarding the cause, including the environment and the mechanical equipment. This becomes part of the **input**. Then, of course in the fatal cases when we do the autopsy and get all the details there, we get together and put the two sets of data together and then from that can predict the morbidity, had the individual survived, that we could expect.

Dr. Levine: I think also using the injury as the input to the research will stop us from spending time—analyzing noninjury accidents. Let's look at the injury accidents and look at what causes injuries. There are a lot of fender-benders that don't do very much. But let's look at the ones that really are meaningful, the ones that cause injury.

Dr. Gennarelli: I think that is a very attractive proposal. There is a lot of NASS information and time and money spent on AIS 1s and 2s. That is not the point, I don't think, that we are trying to address. And maybe your proposal is exactly right.

In my talk yesterday we just made a first cut at defining the head injuries that are bad, subdural hematoma and these so-called shearing injuries. Maybe the accident notification team ought to go out whenever a subdural hematoma comes in or a shearing lesion comes in, either to the pathologist or to one of the hospitals and investigate those accidents.

Dr. Gildenberg: Or at least select that group of patients who is going to be studied in some detail along the line. This is admittedly a select group of patients. But it would give a profile of significant patients.

Dr. McLaurin: That would make more sense to me.

Dr. Gildenberg: For instance, in our place all that would be necessary to identify those crashes that would most likely be rewarding is just to monitor the radio between our dispatcher and the helicopter.

Dr. Levine: That would also enable us to look at other things. What about a head injury from a fall in industry? Because there is not much data on falls. We need other data that might be useful for us to understand head injuries.

Dr. Gennarelli: That would be one way of cementing this marriage between the physician and the engineer that Ayub Ommaya talked about, because other government agencies are interested in falls, e.g., OSHA.

Dr. McLaurin: This is for my own information. How much investigation of an accident, for example, can be done retrospectively? I am not quite sure that I understand that.

Dr. Eppinger: The mechanical event?

Dr. McLaurin: Yes.

Dr. Eppinger: Considerable.

Dr. Liu: You can do a great deal. You can reconstruct the accident with sophisticated techniques so that—Say there is a certain dent on the hood. You can use a reasonable head form and reproduce almost an identical dent.

Dr. McLaurin: And it doesn't have to be done at the scene of the accident?

Dr. Liu: No. All of it can be done retrospectively—the data is there, the tape measurements, photographs, etc.

Dr. McLaurin: By the time he may know that the patient has got a subdural hematoma and so on, it may be several hours later.

Dr. Gildenberg: What happens in our place is that a call comes in to dispatch the helicopter and just a general description of what the injury is may come in from the referring physician or the law enforcement agency. When the helicopter gets to the scene, then the physician and the nurse on board the helicopter will stabilize things. When they lift up to come back, they radio back and they describe the nature of the injury, the cause of the injury, the severity of the injury, how many systems are involved, what treatment has been initiated. And it is on the basis of this information that we mobilize the CT scanner and the operating room before they are ever back.

Now, the average time between trauma or the estimated time of the trauma and arrival back in the emergency room is 38 minutes. So that the dispatch office knows within 10 or 15 minutes and could contact an accident investigation team within 1 hour of the accident.

Dr. McLaurin: I doubt that they have that in very many communities, though.

Dr. Levine: Yes. But, I think we have to select the communities where we can do it. We have got to pick an area which we have got the right people together, so we can get useful data.

Dr. Gildenberg: And there is no reason to believe that the type of injury or the mechanism of injury is going to be any different in Iowa than it is in Texas.

Dr. Ommaya: Agreed that learning more about the injury input is necessary, how about comments from each of us about what kind of measurements of injury in the human need to be made, i.e., what sort of specific techniques do we need? I think that should be addressed because too much irrelevant clinical data collected in an unstandardized manner is as bad as the paucity of data we have now. My own suggestion that we should begin very simply with good clinical neurologic data, CT scan data, neuropsychologic testing data and noninvasive neurophysiologic data obtained sequentially.

Dr. Hurt: We could address that particular question. In the work we are doing on fatal motorcycle accidents we seek to obtain quantitative data on the severity of the injury information in some sort of coherent system that we can all work with. The Abbreviated Injury Scale is one scale we use which offers something that has been used for a long time. There is a considerable amount of past data of fairly high quality. And the Abbreviated Injury Scale can be looked at as an overall view, in assessment of individual and discrete injury, or massaged in various ways in the injury severity scores. The main deficit is that it is usually a one-time measure at the time of injury. I really recommend that we consider some coherent system of measurement of these injuries for the collection of data to include the changes of severity with time which we don't have at this time.

Dr. Gennarelli: NIH is in the process of collecting data at, I think five head injury centers, on severe head injuries. The amount of data that they are collecting is overwhelming. To give you an idea—they are collecting routine physiological data, ICP data, blood pressure, and similar vital sign data sequentially. To give you an idea of how much data is coming in, there is a data collection sheet that has, in the intensive care unit approximately 25 variables being recorded at fairly frequent and short-term intervals, e.g., repeated three times a day, once on each nursing shift, unless an "event" occurs when the frequency of recording is increased. There are a series of events that are defined and those include things like a change in the intracranial pressure, dilation of pupils, that sort of thing. If one of those events occurs, then this data is collected every five minutes for a while and then every hour for a while. So some great computer in Stanford is going to be full of many, many members.

That is one end of the spectrum of data collection. And I guess that is what I would like us to address in terms of what things are really necessary to collect. I am not sure that we have the time to really solidify that and reach a consensus today.

Dr. Ommaya: I agree, but let us all think of this problem and try to be kind to our computers by doing some thinking on what kind of pilot studies should be done before engaging on mammoth data gathering "fishing expeditions."

Dr. Gennarelli: The NIH investigators held an "outcome of head injuries" meeting in Washington during the past summer. Everyone put in their own idea of what to measure for outcome, and including all the neuropsychological tests, some 150 variables were to be measured individually and that were to be called outcome measures. There is, e.g., going to be a **memory** outcome, an outcome of **parietal lobe** damage right hemisphere function, a speech outcome, and so on and so forth, all of which will be quantified to some degree, but not put together in a holistic fashion to say the least.

Dr. Gildenberg: You see, this is one of the problems with that sort of detail. We are looking at some of those things, but we are looking at the Karnofsky Scale. Are you familiar with Karnofsky Scale? This is a 10-level, 100-point scale which goes between "didn't survive" and "a perfect result" and relates to the degree of disability, at intervals of 10 points along the way. "Almost back to normal," "independent," "not quite independent," "requires occasional help" or "requires full-time help" and so forth. So that you have sufficient degrees of freedom to get some sort of meaningful criteria for recovery after neural trauma.

In additional to that, we have an outcome scale that is divided into occupational outcome, social outcome, outcome within the family, and dependency needs. So that we are looking at each one of these separately and then hoping to correlate that with the neuropsychological data to draw some conclusions. If somebody doesn't fully recover, what factors are involved with that lack of recovery?

Dr. Gennarelli: My own view would be that the outcome problem is so complex, at least with regard to head injury, that it ought to be tabled for a while in a very specific sense. I mean we have enough trouble defining in a statistical manner which are the bad injuries, to begin with, based on immediacy of the problem. And I think our ability to look at the subtle nuances of outcome in terms of the grossness of everything else is inappropriate.

Dr. Gildenberg: Yes, but the Karnofsky Scale, though, does contain information not only of medical interest, but also of social interest. Is the patient independent or dependent? And this, or course, allows one to draw other conclusions about the impact of their injury on finances and such.

Dr. Levine: I think outcome is very important. It might be more important than the initial injury. We have got to know what happens with these people in the long term. This is the ultimate cost to society, is the end result.

Dr. Gennarelli: Well, certainly that is true. But in a mechanistic sense it doesn't help you to say that this patient with Injury X had a bad or good outcome, unless you know that it is because of that injury that he had the bad or good outcome. If other extraneous factors, be they social, be they litigation, be they specifics of medical therapy, influence that interface so that what happened to the patient mechanistically in the outcome is no longer directly related, then it is going to muddle our understanding of initial injury mechanisms.

Dr. Levine: But I think this will tend to balance out. You know, you have got the high-need well-motivated achievers and the low-need poorly motivated achievers, those who can get back to work in spite of symptoms and those who, with minimum problems, won't do anything. And I think we can get a big enough group that this kind of thing will cancel itself out.

Dr. Gennarelli: I think that is too simplistic an approach.

Dr. Gildenberg: One of the particular difficulties with analyses of head injury outcome is that the head injury itself affects the psychologic attitude which may provide the motivation to go or not to go back to work. This is a very subtle and very difficult thing to evaluate quantitatively.

Dr. Ommaya: That is why I think the post-traumatic neuropsychological aspects are very important, both for severe and in the lesser degrees of head injury. Again this is a major issue which we will have to table for the present.

I think we have pretty much covered the topic of clinical measurement. The other aspect which I think we should discuss—is the question of what aspects of the physiopathology should be modeled. For example, I can think of two contrasting questions, the contact phenomena induced local brain contusions and the acceleration related diffuse injuries, e.g., concussion and subdural hematomas. I think this subcommittee should come to some sort of recommendation as to what are the important aspects of the human injury response which really should be modeled so that that quantitative data may be obtained. Rolf, do you have a comment?

Dr. Eppinger: I would ask the physicians as to **what** is the trauma response that we should be looking for in the laboratory. We will figure out **how** to measure what it is, whether it be a contact phenomenon, an inertial loading effect or whatever.

Instead of going away from the trauma towards the outcome, can we get as close to the beginning of the traumatic event?

To give you an example in another area, the pedestrian injury area, we have documented accidents where we have x-rays and other clinical data that describe the level of the trauma, with different levels of information qualities, some are more detailed, some are less detailed. We are giving these data to a panel of physicians; each independently has to grade the trauma in terms of his impression of impairment, only given this initial information. Then we gather these opinions from each of the individual physicians; each independently has to grade the trauma in terms of his impression of impairment, only given this initial information. Then we gather these opinions from each of the individual physicians and try to bring it together to see what the scatter is, and then we hope to get everybody in a room and say: How come you have set Injury "x" so high and how come you set Injury "y" so low?

Dr. Gennarelli: Maybe it would be useful in the way of trying to synthesize all the discussions this morning to try to put this in the format of a study and construct it as one would construct a research design project to see if it is feasible to try to assess these questions.

In terms of the things that are most serious from our studies, the acute subdural hematomas and the shearing injury lesions, ("STRICH" lesions) associated with prolonged unconsciousness and coma greater than 24 hours—are the worst. There are other effects that are also injuries, but less so.

If we can prioritize the injuries effect in sort of a list, then the acute subdural hematomas and shearing injuries are first followed by extradural hematoma and long unconsciousness that is not associated with brain stem abnormalities.

Dr. Levine: I would like to just be a little more general and I am going to jump back to AIS. I wonder if we just shouldn't say any AIS 4 or greater head injury that comes in would be selected and then analyzed in both directions, starting from this even more general category as opposed to a specific injury. Then we can see which specific injuries fit into the AIS categories of 4 or 5 and 6.

Dr. Gennarelli: I think it would be cleaner to pick out specific types of injury, rather than a level of severity which is going to comprise many injuries.—From a mechanistic point of view all AIS 4 and 5 injuries may comprise 25 different types of injuries with 25 different mechanisms. But if we can confine it to maybe two or three mechanisms, then it may be possible to approach those mechanisms.

Dr. Gildenberg: I am inclined to lean toward casting a broader net. It depends really on what sort of resources would be allocated. If it is necessary to restrict the study to a very small group of patients or group of accidents, then this would probably be a good group to study. But, on the other hand, if you do identify particular events that lead to these injuries, you still don't know whether those same events may 99 percent of the time not cause these injuries unless you look at the other injuries as well.

And probably what is even more important than what causes the identifiable type of injury is what causes the injury that we can't classify, in hopes that that might provide additional information to help classify that amorphous group.

Dr. Gennarelli: So how would you design a study to answer that? The problem is that the numbers are so great in the lesser injury groups.

Dr. Gildenberg: Well, I don't think you can study all of them. And apparently, from what I gather, there are plenty of data about the very minor injuries.

But perhaps, whether it is an AIS less than 4 or Glasgow Coma score of less than 8, but some arbitrary level based more on severity than diagnosis I think would be more likely to give useful information.

Dr. Gennarelli: Which is your preference? I think from NHTSA's point of view, AIS is where the data are.

Dr. Gildenberg: It depends on who is making the decision to study a particular case.

Dr. Levine: I think we should focus on automobile impact studies where AIS is used. I think it is a good scale right now. I think it is very translatable to many other scales. I think we should pick AIS 4 as a useful level on that scale.

Dr. Gildenberg: But you are going to have to have somebody to identify the patient who is an AIS 4.

Dr. Levine: Yes.

Dr. Gildenberg: And it is necessary to have that individual trained to the use of the AIS classification. (AIS-80)

Dr. Levine: Yes. It is an easy scale to learn.

Dr. Ommaya: I agree, it has been shown that technical staff can use it reliably.

Dr. Gildenberg: Well, it is not a question of just ease of learning; it is a question of having somebody identify the patient, raise his hand and say, here is a patient for you.

Dr. Levine: Again, as we said, at a given center, when they see a head injury patient, they will immediately scale this. It's an AIS 4.

Dr. Gildenberg: That's fine, as long as you have somebody at the center who is going to do that.

Dr. Rehman: In other words, some sort of coordinator would be necessary to do that.

Dr. Gildenberg: And you would have to have some coordinator in order to identify which patients are in which study in order to identify for both groups that here is a patient with common data that you could cross-correlate, cross-pollinate, depending on which metaphor we are using.

Dr. Graham: Can I ask what number of patients you are talking about? And if you have 100 patients admitted consecutively, say, to a head injury unit, how many of them will fall into these various AIS categories?

Dr. Gennarelli: It depends on the center. In our center approximately 75 percent of our admissions are AIS 3, 4 and 5. I think it's something like 45 or 50 percent 4 and 5. And that is because we don't admit as many minor head injuries as a lot of places.

Dr. Ewing: How many people per month like that?

Dr. Gennarelli: Oh, it varies.

Phil's system is three times as large as ours, and it varies from center to center.

Dr. Gildenberg: It really is not a question, I think, of scarcity of opportunities: In other words, we could probably identify more patients than you have resources to study.

Dr. Gennarelli: Yes.

Dr. Gildenberg: And what is needed is just setting up some mechanism to select out of that group, on a random basis, which accidents would be investigated.

Dr. Ommaya: Yes. I am wondering whether we should start at 4. Because minor head injuries are very important also. So we don't want to ignore those.

Dr. Gennarelli: Well, I think ultimately we would all like to see the spectrum involved.

Dr. Ommaya: Yes.

Dr. Levine: I think also if we eliminate severe ones, then the minor ones become more minor. So the whole scale moves down. We have got to get an entry point where there is a reasonable amount of data to be collected. We could spend a lot of time spinning our wheels investigating minor accidents and get slews of data and not know what is happening. We must get to these severe ones with injuries, where we can look at the injuries in the field, we can talk with people in the research labs who ask us to reproduce the injury and we have got something we can reproduce. To reproduce a minor concussion with perhaps five minutes of confusion, in an animal, probably can't even be done.

Dr. Ommaya: That is not true. We have been able to model varying head injury severity from mild to fatal.

Dr. Gildenberg: Well, again it depends on your allocation of resources. If a case with five minutes of concussion is going to make this individual disabled for a year and a half, then it is significant injury from that standpoint. So it depends on what you want to study, once it gets down to the selection basis.

Dr. Gennarelli: Can we agree—I have no problem in defining an injury severity and using that as the independent variable. But can we agree that in most cases it is possible to attribute that severity to one or more lesions, let's say, or problems? Because from NHTSA's viewpoint, they want to protect against something. And if we define specific kinds of entities that would be an AIS 4 who has an acute subdural hematoma, let's say for example, as opposed to a patient who has a little subdural and a little contusion and a little epidural and has eight or ten things, that it is going to be very difficult mechanistically to try to define how those things happen.

Dr. Ewing: We have had a lot a conversation about outcomes and about AIS. Since I am not familiar with the AIS-80 scale nor with the way that this is being done how is the final AIS score for a particular patient determined? Is it determined on the basis of the discharge diagnosis or diagnoses? Is it determined early in the game and then not changed?

Stated differently, if someone goes into the hospital for a subdural suffered during an automobile accident and he dies of intercurrent infection, is that a fatal injury due to subdural? And at what point is that decision made and who makes it?

Dr. Gennarelli: In the AIS 80—let me just explain it in brief terms. The first thing that was done differently with AIS 80 is that skull injuries were separated from injuries to tissue under the skull. The brain injuries are next divided into two categories, anatomical types of lesions and functional or what was called, for lack of a better term, concussive type of injuries.

The anatomical injuries are epidural hematoma, subdural hematoma, contusions, things that the pathologist could see. And the criteria for diagnosis of those have to be some type of anatomical diagnosis; that is, it is either something made at surgery, a CT scan by the pathologist, or something that is verified, so that we don't have a clinical diagnosis of contusion when there may not in fact be a contusion there. That particular example has been very florid amongst neurosurgeons. If somebody is unconscious, it's a cerebral contusion, whether or not there is an actual contusion there. So that is the anatomical section.

The concussive section is based on two factors: the length of unconsciousness and associated neurological difficulties, a hemiparesis, this sort of thing. And, because the length of unconsciousness goes up to 24 hours, that can't be determined until 24 hours after the injury. The anatomical one can be determined whenever the CT scan is done or whenever the pathologist is there and whenever the patient goes to surgery.

We found in our work that the best correlation with overall outcome occurs if one has both of those pieces of information and uses the highest AIS, which usually is the length of unconsciousness.

There are considerable differences with it. But we don't know yet what will happen if people start abusing that system and just look at one piece of information and code the whole patient on that.

So the problem of relating that to death is the problem that Chan mentioned. We don't know if he died of an infection or not.

Dr. Gildenberg: There is another problem, too, that by that definition it wouldn't be possible or feasible to use the AIS scale as the sole criterion for study, since the patient wouldn't be classified until, say at least 24 hours afterward or more, by which time it would be more difficult to reconstruct the events of the accident.

In that case, something like the Glasgow Coma score on admission or some definition that relates to the level of consciousness or severity of injury as the dividing line might be more feasible.

Dr. Ewing: But if at some time we have the accident investigation, the team has done its work, it has identified the bits and pieces that were damaged and tried to associate that with the injury, we then must relate the accident investigation to an AIS number for that patient.

Dr. Levine: Yes.

Dr. Ewing: When is that determined? Is it determined on the basis of the admitting diagnosis, which is the basis for deciding whether he goes into the study or not, or is it determined at the time of the discharge, at which time we may have had several months intervening?

Dr. Levine: Okay. AIS is really determined early in the game. It is a predictability from a given injury, odds of survival basically. As you get severer on the scale, higher on the scale, the percentage of survival drops. And I think basically it predicts along those lines somewhat.

Dr. Ommaya: So it has to be done early.

Dr. Levine: And it is done initially. It is not done a year later, because a year later you may have two deaths that were initially an AIS 3, but they died. They don't become an AIS 6, they are still an AIS 3. But they are an AIS 3, and they happen to be one of those AIS 3's that died because of whatever factor was present.

Dr. Rehman: That AIS scale actually eliminates posttraumatic. . . .

Dr. Ewing: Complications.

Dr. Rehman: Complications. Yes. Because you get your reading immediately or almost immediately.

Dr. Ewing: Yes.

Dr. Rehman: So the additional complications that will develop later on are no longer the concern of the AIS scale.

Dr. Ewing: Well, is that realistic?

Dr. Rehman: I doubt it.

Dr. Ewing: Dr. Ommaya?

Dr. Ommaya: Yes, it is, because it has been found that it is a good predictor in the majority of cases.

Dr. Ewing: Predictor of what?

Dr. Ommaya: Of the mortality and survivability after injury.

Dr. Levine: I am going to jump in here with a research project proposal, that, number one, we have to use as our entry point the injury at the time of admission to the hospital, using possibly an AIS scale, like maybe an initial AIS. It won't be as accurate as the one 24 hours later, but do an initial AIS at the time of admission. Use this to say whether we go further. If we meet our criteria, say of an AIS 4 or greater, then we send the accident team out. The accident team will then investigate the accident. And this accident may or may not fit the kind of accident we want to study. Let's say this is an accident where there is a roll-over and we don't want to look at roll-overs and we say, Okay, this is a roll-over accident, it doesn't fit our current study and we drop this patient out of the study.

If the injury fits the accident, then we go on and do the complete study, with the outcome study. I think this is where we have a feedback from the accident to whether we continue, as well as from the injury. But we are using the injury as our initial entry point to the system.

Dr. Graham: But you need your control population, and the control population is the roll-over. If your one criterion of admission is an AIS of 4, then you have to study all those patients.

Dr. Levine: Okay. Again I will say, if we have limited resources, we may decide the roll-over accidents are so rare that we don't want to study roll-over accidents.

Ms. Pedder: I think what he is saying is using all existing data to decide that, you can use pre-existing data to decide that 98 percent of your accidents are frontal collisions involving passenger cars and only 2 percent are roll-overs. So let's just concentrate on the AIS for frontal impacts, but I think you have got to be very careful about the way in fact the sample is chosen.

Dr. Gildenberg: I have two questions, if I might. The first is whether patients with multiple system injuries should or should not be included.

And the second is how many accidents can a team investigate in the course of a year?

Dr. Gennarelli: It depends on how big the team is, I guess is the answer.

Ms. Pedder: Yes. It depends on how thoroughly the accident is covered, as well.

Dr. Ommaya: Yes. I think Dr. Hurt can answer that.

Dr. Ewing: And how money is available.

Dr. Hurt: The NASS, current NASS teams run about 30 or 40 cases a week

Ms. Pedder: How many cases per person a week do you reckon on, fully covered?

Dr. Hurt: If the cases are fatal cases, these are much more complicated. And it is very difficult for one investigator to handle more than about one-and-a-half cases per week.

Ms. Pedder: Yes, I would back that. I would say one-and-a-half to two per person per week that we thoroughly investigate.

Dr. Levine: I think first of all we have to decide what we want to do, do we want to just take people who have only head injuries and throw everybody else out? Or do we want to do those with head and multiple injuries. I think this is a decision that could be made when we set the project up. And I think that we have got to decide, if we are running a project, how we are going to do it.

Dr. Rehman: You know, that sets up a good question in that if you are going to code them at the start with your AIS scaling, to be repetitious, and you include not only the head, but the neck as well, you can't determine on admission whether there have been additional injuries of a lesser nature, shall we say to the neck, until some degree of examination has been done. Which means that you are faced with a problem initially, if you want to try to code them accurately.

Dr. Ewing: This is my point also.

Dr. Levine: Yes, but we are just coding—we are coding one system. We are not doing an overall AIS. We are talking about doing a head AIS as our entry code.

Dr. Rehman: Are you looking for subdural?

Dr. Levine: No. I am just saying we are doing a head AIS—we are talking about a head AIS.

Dr. Eppinger: There is no region AIS any more.

Dr. Ommaya: Yes, that is correct.

Dr. Eppinger: Each particular trauma gets an AIS category, whatever, 1 to 6. And each identifiable lesion gets a rating. It occurs either in the chest, the neck or the head. But we don't go back any more and make overall assessments of an AIS or average AIS.

Dr. Rehman: Which means that you have got to wait until at least the initial examination has been more or less completed before you can code them.

Dr. Eppinger: But we also monitor everybody at least for 30 days, because that is the definition time of death if it occurs.

Dr. Rehman: Yes.

Dr. Ewing: But at what point do you assign the AIS for that person? Is it on the first day or on the 30th day?

Dr. Gennarelli: The date is retrospectively assessed, isn't it, in the NASS team approach? You go to patient records.

Dr. Eppinger: Yes.

Dr. Gennarelli: What we are talking about doing now is a prospective assessment, done at the time the patient comes to the emergency room or shortly thereafter, and making that AIS determination there as the basis for an accident team investigation and for continuation of medical study.

I think, Phil, in answer to your question that we have to include other system injuries, simply from the fact that if Rolf Eppinger wants to protect against the head and we find that heads do worse when there is a fractured femur, then he has also got to protect against a fractured femur at the same time.

Dr. Gildenberg: Yes. Well, a study can be set up either way, depending on what you are looking for.

Dr. Gennarelli: Yes.

Dr. Gildenberg: It's just to determine at the beginning, are we interested in that particular patient?

Dr. Levine: This is what I'm saying. We can set up our study by how we enter it. And we have got to define our entry point, whether we say AIS head 4 or greater with no other injuries, or AIS 4 or greater with other injuries.

But I think we have to get a reasonable amount of data to analyze. We can get too much data. You know, if we have too many accidents we are looking at, then we get too confused in trying to analyze the data. I think we have got to say, let's get it down to where we can get some usable data, a reasonable amount, that we can come up with something. Rather than trying to analyze 25,000 injuries, let's analyze 5,000 that are bad so we have got something we can work with.

Dr. Gildenberg: Rolf, which is preferable from your standpoint?

Dr. Eppinger: Both. It all depends on what we are looking for. You know, one of the big efforts that have gone into NASS is to make it statistically representative of the total vehicle trauma area. In the past we have conducted very detailed studies called Multidisciplinary Action Investigations where only high severity accidents (in terms of either crash or injury factors) were selected for in-depth study.

In the end, we knew a lot about those cases but what we didn't know was how important they were epidemiologically. What does that mean nationwide? This led to the massive NASS program which will attempt to provide statistical representation of the accident types in the total nation. This is why the data show a bias toward low-injury accidents, i.e., of low crash intensity.

Dr. Gildenberg: So this makes the selection less critical, since you do want to look as broadly as possible.

Dr. Eppinger: Right, for the purposes of the NASS study.

Dr. Levine: Well, you know, that is critical, because how much do we want to spend on follow-up of our patient selection? If we get too broad, we will have an awful lot of patients for a long-term follow-up.

Dr. Ommaya: The point is that we may not need to spend much more money. That is why I was talking about the marriage between the physicians (NIH) and NHTSA: that if we could link up some of the NIH-sponsored trauma centers with some of the NASS teams, then we could have something of broader significance for not much more than what is already being spent by these two agencies.

Dr. Gildenberg: Yes.

Dr. Ommaya: Now that we have decided on the significant lesions, should we discuss the techniques for assessment of the patient according to the chart that Dr. Lindgren presented? Any comments?

Dr. Gildenberg: Tom, do you want to talk about the data base for the multicenter NINCDS study?

Dr. Gennarelli: As I mentioned earlier, we may be gathering too much, but certainly clinical neuroradiological, neurophysiologic and neuropathologic categories should be considered.

What about spine injuries or neck injuries now? Can we use this same type of approach to spine injuries? Can we define either an AIS 4 or 5 spine injury early enough to send out an accident team?

Dr. Frankel: I think so, certainly on the basis of neurological function and x-ray.

Dr. Gildenberg: As a general rule of thumb, there will be 10 percent as many patients with spinal cord injury as with head injury, and probably about two or three times that many who have spine injuries without neurological deficit.

Dr. Frankel: Dr. Gennarelli, what percentage of your head injuries are going to have spine injuries?

Dr. Gennarelli: Less than 10 percent. Ours is about 5 percent.

Dr. Ewing: Does that mean what percent of the head injuries are going to have cord injuries or spine injuries?

Dr. Gildenberg: Five percent or less.

Dr. Frankel: Fifty percent of all the spine injuries that were initially missed in the Johns Hopkins and Baltimore Hospital studies of head injuries were later diagnosed anywhere from 1 day to 1 year after trauma. Everybody had immediate skull x-rays, but very few had neck x-rays. So you have this problem of missing the early spine injuries.

Dr. Gennarelli: You mean isolated spine injuries or those in association with multiple trauma.

Dr. Frankel: No. Isolated spine injuries. They were brought in and seen in the emergency room. In most cases the people were hit on the head, so they all had skull film. But the spine injuries were missed 50 percent of the cases.

Dr. Levine: Hopefully enough cases will be missed in an equivalent manner from all modes of impact to end up with statistically useful numbers. If you are rear-ended, you are more likely to have a neck x-ray than if you have a forward impact.

Dr. Ewing: Dr. Rehman's figure of approximately 12-percent incidence of fracture of the odontoid in his autopsies is to me a very telling figure. I wonder how many people who come in with head injuries, for example, from motorcycle accidents get an odontoid view.

Dr. Rehman: Actually I think there are very few in whom these pillar views that really show up in the odontoid process are obtained routinely.

Dr. Gennarelli: Generally there is an inverse correlation at most centers between the degree to which the spine is investigated and the severity of the head injury. As the head injury becomes more prominent, less attention is paid to the spine.

Dr. Levine: I think there is an important point to be made about the autopsy and the spine. I think we have got to get cervical autopsies because I think there are people coming in DOA of head neck injuries and maybe neck fractures. And unless we get a good autopsy of these people, we are going to lose the details of these important cervical injuries.

Dr. Rehman: That's right. This was rather surprising data to us in our motorcycle fatality study.

Dr. Ewing: You found an incidence of 12 percent. That's enormous.

Dr. Rehman: Yes, but to get such data we had to carry out a detailed dissection of the atlanto-occipital and the atlanto-axial areas.

Dr. Ewing: Well, that brings up a very important point. If you have a DOA from an accident and turn him over to pathology, you are going to get a routine frontal autopsy. You are probably not going to get a posterior approach to the spine and you are probably not going to preserve the brain and cord down to the level en bloc. What you are going to end up with is equivocal information about some of the things that we already know are a significant problem. In other words, the routine hospital autopsy, as opposed to the autopsy that Dr. Rehman is talking about, is not going to show up what he found.

Dr. Gildenberg: That's not exactly true. I think this is one of the problems in the head trauma centers; the quality of the autopsy varies from center to center. In our center we would not miss cervical spine injuries. I agree that the availability of the autopsy varies from center to center.

Dr. Rehman: That's right.

Dr. Gildenberg: I know that in the past we have had a difficult time getting any information at all from the medical examiner's office. Now that has improved, and we are starting to get some information. But those data were just lost to us before. And I am sure this is a common problem.

Dr. Rehman: It is going to require an educational program really as to what you are looking for.

Dr. Ewing: For pathologists.

Dr. Rehman: For pathologists, yes.

Dr. Levine: We should work in certain areas where there is a high incidence of these accidents and talk to those examiners and let's set up teams with the examiners and have them working with us. We have a medical examiner doing a lot of our cadaver autopsies right now, which are great.

Dr. Rehman: Does he dissect about the clavicle, though?

Dr. Levine: He takes the neck out en bloc, takes the cord out.

Dr. Rehman: This is what we have been doing for years. In other words, go in there and take the tongue, trachea, esophagus, pharynx and larynx as a unit. But what do you see? Nothing. The only thing you will see there is if there is damage to the hyoid bone or the cricoid or if there is hemorrhage on the wall of the pharynx or in the larynx. But you don't see anything lateral; you don't really; they never look at the vertebral column.

Dr. Levine: Okay. Our medical examiner doing our experimental autopsies is looking at the vertebral column also.

Dr. Rehman: Oh, he is? Then that is a different approach.

Dr. Levine: I will show you our odontoid fractures, ligament tears between C1 and C2 on our cadavers. But it is a special case. He knows what to look for, and he is doing it. But he says he has seen it in real life, too. So I think there are some examiners doing this.

Dr. Rehman: Not very many.

Dr. Ewing: My point is this. You are going to have people studying the accident, NHTSA teams that really know their business; they probably really like what they are doing and they will come up with the data that are comparable, at least for a given team, between weeks and between months and between accidents and so forth. But at the time those teams are going to have to relate the findings from the accident itself, to the injury suffered in the accident, and if we don't have the same type of competence in the medical and pathological examinations that we have in the engineering examinations of the inertial events, we are going to end up with two qualities of data, one high-quality accident investigation and one low-quality human investigation.

Dr. Gennarelli: I don't see that as an insoluble problem, Channing.

Dr. Ommaya: I agree, I have advised NHTSA on how we can obtain improved medical data.

Dr. Gennarelli: I think if we can identify centers in which the pathology is done superbly, such as in Los Angeles, then they should be the ones to study the DOAs, as they are doing. And in centers like some of ours where it is hard to extract information, where the pathologists are not necessarily interested in it, then those centers should concentrate on the non-DOAs.

Dr. Graham: My experience is such that I don't think I am missing very many cervical injuries in patients who have essentially died from severe head injury. I think the figure of 12 percent is remarkably high. And I would doubt that is generally correct.

Dr. Gennarelli: But those are DOAs.

Dr. Graham: Yes. I would think the ones that die in hospitals are less than 1 percent.

Dr. Gildenberg: Yes. I think it is important to note that this work of Dr. Rehman's group at L.A. set of patients with partial motorcyle injuries as compared to other types of head injuries.

It is not, however, necessary to look at those people in the same centers as these other people are being followed more comprehensively.

So, it may be appropriate to have some of the teams interrelating with the head trauma centers and other teams interrelating with the medical examiners' offices who are competent and doing a good job on the autopsies, as a separate consideration.

Dr. Rehman: I think in defense of our 12 percent incidence cervical spine injuries I should emphasize that firstly, we are dealing with strictly motorcycle accidents, where as a general rule once their motorcycle stops on impact, they are still continuing.

Dr. Ewing: Right.

Dr. Rehman: We have had cases where they had continued through the air for 20 feet and then they land up against a lightpole, using their head as a battering ram or they hit the side of the guardrail, so that there is a direct contact there. I think it is a selected group from the point of view of injuries to that area. They are not typical of a motor vehicular type of accident.

Dr. Graham: In this system in L.A. such that you are peripatetic in that you could travel to other mortuaries and do the same dissection of patients who have died after a period of time?

Dr. Rehman: In L.A. any case of trauma must be handled through the Coroner's office. That is the law.

Dr. Graham: So you have access to patients who have died, say, having been in your surgical units.

Dr. Rehman: Yes, if death has occurred within 10 days of the injury.

Dr. Ewing: All right. But the point I'm making is that I think the team approach to accident investigation in injury quantification is essential and needs to be done with great care so that the people on the injury quantification team can be shown to be qualified to make the judgment.

Dr. Rehman: Oh, yes.

Dr. Ewing: Otherwise, you are going to end up with mush on one side and hard data on the other. And that does not serve to solve or even identify the problem.

Dr. Rehman: That's true. Because even at our place some of the death reports in fatal cases go in as massive head trauma, period.

Dr. Ewing: Right.

Dr. Rehman: And that is all that it is. That's the cause of death. And that doesn't tell us anything about the case, other than the fact that the individual died.

Dr. Ewing: Yes.

Dr. Rehman: So it requires basically what we have talked about, not only a team approach, but an education of the team to bring them up to the level of competence.

Rolf, what is the best kind of mechanical data that can be reconstructed? How closely can one approach an acceleration and time history, let's say from reconstructed data? Are we talking about never or maybe one out of a hundred times?

Dr. Eppinger: You are never going to get an exact reproduction. The techniques they use now go to retrospective, even with the velocity estimates within plus or minus 5 miles an hour. If, for example, I'm at 30 mph plus or minus 5, then the total energy in that event is the square of that already.

And then if you are saying going back to reconstruct that on an individual basis, the accuracy that you have in that is very low. And the only way that we could usefully use reconstruction is in vast numbers, because you have to say, I am going to first reconstruct it. If I am going to put a dummy back into the vehicle to assess the validity of the dummy versus what the actual victims say, you have to do a sort of paired statistical study. I run this test, the dummy says this, the actual victim says this. And is it high versus low? By one test I can't tell you anything; I have to do pair after pair after pair.

Right now we are trying to make our dummies sense and read out an output index like the AIS. I have done some rough calculations that even if the dummy is predicting inaccurately by one AIS, you would have to go through 11 tests where you consistently were off by one AIS to say that the dummy is actually wrong, because there is so much variance within the data itself.

So it comes back with disproving, to disprove the validity of the device, is a lot of tests away.

Dr. Gennarelli: I think what we could provide from the medical point of view is a prospective view that we can define the extent, entry and outcome in patient relatively quickly after the injury; that this is a patient with an AIS of 4 or 5 who has any one of a number of specific lesions, say a subdural hematoma, and we can provide an estimation at an impact point of the head or contact point in a prospective fashion.

But that is about the data that we can provide to you on an immediate basis, and then eventually some measure of outcome.

Now, the question is: Are you going to be able to do enough with that to make the whole thing worthwhile?

Dr. Eppinger: Well, let me give you an example. If the hypothesis of this diffuse white matter shear is sustained—and your data suggests that—what do I do with that? I say, Can I identify that lesion in some sort of experimental environment, animals, cadavers, other techniques to identify it in these various surrogates? Can I then go through and construct a sequence of experiments that can tell me the mechanical environment that would indeed produce that trauma?

And if I know that trauma, through your other studies, consistently leads to a poor recovery, in other words there is another trail of evidence that says that the recovery, given this type of trauma, is consistently either death or persistently vegetative or something of that nature, it justifies us going the other way and saying, I would like to prevent that in our crash environment, and trying to devise our test with the dummy to be sensitive to that measure and the mechanical environment that produces it.

I would like to go down this list of causal events: Can you identify essentially on initial entry into the hospital those conditions that you think are very, very serious that we should eliminate? In other words, we have some attempts at it with this AIS and the revision of the AIS. Some of them are actual trauma identification, physical lesions, and other things are clinical manifestations that consistently lead us to a poor outcome.

And in some of those where we can't identify physical lesions, I would have to use more of an animal type of model. If I can go back to the trauma type, I can use the cadaver model or the animal model.

Dr. Gennarelli: I guess the question I would have, though, is—suppose we have in various head injury centers identified in a prospective fashion, let's say, the diffuse white matter kind of problem, the shearing injury, and let's say just for clarity that there are no other injuries to the body, so this is a pure head injury. And we have 100 of those accidents that are investigated by the NASS team type approach. Wouldn't you expect to find some percentage of those accidents that are relatively clean? Somebody runs into a telephone pole where you could make closer approximations than a six-car crash where occupants are spinning around and flipping and rolling and that sort of thing. I mean really ball park, to correlate with the experimental data in animals or computer models to say that, e.g., the pulse duration must have been somewhere between 15 and 20 ms as opposed to between 2 to 3 ms and that the acceleration seen must have been somewhere between x and y—then the question is: Can those confidence limits be small enough to be useful? Or can you not say anything about those kinds of confidence limits?

Dr. Eppinger: That is sort of the third step.

If you identify, let's say the shearing lesion, then we have to try to see what mechanical environment produces that. And we have to try to incorporate that into the test device. And then you are saying, physically now I would like to validate that test device. That is when we finally come back to the detailed reconstruction. Because if I put a nonaccurate device in there, suppose I would just put a big rigid block in here rather than even our articulated dummy right now, any reading I would be getting off that device is an incorrect reading from what the actual victims saw.

Dr. Gennarelli: The problem is that it is the third step only conceptually. But it has to be—in order to collect the data, it has to be done at the same time.

Dr. Eppinger: We collect as clean data as we can about the event. And we could actually go back through that and say, given this data, what kind of confidence do we have in, let's say, the initial conditions of the vehicle?

Dr. Gennarelli: The whole point of the question was really: Is it worth collecting the NASS type of data in these patients?

Dr. Eppinger: Yes.

Ms. Pedder: Could I just comment on the fact that one shouldn't forget the immediate use that the data could be put to. Some of us are involved every day in regulation committees, committees making decisions of standards, where we are asked, what do we want to protect the motorcyclist's head against?

Now, unless there is a good supply of immediately available representative medical data, where we can see, e.g., that 80 percent of our seriously injured motorcyclists suffer a type of brain injury, which we believe is caused by rotation or even if you can identify the problem for us in simpler fashion we don't know where even to start. I totally agree with you. I think the long-term aims and the goals are to develop and consider the sum of medical information in the consideration of improved experimental models, cadaver work, animal experimentation. In Europe and England and no doubt here in the U.S.A. as well, obviously there are immediate day to day decisions being made on standards. At the moment these decisions are being made on a tremendous paucity of well-documented and representative samples of medical information. And I would say, if you gave us that information tomorrow, it would be wonderful and it would be used straight away, immediately. Okay, not in the best form and not in the most ideal fashion, and, sure we want to set human tolerance limits and a lot of long-term ambitions that we all have. But in the immediate future, like tomorrow or next week, many of us here are going to be involved in sitting down and writing a standard. And if we have got a good medical base, that is what we would use it for.

I would like to feel that one or two optimists like myself do remain in the field, where I really believe that your information could be used.

Mr. Black: Let me interject a point on medicolegal aspects. Mr. Rick Ball and I were raised on automobile accident litigation and also do work in helmet cases. We deal with automobile accident reconstruction people. They are very scarce. There are very few Darwin Severys around. We need more.

I am concerned about the availability of these investigators. I am not sure you are going to have this high level of mechanical investigation that you are speaking about. I think it's going to be the other way, i.e., your medical data may be superior to the engineering data.

You may have to consider the necessity for training people who presently aren't around to do these investigations. And then you have got to give them incentives to keep them working.

I'm sure there are answers to these problems. But I think there is going to be a need for some serious training centers where a lot of research work is done. The average policeman doesn't have the time and doesn't have the technical ability.

Dr. Hurt: The NASS team personnel are far above the average traffic officer in qualifications. They are no Darwin Severys. But they do a very credible job with a great variety of skills required. They are collecting the data, reconstructing accidents, collecting medical data, getting it in a proper format for a later detailed examination in the National Center for Statistics Analysis.

Mr. Black: Do those teams exist now?

Dr. Ommaya: Yes, we heard a brief review of the NASS program yesterday.

Mr. Black: The NASS teams are out there in the real world.

Dr. Hurt: They're out there and working hard.

Dr. Eppinger: They're on line right now.

Dr. Digges: Yes. There are not many of them, there are some there, about 50 teams and more are planned.

Dr. Hurt: And there are even special studies where the people get additional special training for side impact intrusion and motorcycle studies and such.

Mr. Black: When you talk about 50 NASS teams, I think this may offer a great potential for guys who are studying to get their Ph.D. You've got a lot of bright guys, who if they could have some sort of program like this to work with, I think that is where you could seek to find your candidates for a future training.

Dr. Ommaya: We are running short of time. We have about 10 or 15 minutes more. I would like Dr. Ewing to comment on the use of human volunteers. We have talked about the medical-engineering "marriage" interests. The question I raise now concerns how we can use human volunteers in these studies.

Dr. Ewing: The approach that we have taken, as I am sure most of you are aware, is to use as variables initial position of head relative to neck, peak acceleration, rate of onset of acceleration, duration at peak acceleration, and anthropomorphic variables.

We have gone through minus x, plus y, and minus x plus y. I believe that we now have sufficent information for the head and neck to develop a head and neck dummy at least covering from plus y to minus y in the horizontal plane.

Obviously that is just a beginning. What is required is plus x, plus minus z, and a number of off-axis vectors.

But the question is, the important question is, to what level can we take human subjects? We cannot test human subjects beyond the limit of their voluntary tolerance. When the subject is ready for the test and if he does not want to make the run, all he has to do is open his hand, which dumps the firing switch, and that is the end of the test. We have never had any of the subjects refuse to make a run. So we have to have a doctor to protect the subject, to see that the subject does not voluntarily undergo something that might conceivably be injurious. And in our experience, it has been the physician who has stopped the run if the subject faints, for example.

We have gone up to 15 g minus x. We stopped at 15 g because we did not have any capability for determining the onset of potentially injurious conditions such as changes in the cortical evoked potential; we had no way of looking at performance, for example, of memory. So we couldn't determine whether we were getting into an area that was potentially injurious.

We have developed or are developing as a result of our animal experiments criteria for exposure of humans based upon audiovisual evoked potential, which is a lot more complex than the somatosensory, simply because you have to do it on human subjects and you have to monitor during the run. However, we expect to make exposures of human subjects using this equipment to determine the changes in evoked potential sometime within the next three months.

If we are able to get correlation between the audiovisual evoked potential and the cortical evoked potential that we have measured in animals, then we intend to go on up to peak accelerations that are considerably higher than we have presently reached, simply because we feel that we will have enough data to make sure that human subject is not unknowingly subjected to an injurious pulse.

So I think that the volunteer testing business is getting set up for a new step to higher levels.

The approach that we have taken on a theoretical basis in the past has been to measure the dynamic response of the volunteers up to the limit of the voluntary tolerance or until we are concerned about potential hazard, to subject sub-human primates to the same levels of acceleration and the same vector directions, make a model of the comparison between the dynamics response of the two, up to the limit of voluntary human tolerance, then extend the animal work out to points where injury occurs and use the model of correspondence between human and primate to extrapolate what the human response would have been, giving the primate response and the model correspondence. The problem is that all of these things take time. You have to take great pains with the primate work. We have had a hiring freeze in the Federal Government, at least in our laboratory, since October 1, 1979. That was relieved two weeks ago. It is going to take two months to hire the people back to the point where we were in September 1979.

We do have 21 full-time volunteers. We are going to be having a fairly high run rate, but that is after we find out whether the audiovisual evoked potential will work.

We found in the human runs on plus y that the man's ear came within about one-eighth of an inch of impacting his shoulder. That is at 7.5 g, high onset, long duration. We considered that that represented an end point, at least with that particular restraint configuration, because he would suffer impact of the head against the shoulder, and that might be very dangerous.

So we started doing primate runs, with 20-pound Rhesus monkeys. We started at 10 g, no contact, no injury. 15 g, no contact, no injury. Then 20 g. We knew that would do it. No contact, no injury. We went up in increments to 90 g. No injury and no contact. The primate was perfectly all right in this plus y series. I don't know how to explain it.

Provided we continue to get the funding and provided that the Navy continues to function, I presume that we are going to continue to do this work until it is completed. We are looking at a long program extending some years in the future, because it costs us about $100,000 per primate run. To support a crew of 28 or 30 people to run one 20-pound Rhesus monkey. But if you are going to get the kind of extensive data that are the reason for the run, you have to have such a large group.

Any questions?

Dr. Ommaya: Is there any other human volunteer group being tested in any other laboratory?

Dr. Levine: Yes. We run one a week, not quite as high as Dr. Ewing's group. Our approach is different. We like to use cadavers prior to volunteer runs. I put my cadavers in the same mode as my volunteer is going to be in and go to twice the g level that I am going to allow for the volunteer. If the cadaver comes out uninjured, then I will let my volunteer go, and we start out low and work up higher.

I think we have to look at cadavers also. I think we can use human volunteers at low g levels, cadavers at low g levels and compare the two, and take our cadavers to injury levels and then try to go to what our volunteers would do.

There are differences between cadavers and the living, but I think we can extrapolate between the two within certain parameters for certain types of injuries.

Dr. Ewing: There is one other point I would like to make. We have requested funding on two separate occasions to do a long-term follow-up on our human volunteers that were run in 1967, 1968, 1969 and 1970, to find out if there are any long-term effects from these multiple exposures to impact acceleration. It was turned down every single time.

And then an admiral came through our laboratory and said, "Why haven't you done this study yet?" We showed him the rejection letter and he said, Okay, now you have got to do it! I am ordering you to do it. So we submitted a proposal at the present time that has been rattling around between Washington and New Orleans for nine months. We still do not have an approved experimental design. Some day we may have one.

Now, if we find that there are injurious effects to the volunteers run 12 years ago, then that will cause a rethinking of many of our present tenets.

I didn't expect that any such study will be completed for at least two years. But I want you to know that we are concerned about the problem.

Mr. Black: Send me their names (Laughter).

Dr. Rehman: Are you worrying about malpractice?

Dr. Gildenberg: Is the reticence perhaps a need not to know?

Dr. Ewing: No, not on our part.

Dr. Gildenberg: Have you looked at pilots who have been catapulted multiple times?

Dr. Ewing: No, we really haven't. We examined Col. John Paul Stapp about six years ago, and we were unable to determine that there were any injuries as a result of all the very high acceleration runs that he had made. We got in some of the other people who had gone through very high acceleration runs. Ellis Taylor, for example, went through a 100 g plus x exposure with fitted couch and in a vertical direction, and it turns out that he had no permanent injuries of any kind.

One thing that both John Paul Stapp and Ellis Taylor told us, once we talked to them a little bit, was that both of them had suffered cardiac arrythmias for a year after their highest acceleration runs and they didn't tell anybody. They didn't even tell each other. They both found out in our laboratory that they had both suffered cardiac arrhythmias lasting about a year after the runs. We didn't know it.

Dr. Levine: I think we have one more group we should look at. What about parachutes? From the movies we saw yesterday, they sustain fairly high accelerations. I think they are groups who are going through acceleration voluntarily. We should be looking at these people also and see if useful data can be obtained. Also let us not forget boxers. It may be worthwhile to study people who are readily available and who are voluntarily submitting to such impacts.

Dr. Ewing: But how are you going to measure input?

Dr. Ommaya: I would like to answer briefly that with reference to a planned boxer study. This study is part of the NHTSA program, and is at the stage of testing the feasibility of implementing a set of 9 rotational accelerometers in the mouthpiece of boxers.

The instrumentation package has to be practical in terms of measuring angular acceleration and that is where the state of the art is.

Consensus Process

Dr. Ommaya: I think the discussions have progressed very well. We're all slightly ahead of the Session IV reporters who are still on their way. They should be here quite shortly. The format will be that each of them will present a summary of the deliberations of the group which will then be thrown open to the floor for discussion.

I have asked Dr. Eppinger to sit up here along with the presenters of those two documents and then we will discuss it further and come up, hopefully, with a list of recommendations, either accept the recommendations as written or modify them or bring up any ideas that you may have which are still festering in the back of your mind that you haven't had a chance to bring out and then, hopefully, we'll end up with something very useful.

We will send you copies of these recommendations, I think fairly soon, and then the plan is to try to publish the proceedings of this conference, including the papers. We would also like to invite those who have not submitted manuscripts to make sure they submit these or even those who have not given a paper but wish something to be included which they think is very important and which we have overlooked. We want to make this, I think, a useful source book for the present state of the art and for the future research plans. So not only the work that has been accomplished, up-to-date work that's available, summaries of your work but also in terms of description of what facilities are available.

If you feel that you are in an area or you know of somebody who has some kind of facility, either a medical facility or an engineering facility or any kind of facility that would enable this work to be done in a better manner, then I think we would like to hear about that also and we will put that all in some kind of listing.

I see the people are here. I think we should start with the clinical side first and then go on to the modeling Dr. Gennarelli.

Dr. Gennarelli: We've been trying to furiously write up the 4 hours of deliberation. What we did in the Human Studies Committee was to discuss generally the problems that the various investigators felt were important and in general fashion attack the question that Dr. Digges provided for us. It became clear as the talks became more systematic that individual investigators had a pretty good idea specifically about the nature of the head and neck injuries, the specific mechanisms that were proposed, which types of injuries are important, and generally speaking, how to measure what was felt to be important.

Much of this was very similar to what I presented yesterday in terms of the kinds of head injuries particularly that are bad, those that are less bad and proposed mechanisms for them.

What we really spent our time on was what we felt was the weakest link in understanding the whole human situation, and that's the link between the engineering groups and the medical groups. We felt that there was still poor communication between these two groups, and meetings like this, I think, are very helpful.

One of the problems is that those attempting to field studies, accident investigations, were observing a serious mismatch of the information that was available. That is, the engineering aspects of those studies were voluminous and very discrete and very well done, whereas the medical correlations to those were, generally speaking, of lesser caliber. The converse was true from those of us in the head injury clinical business. Whereas we measure volumes and volumes of physiological data and radiological data, things like this, but really have very little appreciation and certainly very little sophistication in measuring the accident input variables. We felt that this was clearly the weakest link in understanding the human situation.

We felt that a very specific proposal could be developed and it was the consensus of this committee that we recommend strongly the following proposal:

That a prospective cooperative study be accomplished utilizing the best talents of field investigation accident work and the best talents of those involved in the medical aspects of head and neck injury.

Specifically, as I have mentioned, this would involve a marriage of existing investigations in this country and specifically the NASS investigation teams or their counterparts funded, as you know, by NHTSA and the head injury centers, which are the 6 to 8 centers in the United States funded by the National Institutes of Health. Currently there is no communication whatsoever between these two groups. Both are interested in the same problem and are approaching it from a very systematic fashion but that interface between the two is nonexistent.

We felt that the best way to approach this would be to have a NASS type team associated with the various head injury centers in the United States and to set about to coordinate these two data sets in a systematic fashion and it would work something like this:

The neurosurgeon at the head injury center would identify the injury severity at the time of the presentation of the patient. It might be necessary to begin with the severely injured patients, at least in terms of defining death and disability.

Utilizing an injury scale, probably the AIS, determination would be done prospectively as soon as the patient is stable. The accident investigation team then would make their systematic approach to the accident variables while the head injury team would continue its systematic approach to defining the injury, its magnitude, its severity, its distribution by the systems that have already been developed by these NHTSA workshops in the last 3 or 4 years. Those systematic data collections are not being utilized by the NIH groups. They don't know about them. Those who do know about them I think would have no reluctance to use these systems.

We felt that it was only in this manner that we could get two very good data sets merged so that we could define in a very systematic fashion what are the bad injuries that produce death and disability, what are the real-world situations that cause those and from that infer injury mechanisms and ballpark ideas of the magnitude of input that's important and then play that back onto the investigative efforts, the experimental investigative efforts, either in analytical, physical or surrogate modeling and then close the loop and play back the results of experimentalists' work onto this data set from real-world situations, to in essence validate the data from the experimental groups.

So that came out as the main specific proposal to bridge what is felt is the most critical problem on the human side of head injury work, and that is the interface between engineering and medical types.

Dr. Ommaya: Thank you. Any clarification questions at this stage?

Dr. Alem: I don't know whether you people have addressed the adequacy of the AIS rating system at this point. Do you think the AIS–80 or a revised version is going to be an improved version? Have you addressed the question?

Dr. Gennarelli: Yes. The question was addressed as well as other approaches to injury severity. I think if we can show you some actual data later that might help to answer that.

Dr. Ommaya: I will now ask Prof. Goldsmith to present his report.

Prof. Goldsmith: This is the report of the Committee on Human Surrogate Research. Myself and John Melvin were co-chairmen. We decided that there would be too many people in one committee to try to get anything done effectively so we split the group into two. The committee was divided into the following groups: A—Cadavers and Physical Models, and this was subchaired by Larry Thibault, and B—Animals and Theoretical Models subchaired by Albert King.

Now I am going to read the list of the participants for only one reason. I know this list is incomplete and I would very much like any of you who participated in either group whose name is not on here to come up afterwards and supplement your name on this list.

In Group A there were:

Dr. Claude Tarriere	Dr. Nahib Alem
Dr. Richard Stalnaker	Dr. Bertil Aldman
Mr. Nils Bohlin	Mr. Herbert Lee
Mr. Aldo Fozzati	Mr. Shermon Henson
Mr. Jeff Marcus	Mr. Yoshiro Goi
Mr. Stan Backaitis	Mr. Roger Saul
Dr. Peter Niederer	Mr. Charles Gadd
Mr. D. Cesari	Dr. Alan Nahum

In Group B there were:

Dr. Jack Lennox	Dr. Christen Ljung
Mr. Guy Nuscholtz	Dr. Eberhardt Privitzer
Dr. Daniel Thomas	
Dr. Carley Ward	Dr. Pria Prasad
Mr. Richard Morgan	Mr. Joseph Haley
Mr. Y.G. Kulkarni	Mr. John Kotwick
Dr. James Newman	Mr. David Bliss
Dr. Panjabi	Dr. A. Mamarou, and
Dr. H.E. Wong	

I'm going to add Dr. Y.K. Liu because he did join the group later. And it was co-chaired by Dr. John Melvin and Dr. Albert King.

I am going to give the report of Committee A and then Dr. Melvin will give the report of Committee B and then I am going to close out with about four sentences, which represents the sense of the joint committee.

The committees attempted to address the following questions:

A—What is the state of the art and what are we satisfied with, any particular part of this area?

B—What further research and investigations need to be done, and what, if possible, is the priority and reasonable time scale for this?

C—How does this fit in with DOT objectives?

So we thought we were boiling down the 8 questions that we were being asked to address into these three categories.

There was a general consensus within Group A that no area was at a satisfactory level of development or knowledge but that, with certain specific exceptions, the most nearly satisfactory domain was that of instrumentation.

Unfortunately, all items discussed were given top priority; and, hence, it is not possible to distinguish among their importance, although some items obviously require the satisfactory resolution of other problems before being tackled. However, this need not be an indication that these items are of secondary importance.

There was absolutely uniform agreement that basic research needs to be urgently done and that it be properly funded. All activity should keep in mind the need for cross-correlation between animals and physical, cadaver and theoretical models and their relation to the real world.

The following is a list of special items to be addressed within the field of human surrogate research involving cadavers and physical models, that's Group A:

One—Standardization. This is to be done immediately by setting up a uniform set of forms and/or specifications of a protocol. One suggestion was that this be undertaken at perhaps 3 to 5 locales with a meeting of the workers afterwards for a uniform output. However, a majority of the group felt that this should be done through one of the major agencies, such as ISO at the international level, considered to be important to minimize regional differences in human characteristics. Another possibility would be the undertaking of this by NHTSA, the SAE or a working group of the NAS/NAE. DOT could push this project by providing adequate funds. There was some substantial disagreement as to feasibility of employing this mechanism because each individual group would want to define their own object in their own way. The time scale for this endeavor was estimated at something of the order of 6 months to 1 year.

Two—Characterization. This was considered on a time scale of 5 years. What is needed is a better definition of both geometry and properties of the head-neck components, including statistical evidence concerning the 10th and 90th percentile values over the population, if this can be ascertained with any degree of confidence. It was pointed out that HSRI at the University of Michigan is currently under contract to define what anthropomorphic measurements should be used in dummies, however, no properties were included in this. Furthermore, additional work is needed in ascertaining the mass distribution in dummies, particularly with respect to soft tissue injuries.

Much more work is needed on brain properties, particularly with regard to failure, and this means both what type and at what level and under what circumstances, and loading rates. This part, the failure criterion, is open-ended in time in the opinion of the group.

Further properties of the vasculature need to be explored with respect to strength, mechanical properties and post-mortem changes. All such work should be correlated with previous data, if available and if sufficiently reliable.

Work needs to be done on animals in these areas and tied in with human measurement where such can be effected. The methodology with regard to measurements in humans, possibly even partly in living persons, needs to be urgently addressed, but is not yet sufficiently defined to permit a suggestion as to how to proceed. There also needs to be a proper correlation of loading histories with proper measurement.

Three—Neck Development. This was divided into two categories:

A—Mechanics of the neck, with particular reference to musculature, and

B—Development of a suitable surrogate. The latter should be intimately tied in with the head to produce an appropriate single unit for the head-neck system.

Part A was considered to be performable with a time scale of approximately 2 years, followed by a 3-year period for part B.

Four—Specific Injury Criteria. There was agreement that this should be divided into noncontact and contact events, with a time scale of 2 years, but there was disagreement as to the applicability of the HIC criterion for noncontact events. Beyond this subdivision, it was agreed that the criteria should sooner or later address specific trauma situations, that is to say skull fracture, epidural hematoma, coup and contrecoup injuries, etc.

A rotational injury criterion is urgently needed but this must await the development of suitable instrumentation and methodology for the measurement of brain rotation. The development of such a criterion is considered to be 2 to 3 years beyond the development of suitable instrumentation.

There is a need for a better definition of specific criteria in all areas, perhaps including the replacement of current standards, but the group felt that the discipline is not currently ready to implement such a change. This phase of the subject is and probably aways will remain open-ended.

Five—There is currently a committee involving the various departments of the government on rehabilitation and prosthetic and orthotic devices. A comparable committee should be set up in the area of prevention, involving interagency coordination. This was felt to be of urgent priority and relatively easy to achieve, with DOT providing the impetus. As a minimum, it should involve the DOD, NIH, HIOSH, OSHA and DOT, as well as perhaps some other agencies such as the Insurance Institute for Highway Safety and some other semi-official or private organizations.

Six—Measurements of Localized Loading. The instrumentation for the adequate measurement of the physical parameters within the contact zone was considered to be of the same high priority as the development of an angular accelerometer. In fact, some of the members of the group felt that a lack of understanding of the contact phenomena is an absolutely crucial deficit in an analysis of head and neck injury. The rapidity of the changes in pressure and deformation within this zone pose particular instrumentation difficulties but must be pursued. The same applies to measurement of localized pressure within the brain.

Seven—Instrumentation Development for Neck Phenomena. This field is virtually unexplored, particularly for cadavers, and needs to be strongly addressed.

I hope that I have properly reported the input of all the people that were in Group A and I will now turn this over the John Melvin for the Report on Group B.

Dr. Melvin: The format of my report will be a little more directly along the lines of those questions. I think we will find that many of the comments that we made in our session on Animals and Theoretical Models overlaps with what Werner has already mentioned in the other group.

With regard to the question of what is the nature of head and neck injury and what mechanisms are important, and what observations are important: with respect to the head, the creation of injury in the brain appears to be related to pressures and deformations that occur in the brain tissue itself and it is possible to measure these quantities in a limited sense in animal experiments. It is not possible to measure it in the complete field sense. Therefore, theoretical models may be necessary to extend these limited types of measurements that are available in the animal to be able to relate what's going on in the entirety of the brain to the subsequent dysfunctions and injury that are observed, since experimentally you just can't measure everything everywhere, but the models do purport to have that ability. Obviously, the validation of models to achieve these effects is still a question.

In the area of the neck, although spinal cord damage is the injury end point of concern, the loading of the bony elements of the neck and their subsequent loadings are the means by which the cord is damaged and the measurement of neck loading, motions of individual spinal elements and overall spinal configuration changes must be made in the experimental situation, if we are to describe what is going on.

With regard to the question of what are the important parameters for researchers to measure in the experimental environment, the answer we feel is that theoretical modeling can aid in guiding the experimentalist in the design of his experiments and, therefore, the kind of parameters that the experimentalist will measure.

Both head impacts, and head and neck motions, in accident situations are three-dimensional in nature and future experiments should reflect this. In addition to *in vivo* and post-mortem system testing, that is whole body or head-neck testing of the entire system, in *vitro* determination of component mechanical properties of soft tissues such as ligaments and brain tissue is necessary and was discussed to some extent with respect to implementation in advanced models.

Experimental techniques should quantify inputs to the subject as well as measure the responses. This was brought up a couple of times.

What are the benefits and deficiencies of existing criteria and the head injury criteria, and there are a number available, of course? The present criteria are simple and easy to use but are of doubtful applicability in noncontact phenomena. Some of the peak acceleration limits and other element tests methods may be producing inappropriate shell and liner properties for optimum protection but, because of the limited data base with which all of this has been developed, it was severely hampered in terms of covering some of these additional factors of injury.

Another question was: "Are there presently available alternatives which are better than the HIC?" And the answer is at this point, I guess, no. There certainly are some suggestions, but the research really hasn't been done yet to point any one criteria that would be better than the HIC.

With respect to a criteria for neck injury, there just isn't really anything at this point. The neck is really something that has not been studied very extensively. It was very obvious in our discussions that it was discussion of the head and brain that predominated, primarily because we don't know that much about the neck and, therefore, there's not much to say yet, other than that we don't know very much.

What additional data needs to be developed to improve head and neck injury criteria? The primary concern there is the need for cervical spine response and injury data. This includes force deformation data and soft tissue interaction, muscle, tendon, ligamentous structures.

There are virtually no existing injury or tolerance data in any vector direction or bending mode. It is also necessary to establish the appropriate animal surrogates for neck injury research and to define a tolerance level. Geometric and material properties should also be ascertained for modeling purposes.

For head injury data, one needs to clearly delineate contact and noncontact types of loading and to establish separate injury mechanisms, tolerances and criteria.

The methodology would involve the measurement of various input parameters which have to be correlated to intracranial pressures in brain motion.

For the noncontact mode, the injury criteria may be controlled by the shear stress in the brain or cord and brain stem or both criteria, both phenomena would be the limiting criteria.

In terms of what combination of approaches offers the best way to proceed, some of the approaches that were suggested for developing the needed data include the following, and these are in some order of priority:

Testing of live anesthetized and freshly killed and unembalmed animals for the purposes of translating cadaver data to the living human. It is felt that one of the most useful functions of the animal experimentation is to bridge that gap between the living and the dead, since the only available human data in the injury, high-level range is the dead subject.

Another step after testing of the various states of the animal is pressurizing the vascular system of the dead animal to ascertain if a better simulation of response is obtainable. In other words, can we recreate, once we know the differences between the living and the dead, can we recreate the living situation, as is now being attempted in cadavers but has not been validated?

Another technique is the use of the CAT-scan technique to determine animal injury in the acute and chronic recovery states to allow additional experimenting to be done without the necessity to sacrifice the animal to obtain the injury information.

Another subject would be generating data on longer duration noncontact animal impact. Most of the data so far has been on very short-duration contact type impacts.

Finally, developing discrete parameter cervical spine mathematical models which could provide input data to finite element skull and brain models is another item of development that should be approached in the near future.

These are all subjects we felt that could be attached within a 5-year span.

Finally, item 8, which was: What mechanisms are required to achieve a continuing dialogue and coordination of head and neck injury research? We felt that NHTSA should take the lead in coordinating efforts at establishing standards in injury criteria. It should have a continuing dialogue with other standards organizations, however, and the research community. NHTSA should also establish uniform methodology in data gathering, presentation and the use of models in order to keep the consistency of the various research results.

Prof. Goldsmith: As you can see, there was some substantial overlap, as was to be expected, between the two groups. We feel that this is not at all undesirable because it underscores the points that both of our groups considered.

Finally, in conclusion, it is recommended that DOT consider all of these areas and, if possible, support work in all of them, but, since this is clearly a Utopia, it's going to have to make its own choice if priorities are to be given in the way of funding.

DOT standards should not be encased in concrete because the community even now has very, very serious reservations about these standards, but there is currently not enough information to supplant existing edicts.

It should be emphasized that any changes and construction of future standards, however, should be based on sound principles of mechanics, proper methods of experimentation and measurement, and acceptable procedures of correlation between these and with real-world experience.

Dr. Ommaya: Thank you, Werner.

Tom, did you have some slides to show of the AIS?

Dr. Gennarelli: Questions about the AIS have been occurring both yesterday and today and I thought I'd show you some real-world data that we put together using the AIS-80 and this was this same group of 434 hospitalized head injury patients, looking at the correlations between outcome as defined on 5-point scale.

(Slide) The AIS-80 has some major differences than the '76 revision. One principal difference is it has a separate AIS code for skull and a separate code for brain and that's AIS-B, the brain code, on the left. We had no sixes in our group because they all went to the medical examiner's office. But this correlation with outcome, as you can see, is relatively good. All the patients with AIS-1 injuries had a good outcome and as you go down the good recovery group, as AIS increases, the percentage of good recovery progressively decreases till you get to AIS-5 and there's only 10 percent of the patients having a good recovery there.

If you go to the other end of the slide, the patients who died, almost all of the patients who died ended up with an AIS-5 score.

I think that comprises, the AIS-5 group comprises something like 85 percent of all the deaths. There was an occasional death in AIS-3 group, 2 percent of the 3's and 4 percent of the 4's. So this study tended to develop the AIS-80 as a reasonable injury scale. I've not been privy to studies in the past making these kinds of correlations, but I think these are the kinds of correlations that are necessary with perhaps the spine and other parts of the AIS to really put it on solid grounds.

(Slide) Just to correlate this to other independent measures of outcome, we looked at several things. We're looking at the cumulative percentage of patients within each AIS category versus, in this case, the days spent in the intensive care unit, as another measure of injury severity independent of whether we would categorize the result good, moderate, severe or dead, and what you see in the upper left hand corner is that virtually all of the patients who are AIS-1 were out of the intensive care unit by one day. Of course, most of those never got to intensive care unit but the numbers along the curves refer to the AIS numbers and, as you can see, as AIS increases, you progressively get longer and longer days in the ICU. So that indirect measure of injury severity also fits with AIS.

(Slide) We looked at a few other things. These are all plotted the same way. This is total hospital days and again you can see that there is excellent correlation between days spent in hospital as an injury severity measure and the AIS and, finally, on the last slide (Slide) cost, which had been brought up in our committee meeting and AIS does correlate well again with, in this case we're talking about total hospital charges per patient and it does not include any indirect costs, disability costs or anything. These are just what it cost to be in the hospital for the injury and again, as you can see, as you go to higher AIS levels, it costs you more, even if you exclude the patients who died. Many of them died quickly and, therefore, did not have this high cost as those who died later.

So I think this study just helped solidify that as far as brain injury is concerned the AIS-80 does the job.

Prof. Aldman: I find that the problem of age has not been discussed at all and, if we look at the population at risk, it spreads from infants to the very old and I think the tolerance and possibly also the injury mechanism may not be the same over the whole age again.

Dr. Ommaya: Yes. I think that's a very important question. I think Dr. Eppinger might answer that in terms of what we are trying to do to get some child data or is it possible to get the children data?

Dr. Eppinger: I think we try to experimentally cover the age range from the child through the adult. In the cadaver-type test programs we've made special attempts to span the range and make the age more reflective of the population at risk. There are obvious limitations in attempting to do that in terms of just where specimens occur. So within our practical capability, I think we attempt to address those things.

The other difficulty we find is in the number of the experiments that we can conduct. To understand a variety of independent variables and their influence on the outcome requires a large amount of tests. Initially we have to ignore some of those facts because we don't have sufficient data to support a more complicated relationship. Hopefully, if everyone working in this area will accept standardization of instrumentation and documentation these data will become available to address the variety of factors that do influence the injury.

Dr. Ommaya: We may get useful data from the kind of study that was proposed by the first committee, that is to develop a good correlation between the input data reported by the accident investigation teams and the clinical data in which age is always recorded. We know at this time that in terms of morbidity and mortality age is a very significant variable. I think the mortality decreases by more than 20 percent below the age of 15. It's a very significant age increase for mortality especially. Of course we would get that information from the victims of accidents, I think, both for mortality and morbidity, if we had this kind of good correlated study.

Dr. Gennarelli: As Dr. Eppinger pointed out, the influence of age is multi-dimensional, as we all know. I think, for instance, it is not well known what this age influence is. It is simply that the younger brain recovers better or doesn't get as badly injured or is it that younger patients get different injuries? There are various camps of feelings on that but my own inclination is that the younger patients get different injuries than the older patient.

Certainly the incidence of acute subdural hematoma is far and away higher in the older population, over 45 years of age, which is where the mortality goes up. It goes up in parallel with the incidence of subdural hematoma, whereas, it's very uncommon particularly in either pedestrian or motor vehicle accidents to have subdural hematoma in someone less than 10 years of age.

So it's a multi-faceted problem and the answer is not going to come easily but, as Dr. Ommaya says, if the data are gathered with all these contingencies in mind, it's an answerable problem.

Dr. Ommaya: There is, as far as I know, only one good paper on the difference between child brain and adult brain in terms of the lesions. That's by Lendenbery in which he showed that, in addition to this difference of the hematomas, there is a very specific kind of lesion in the child brain, which is a splitting. He described this as almost a sudden split in the brain substance which was a type of lesion he did not see at all in the adult brain.

If Dr. Graham is here, I wonder if he would comment on that. Have you seen that at all, David?

Dr. Graham: I think the description is accurate. The brain is responding in a different way to the trauma but I think it's not restricted to children. We have not put an age on this, but I think a child is someone less than about 18, and we're talking about children and young adults also that responded like this.

Dr. Tarriere: This is not a question, but I have the feeling that because for the neck we have no knowledge equal to the head, and because there is no protection criteria for the neck, I think that we have the natural tendency to ask for something for the neck for future protection criteria without contemplating the statistical—the real world of accidents. My feeling is that for 50 percent of the brain or head injuries that may be AIS 6, we see no more than about 7 percent with neck injury, and I am afraid that we have not contemplated such statistics during these two days.

At the EEC, we defined the priorities. The priorities were the head, the heart, the abdomen, the lower limbs for the pedestrian but the neck was a low priority.

So perhaps we are overly emphasizing the importance of the neck.

Dr. Ommaya: That's the general impression but I would like to remind you of the data presented by Dr. Rehman in terms of his fatal motorcycle head injuries. There are 100 cases—these are fatal head and neck injuries—they were just fatalities. Of those 100 cases there were only 6 or 7 broken necks but 70 to 80 percent had soft tissue injuries in the neck. This is real-world data. It's very new but that to me is very important data.

Dr. Tarriere: These data relate to motorcyclists, and a car occupant would be quite different and I was speaking of car occupants.

Mr. Hirsch: I think, Claude, the problem, and perhaps Dr. Rehman might comment on this, is the fact that the neck autopsies are neglected in accidents. No one looks at the neck because the coroners don't know how to autopsy it or it's too difficult, or they don't want to damage the neck for viewing of the corpse.

Dr. Rehman: I think Arthur has hit upon a rather sensitive aspect of this and that is that when we do an autopsy the usual Rokitansky incision means staying below the clavicle and doing everything below the clavicles but the modification that we've added, and this is done by some, is to turn the skin up above the chin so we have the total neck exposed. Now, if inadvertently we nick the skin, that is a no-no because of exactly what Mr. Hirsch is pointing out. In other words, the body has to be viewed later on by relatives, etc.

But when we do this autopsy it is quite different from the usual autopsy. It's completely different from the type of autopsy that a hospital pathologist does in that they do not go up into the head and neck area unless they absolutely have to, unless there is some definite indication of trauma.

But in the forensic pathology field usually, if they do go up into the head and neck, it is merely to remove the tongue, pharynx, larynx, trachea and esophagus as a unit. If we do that, what we can see then is hemorrhage or hematoma on the trachea, on pharyngeal wall posterior. We split open the pharynx and larynx. We can see whether there's hemorrhage inside. We can see whether there's edema there and indication as to whether the individual had been in the hospital but this is very gross when you get right down to it. It gives us no real indication. They do not look at the vertebral column. They do not look at the posterior aspect of the posterior triangle, the supraclavicular triangle, in other words, the structures that will lead to subsequent morbidity, should the individual have survived. That is not examined.

So the thing that Mr. Hirsch has pointed out is that a few years back when our NHTSA-supported program was set up we attempted to devise a method of doing an autopsy of the head and neck without deforming or doing any damage to it superficially and to obtain not only the anterior aspect of the neck in detail but the posterior as well, which turns out to be extremely important because that is where we have picked up, particularly in sub-occipital area, with the atlanto-occipital, with the odontoid process and so on, we've been able to pick up hemorrhages there, hematomas, you can't see from the surface.

We can do the hyperextension and hyperflexion tests and so on but that still does not give us a true indication of what is deep and, or course, the additional aspect of the autopsy to remove the brain and cervical spinal cord as a unit. This came up at the last DOT meeting. It became very important to know what happens at that junction between the brain stem and the cervical spinal cord.

So this is one of the reasons I feel that our data, even though it's limited to motorcycles, is quite different from what we normally find. Theoretically, in a car, I would think much of this occurs as well. So, of course, if I sound biased, I think I am.

Dr. Ommaya: There is a paper by Sabina Strich and somebody else published over 10 years ago, I think in the *Lancet,* in which she did autopsies on patients dying of severe head injuries, I think most of them were automobile but this I'm not sure of, what the source was, but they were not motorcycle injuries as far as I recall, and she examined the cervical spine and the nerve roots, as well as the brain. For the same reason, she said usually nobody looks at the neck, and she found significant hemorrhages around the cord and also along the nerve roots and in the ganglia, especially in the sensory ganglia, they had hemorrhages in them, which she then correlated with persisting shoulder and arm problems in patients with head injuries to explain how these patients kept on complaining.

So I think it's a matter of maybe we're missing this. Maybe a lot of these—they may not be significant only in motorcycle but maybe in automobile.

Dr. Eppinger: We recently, about 6 months ago, went back through our NCSS data, National Crash Severity Study, and where we would rank order all the different trauma in terms of the probability of fatality and we coarsely did this similar to the way Tom Gennarelli presented it; but there are percentages in each AIS category of the percentage of fatalities, even if the AIS is the highest AIS. So that when certain patients or victims are categorized as an AIS 3, there is still a certain percentage that die and as I recall that came out to be 1 or 2 percent at the AIS 3 level, and at the AIS 4 level about 20 percent at the AIS 5 level.

If you go back and then address all the types of trauma that you see in the automotive environment and take the frequency times the severity, neck injury comes up very high in the total effect. In other words, we don't have as many neck injuries but when they occur they tend to occur at the high AIS levels, and therefore, they have a strong influence on the ultimate outcome and are a major contributor to the fatality picture in the automotive environment, not so much on survivor.

I think with that information, the emphasis leads us into the neck area also.

Could I make another comment on one of the workshops?

We said we had no neck data at all and I was just wondering why you've excluded Mertz's data and his proposed corridors and also the device within a physical surrogate that attempts to mimic those and monitor that.

Prof. Goldsmith: I brought up this point in the committee and I mentioned the fact that we have the Mertz data, it's in my survey paper of 1979, and it was pointed out that these are motion data, not tolerance data and I do not know really what the difference was, but I deferred to the people who seemed to be very emphatic about it.

There was, however, one other point that I would like to make. It was said that there were no neck models available. I regret that I would have to disenfranchise two Ph.D. students if this were true. We do have artificial necks. I am not sure whether they have been adequately validated, but I attempted to present at least some of the physical and some of the experimental results obtained there from the other day.

Now, they cannot be mass manufactured. That I can tell you. So perhaps we need to go to something that is a littler easier to produce than to spend 3 years in development.

Dr. Melvin: One comment with respect to Dr. Tarriere's comments on the occurrence of neck injuries. Your data is retrospective. If we are going to change what automobiles are like to protective systems are like, then you may have a problem and it may be the neck is the limit.

In our group's discussion, it was felt that maybe the noncontact head injury criteria may in fact be a neck injury criteria. This may be one and the same. That's a possibility. That there are limits, as Dr. Thomas has talked about, that the upper limit of restraint system performance may be the neck and as we approach that in automotive design we may enter into that phase and to wait until we see that happening in the world of accidents before we do something about setting it is probably way to late.

Dr. Tarriere: You agree at least for lateral impact.

Mr. Backaitis: The NCSS data, John, also indicates that neck injury with a noncontact type of interface is not very high. It seems when you have contact that it becomes very serious.

Dr. Melvin: Yes. The point is if you change the crash pulse significantly and try to hold onto them you may find that you begin to have the problem. If we're approaching the threshold, it would be nice to know that we're approaching it, not after the fact finding out that we have passed it.

Mr. Hirsch: I would like to add one more point to what Rolf Eppinger said about the neck injury. While they may not indeed come out to be all that many, which we don't know, of course, because my contention is that they don't look for them, the fact is that the neck injury, aside from the fatalities occurring from them, are very serious, and very, very expensive. In terms of societal costs they are among the most expensive of the injuries.

Mr. Backaitis: Perhaps this is the problem with the AIS description of neck injury. Perhaps it's being sort of overlooked in the AIS as far as the financial consequences go.

Dr. Ommaya: That's right. Maybe there should be a further revision of the AIS for neck injuries to expand the rating of AIS 1–4 injuries to reflect these opinions.

Mr. Hirsch: An AIS 4 for one type of injury and an AIS 4 for the neck injury may not be the same. There may be several orders of magnitude in terms of the societal costs associated.

Dr. Lennox: For the industrial air cushion "out of position" work the attempt was made to grade all injuries in terms of their threat to life potential under a 0 to 6 score, and also their permanent impairment potential and so, for instance, you could have a neck injury which had a threat to life of, let's say, a grade of 2 which might have a permanent impairment that is quite significant over a period of time. The question is, is it better to have a threat to life injury of, let's say 4 with a permanent impairment of 0 or a threat to life injury at the level of, let's say 2 that has a long-term sustained permanent impairment?

If you grade neck injuries within the AIS code going back to the '76 book which gave you other alternatives I think that this could be reflected.

Summary of Major Results

A. K. Ommaya, M.D.

The theme of this workshop was Accidental Injury to the Head and Neck, particularly as they occur in the automotive and transportation environment. Evaluations of existing national and international criteria and reviews of head/neck injury mechanisms were completed. This effort provided the basis of recommendations for what type of work must be done to improve the scientific merit of injury criteria now in use as basis for standards and regulations. Attendees included scientists and other individuals from the United States, United Kingdom, Canada, France, Sweden, Germany and Japan, representing major universities, government agencies and manufacturers.

The most important fact that emerged was the recognition of a serious mismatch now occurring between the quantity and quality of **engineering** and **medical** data being collected in various studies. For example, the National Crash Severity Study (NCSS) data files of the National Highway Traffic Safety Administration (NHTSA) contain voluminous data of superior quality concerning the crash circumstances, but quite often this superb engineering data base is accompanied by imprecise or inadequate medical data concerning diagnosis and outcome of the injuries. Conversely the Head Injury and Spinal Cord Injury Centers supported by the National Institutes of Health (NIH) [NINCDC] are gathering excellent medical data which unfortunately is often unaccompanied by useful physical and engineering data on the accident circumstances. This mismatch of two important sets of data could be corrected by assigning NASS investigation teams to the head and spinal cord injury centers by developing an interagency collaborative program between NHTSA and NIH. Such collaborative study would add little expense since both agencies are already funding such studies and indeed, collaboration could lead to long-term cost benefits.

The current Head Injury Criterion (HIC) was recognized as being characterized by magnitudes derived from the temporal variation of a single mechanical parameter, the linear head acceleration (presumable of the mass center) for all types of head injury. The "dosage" or "tolerance level" thus defined has evolved on the basis of a description of the impacts process to the head in terms of rigid body mechanics, obviously an unsatisfactory idealization. Recognizing the widespread acceptance of the HIC and its relative simplicity in use, participants also noted the doubtful applicability of the HIC to noncontact head injuries, its inaccurate extrapolation temporally at both ends (because it would predict infinite permissible accelerations in the short duration limit and infinite velocities when the loading is essentially quasi-static) and its failure to address the problem of brain injuries caused by rotational acceleration or associated with the occurrence of skull fractures due to contact phenomena when stresses in excess of the fracture limit (10,000 ± 5,000 psi) are achieved. No other alternative criterion for head injury has gained acceptance and the consensus amongst the participants was that a considerable amount of new research was needed before more rational criteria can be developed and recommended as national or international standards. Qualitatively, it would certainly appear that a set of head injury criteria for the different manifestations of head injury may be required.

The proceedings contain numerous suggestions for new research programs which should result in an integrated series of studies using more sophisticated observations on human accidents and data from theoretical, physical, animal and cadaver models. Until such data are available and a set of new rational head injury criteria are developed the HIC should be evaluated in comparison with the above-mentioned NHTSA suggestions for criteria as a guide to the design and construction of countermeasure devices and standards. It is not recommended however that the HIC be used to delineate actual human head injury tolerances in individual human cases for the reasons given above as well as for the reason that common individual and age-related variables in the structures and functions of the component of the human head are highly significant factors in influencing tolerance level.

Finally, it was clearly recognized that currently suggested criteria for neck injury are weak and that much more work needs to be done on neck and head/neck interface injury problems, specifics of which are given in the proceedings.

The most significant overall achievement of this workshop, apart from the interim criteria recommendations and clarification of the type of work that must be done, was the clear recognition of the necessity for an open communication channel between medical and engineering workers in this field. Interdisciplinary collaboration of this type is absolutely essential in order that medical as well as engineering aspects of the complex and highly important public health problem of head and neck injuries may be properly investigated. The major responsibility of the lead agencies in encouraging and facilitating such collaboration cannot be sufficiently emphasized.

Participants

Bertil Aldman, M.D.
Professor and Chairman
Chalmers University of Technology
Dept. of Traffic Safety
Fack S-40220
Gothenburg 5, Sweden

S. W. Alderson
17022 Montanero St.
Carson, CA 90746

Nahib M. Alem, Ph.D.
Highway Safety Research Institute
University of Michigan
Ann Arbor, MI 48109

Stanley Backaitis
NHTSA
400 Seventh St., S.W.
Washington, DC 20590

Richard T. Ball
141 E. Palm Lane
Suite 205
Phoenix, AZ 85004

David Biss
NHTSA
400 Seventh St., S.W.
Washington, DC 20590

Richard A. Black
3003 N. Central Ave.
Suite 2305
Phoenix, AZ 85012

John Bogdanski
Howd & Ludorf
67 Russ Street
Hartford, CT 06106

Nils Bohlin
Volvo, S-40508
Goteborg, Sweden

August Burgett
NHTSA
400 Seventh St., S.W.
Washington, DC 20590

Albert Burstein, Ph. D.
Department of Biomechanics
Hospital for Special Surgery
535 E. 70th Street
New York, NY 10021

D. Cesari, Ph. D.
Organisme National de Sécurité Routière
109 Salvador Allende Ave.
Bron, France

Conrad Cooke
NHTSA
400 Seventh St., S.W.
Washington, DC 20590

Robert Crone
NHTSA
Rulemaking
400 Seventh St., S.W.
Washington, DC 20590

Dianius J. Dalmotas
Transport Canada
Surface, Road Safety
Place de Ville
Ottawa, Canada K1A ON5

Leon Delarm
NHTSA
Crash Worthiness Rulemaking
400 Seventh St., S.W.
Washington, DC 20590

Kennerly Digges, Ph. D.
NHTSA
400 Seventh St., S.W.
Washington, DC 20590

Rolf Eppinger, Ph. D.
NHTSA
400 Seventh St., S.W.
Washington, DC 20590

Channing Ewing, M.D.
Naval Aerospace Medical Research Laboratory
Michoud Station
Box 29407
New Orleans, LA 70189

Dean Fisher
15301 Shoemaker
Norwalk, CA 90650

Aldo Fozzati
FIAT
Suite 1210
Dearborn, MI 48120

Victor Frankel, M.D.
Professor and Chairman
Dept. of Orthopaedics RK-10
School of Medicine
University of Washington
Seattle, WA 98195

Charles Gadd
3773 Indian Trail
Orchard Lake, MI 48033

Thomas Gennarelli, M.D.
Division of Neurosurgery
University of Pennsylvania Hospital
3400 Spruce St.
Philadelphia, PA 19101

Phillip Gildenberg, M.D.
Professor and Chairman
Dept. of Neurological Surgery
University of Texas Medical School
Houston, TX 77030

Yoshiro Goi
Technical Manager
Mitsubishi Motors
300 Town Center, Suite 1960
Southfield, MI 48075

Werner Goldsmith, Ph.D.
College of Engineering
Mechanical Engineering Department
University of California
Berkeley, CA 94720

David Graham, M.D.
Department of Neuropathology
Institute of Neurobiological Sciences
Southern Glasgow Hospital
Glasgow, G51 4TF Scotland

Ms. Cynthia Gross
Office of Biometry
National Institutes of Health
Federal Building 7A08
7550 Wisconsin Ave.
Bethesda, MD 20205

Mark Haffner
NHTSA
400 Seventh St., S.W.
Washington, DC 20590

Joseph L. Haley, Jr.
Biodynamics Division
Army Aeromedical Research Laboratory
Fort Rucker, AL 36362

Benjamin Harris III
NTS Research Corporation
2634 Chapel Hill Blvd.
Durham, NC 27707

Rodney Harris
Research Engineer
Motor Vehicle Manufacturing Association
300 New Center Building
Detroit, MI 48202

Shermon E. Henson
Principal Staff Engineer
Ford Motor Co.
Impact Department
Dearborn, MI 48121

Arthur E. Hirsch
Chi Associates, Inc.
956 N. Monroe St.
Arlington, VA 22201

Voigt Hodgson, Ph.D.
Director of Gurdjin-Lissner Biomechanics Laboratory
School of Medicine
Wayne State University
540 E. Canfield Ave.
Detroit, MI 48201

Hadleigh Howd
Howd & Ludorf
67 Russ Street
Hartford, CT 06106

H. K. Huang, Ph.D.
College of Engineering
University of Iowa
1214 Engineering Building
Iowa City, IA 52242

Professor Hugh H. Hurt, Jr.
The Traffic Safety Center
University of Southern California
University Park
Los Angeles, CA 90007

Albert King, Ph.D.
Biomechanics Research Center
Wayne State University
Detroit, MI 48202

John Kotwick, M.D.
Sports Medicine Center
University of Pennsylvania
235 South 33 Street
Philadelphia, PA 19104

Martin Krag, M.D.
Department of Orthopaedics
University of Vermont
Burlington, VT 05405

Y. G. Kulkarni
NHTSA
400 Seventh Street, S.W.
Washington, DC 20590

Herbert Lee
AVRADCOM
ATTN: DRDAV-EDG (Lee)
4300 Goodfellow
St. Louis, MO 63120

Jack Lennox, M.D.
Southwest Research Institute
6220 Culebra Road
P.O. Drawer 28510
San Antonio, TX 78284

Arnold Levine, Ph. D.
Dept. of Physics
West Virginia University
Morgantown, WV 26506

Robert S. Levine, M.D.
Bioengineering Center
Wayne State University
418 Health Sciences Building
Detroit, MI 48202

Sten Lindgren, M.D.
Professor and Chairman
Department of Neurosurgery
University of Gothenburg
Salilgrenska Sjukhuset
S. 413 Göteburg
Sweden

J. J. Liu
NHTSA
400 Seventh Street, S.W.
Washington, DC 20590

Y. King Liu, Ph. D.
Professor and Director
Center for Materials Research
1214 Engineering Building
University of Iowa
Iowa City, IA 52242

Christer Ljung, Ph. D.
Division of Solid Mechanics
National Testing Institute
Box 857, S-501-15 Boras
Sweden

Jeff Marcus
NHTSA
400 Seventh St., S.W.
Washington, DC 20590

Robert McLaurin, M.D.
Professor and Chairman
Division of Neurosurgery
231 Bethesda Ave.
Cincinnati, OH 45267

John Melvin, Ph. D.
Highway Safety Research Institute
University of Michigan
Ann Arbor, MI 48109

Richard Morgan
NHTSA
400 Seventh St., S.W.
Washington, DC 20590

Alan Nahum, M.D.
Department of Surgery
University Hospital
225 W. Dickenson
San Diego, CA 92103

Norio Nakamura, M.D.
Department of Neurosurgery
The Jikei Univ. School of Medicine
3-25-8, Nishi-Shinbashi
Minato-Ku, Tokyo
Japan

James A. Newman, Ph.D.
1481 Cyrville Road
Ottawa, Ontario
Canada KIJ 3L7

Peter F. Niederer, M.D.
Institute of Forensic Medicine
University of Zurich
CH-8028 Zurich, Switzerland

Guy Nuscholtz, Ph.D.
Highway Safety Research Institute
University of Michigan
Ann Arbor, MI 48104

Gerald W. Nyquist, Ph.D.
Engineering Analysis Department
Engineering Staff
General Motors Technical Center
Warren, MI 48090

Ayub K. Ommaya, M.D.
Chief Medical Advisor, NRD-10
NHTSA
400 Seventh Street, S.W.
Washington, DC 20590

M. M. Panjabi, Ph.D.
Director, Bioengineering Research
Yale University School of Medicine
New Haven, CT 06510

Ms. Jocelyn Pedder
Accident Research Unit
University of Birmingham
P.O. Box 363
Birmingham, B15 2TT England

Daniel Petterson
444 Capital Mall
Sacramento, CA 95814

Pria Prasad, Ph. D.
Senior Research Engineer
Automotive Safety Office
Ford Motor Co.
Village Road
Dearborn, MI 48121

Eberhardt Privitzer, Ph. D.
ASAMRL/BBM
Wright Patterson AFB
OH 45433

James Pugh, M.D.
Hospital for Joint Diseases
Orthopaedic Institute
301 East 17th Street
New York, NY 10003

V. Radovich
NHTSA
400 Seventh St., S.W.
Washington, DC 20590

André Rausch, Ph. D.
Insurance Institute for Highway Safety
Watergate 600
Washington, DC 20037

Irving Rehman, M.D.
5228-1 Lindley Ave.
Encino, CA 91316

Gerald Sack
Howd & Ludorf
67 Russ Street
Hartford, CT 06106

Roger Saul
NHTSA
Safety Research Laboratory
East Liberty, OH 43319

Henry Schmidek, M.D.
University of Vermont
College of Medicine
1 South Prospect St.
Burlington, VT 05401

William Scott
Head, National Accident Statistics Division
NHTSA
400 Seventh St., S.W.
Washington, DC 20590

Russell Smith
NHTSA
400 Seventh St., S.W.
Washington, DC 20590

John Smreker
Volkswagen
7111 E. 11 Mile Road
Warren, MI 48090

Richard Stalnaker, Ph. D.
Southwest Research Institute
6220 Culebra Road
P.O. Drawer 28510
San Antonio, TX 78284

Claude Tarriere, M.D.
Laboratoire de Physiologie et de Biomécanique
Association Peugeot-Renault
18 Rue de Fauvelles
92 La Garenne
Colombe, France

Daniel Thomas, Ph. D.
Naval Aerospace Medical Research Lab.
Michoud Station
Box 29407
New Orleans, LA 70189

Larry Thibault, Ph. D.
Division of Neurosurgery
University of Pennsylvania Hospital
3400 Spruce Street
Philadelphia, PA 19104

Joseph Torg, M.D.
Professor and Director
University of Pennsylvania
Sports Medicine Center
235 South 33rd Street
Philadelphia, PA 19104

Nick Tsongas
NHTSA
400 Seventh St., S.W.
Washington, DC 20590

David Viano, Ph.D.
Biomedical Science Department
General Motors Research
Warren, MI 48090

Ivan Wagner
3513 Garysby
San Pedro, CA 90732

Carrie Walters, M.D.
Department of Neurosurgery
University of Vermont
Burlington, VT 05405

Carley Ward, Ph.D.
705 Hampden Place
Pacific Palisades, CA 90272

Robert Wishner
611 W. 6th St., Suite 1600
Los Angeles, CA 90017